ATLAS OF
Atherosclerosis

RISK FACTORS AND TREATMENT
Third Edition

ATLAS OF
Atherosclerosis

RISK FACTORS AND TREATMENT
Third Edition

Peter W. F. Wilson, MD
Editor

Professor of Medicine
Boston University School of Medicine
Boston, Massachusetts;
Director of Laboratories
Framingham Heart Study
Framingham, Massachusetts

CURRENT MEDICINE, INC.
PHILADELPHIA

CURRENT MEDICINE

400 MARKET STREET, SUITE 700 • PHILADELPHIA, PA 19106

Developmental Editor . . . . *Elise M. Paxson*

Editorial Assistant . . . . *Annmarie D'Ortona*

Design and Layout . . . . *Jennifer Knight, John McCullough*

Illustrators . . . . *Wieslawa Langenfeld, Maureen Looney*

Assistant Production Manager . . . . *Margaret La Mare*

Indexing . . . . *Holly Lukens*

Library of Congress Cataloging-in-Publication Data
Atlas of atherosclerosis : risk factors and treatment / editor, Peter W.F. Wilson ;
developed by Current Medicine, Inc.-- 3rd ed.
      p. ; cm.
   Includes bibliographical references and index.
   ISBN 1-57340-187-0
     1. Arteriosclerosis--Risk factors--Atlases. 2. Arteriosclerosis--Treatment--Atlases. I.
Wilson, Peter, 1948- II. Current Medicine, Inc.
   [DNLM: 1. Arteriosclerosis--pathology--Atlases. 2. Arteriosclerosis--therapy--Atlases.
3. Lipoproteins--metabolism--Atlases. 4. Risk Factors--Atlases. WG 17 A8808 2002]
RC692 .A745 2002
616.1'36--dc21

                                               2002067490

ISBN 1-57340-187-0

For more information please call 1-800-427-1796 or e-mail us at inquiry@phl.cursci.com
www.current-science-group.com

Printed in Singapore by Imago Productions (FE) Ltd.

10 9 8 7 6 5 4 3 2 1

Although every effort has been made to ensure that drug doses and other information are presented accurately in this publication, the ultimate responsibility rests with the prescribing physician. Neither the publishers nor the author can be held responsible for errors or for any consequences arising from the use of the information contained therein. Any product mentioned in this publication should be used in accordance with prescribing information prepared by the manufacturers. No claims or endorsements are made for any drug or compound at present under clinical investigation.

PREFACE

We are in the early years of a new millennium and atherosclerotic disease is now thought to underlie more adult deaths than any other disease on the planet. The lifetime burden of risk is high, and Framingham data suggest that approximately 50% of men and 30% of women will experience coronary heart disease during their lifetime. This process begins at a young age, and autopsies of casualties from the Korean and Vietnam wars as well as accident victims in more recent times have shown that fatty streak lesions are very common in young adults. Recent research has extended these pathologic studies to investigate the dynamics and milieu that foster the creation of these early lesions. Increased concentrations of low-density lipoprotein (LDL) cholesterol lead to changes in the endothelial surfaces of arteries, expression of cellular adhesion molecules, and binding of monocytes to the artery surface. A complex series of cellular events ensues, including recruitment of monocytes and macrophages in the subendothelial space. These cells subsequently ingest cholesterol molecules and become foam cells, and the latter secrete growth factors and chemokines, eventually leading to more mature lesions.

Tremendous interest is now focused on the characteristics of atherosclerotic plaques, as we recognize that many clinical coronary events are attributable to unstable lesions that do not cause severe stenoses but are prone to rupture and precipitate angina pectoris or a myocardial infarction. A variety of factors are under study to help determine what affects the balance between plaque stability and instability. Some of this research is fueled by the fact that therapy for dyslipidemia often has effects that are not related to the lipoprotein cholesterol alterations, but stem from the pleiotropic effects of such medications on hematologic and inflammatory mechanisms.

The current volume focuses on the breadth of atherosclerosis, considering its beginnings at a cellular level and the biologic mechanisms underlying the development of clinical atherosclerosis. We have provided critical updates since the last edition. Certain fields, notably endothelial research, novel risk factors, and clinical trials, have charted new territories. This edition presents information on a variety of topics, including vascular biology and lipid metabolism, risk factors, lipid pharmacotherapy, and costs to treat and prevent atherosclerotic disease.

Peter W.F. Wilson, MD

CONTRIBUTORS

G.M. Anantharamaiah, PhD
Professor
Department of Medicine and
  Gerontology;
Atherosclerosis Research Unit Co-Director
University of Alabama at Birmingham
  School of Medicine
Birmingham, Alabama

H. Bryan Brewer, Jr., MD
Chief, Molecular Disease Branch
National Heart, Lung, and Blood
  Institute/National Institutes of Health
Bethesda, Maryland

W. Virgil Brown, MD
Professor of Medicine
Emory University School of Medicine
Atlanta, Georgia;
Chief of Medicine
Atlanta Veterans Affairs Medical Center
Decatur, Georgia

Alan Chait, MD
Edwin L. Bierman Professor of Medicine
Head, Division of Metabolism,
  Endocrinology and Nutrition
Department of Medicine;
University of Washington Medical School
Seattle, Washington

David W. Garber, MD
Assistant Professor
Department of Medicine and Gerontology
University of Alabama at Birmingham
  School of Medicine
Birmingham, Alabama

Henry N. Ginsberg, MD
Irving Professor of Medicine
Columbia University College of
  Physicians and Surgeons;
Attending Physician in Medicine
New York Presbyterian Hospital
New York, New York

Noyan Gokce, MD
Assistant Professor
Department of Medicine
Boston University School of Medicine;
Staff Cardiologist
Boston Medical Center
Boston, Massachusetts

Ira J. Goldberg, MD
Professor of Medicine
Department of Medicine
Columbia University Medical School;
Attending Physician in Medicine
New York Presbyterian Hospital
New York, New York

Michael B. Gravanis, MD
Professor of Pathology and Cardiology
Emory University School of Medicine
Atlanta, Georgia

Paul A. Heidenreich, MD
Assistant Professor
Department of Medicine
Stanford University School of Medicine
Palo Alto, California

Harlan M. Krumholz, MD
Associate Professor of Medicine
Department of Medicine
Yale University School of Medicine
New Haven, Connecticut

Ngoc-Anh Le, PhD
Associate Professor
Department of Medicine
Emory University School of Medicine
Atlanta, Georgia;
Laboratory Director
Lipid Research Laboratory
Atlanta Veterans Affairs Medical Center
Decatur, Georgia

Peter Libby, MD
Chief, Cardiovascular Medicine
Brigham & Women's Hospital;
Mallinckrodt Professor of Medicine
Harvard Medical School
Boston, Massachusetts

Alice H. Lichtenstein, D.Sc.
Stanley N. Gershoff Professor of Nutrition
  Science and Policy
School of Nutrition Science and Policy;
Director and Senior Scientist
Cardiovascular Nutrition Research
  Program
Jean Mayer USDA Human Nutrition
  Research Center on Aging at Tufts
  University
Tufts University School of Medicine
Boston, Massachusetts

Joseph Loscalzo, MD, PhD
Wade Professor and Chairman
Department of Medicine
Boston University School of Medicine;
Chairman, Department of Medicine
Boston University Medical Center
Boston, Massachusetts

Sampath Parthasarathy, PhD
Professor
Department of Gynecology and Obstetrics
Emory University School of Medicine
Atlanta, Georgia

Michael E. Rosenfeld, MD
Associate Professor
Department of Pathobiology
University of Washington School of
  Medicine
Seattle, Washington

Jere P. Segrest, MD, PhD
Professor
Department of Medicine
The University of Alabama at Birmingham
  School of Medicine
Birmingham, Alabama

Clay F. Semenkovich, MD
Professor
Department of Medicine
Washington University School of
  Medicine
St. Louis, Missouri

Evan A. Stein, MD
Medical Research Laboratories
  International
Highland Heights, Kentucky

Nanette K. Wenger, MD
Professor
Department of Medicine
Emory University School of Medicine;
Chief of Cardiology
Grady Memorial Hospital
Atlanta, Georgia

Peter W.F. Wilson, MD
Professor of Medicine
Boston University School of Medicine
Boston, Massachusetts;
Director of Laboratories
Framingham Heart Study
Framingham, Massachusetts

CONTENTS

HISTOPATHOLOGY OF ARTERIOSCLEROSIS

Michael B. Gravanis

Both denuding and nondenuding endothelial injury have been proposed as pathogenetic mechanisms in atherogenesis. Conversion of a nondenuding injury to a denuding one, however, is not considered to be a rare event. Although both mechanisms initiate different molecular pathways, they ultimately lead to 1) proliferation of smooth muscle cells; 2) synthesis of connective tissue matrix; 3) focal accumulation of monocytes/macrophages; 4) lymphocytic infiltration; and 5) variable intracellular and extracellular lipid accumulation and eventually stenotic lesions [1].

Recent publications have stressed that the endothelium has a wide range of important homeostatic functions. Such functions include control over thrombosis and thrombolysis, platelet and leukocyte interactions with the vascular wall, and regulation of vascular tone through the secretion of vasorelaxing (*eg*, nitric oxide) and vasoconstricting (*eg*, endothelin-1) substances.

Dysfunctional endothelium in a nondenuding injury may display altered expression of leukocyte adhesion molecules, as is the case of the intact endothelium overlying a fatty streak in which monocyte chemotactic protein-1 and vascular cell adhesion molecule-1 are detected [2]. Although normal endothelium is nonthrombogenic, a dysfunctional one may promote thrombosis by upregulation of thrombogenic proteins.

Recent studies have shown that endothelial dysfunction may be reversible, which raises the hope that slowing the progression of atherosclerosis may indeed be feasible [3].

Various mechanisms may be involved in inducing endothelial injury (denudation), including hypertension, hypercholesterolemia, immune complexes, viral infection, tobacco (chemical irritants), diabetes mellitus (hyperglycemia), vasoactive amines, and hemodynamic factors (shear stress). Exposure of the subendothelial matrix to blood in a denuding injury is followed by platelet deposition because of interactions with glycoprotein receptors and von Willebrand factor. Activated platelets will release growth factors from their alpha granules. Depending on the extent of the denuding injury, activation of the coagulation system leads to increased thrombin activity, platelet aggregation, and fibrin formation. Furthermore, thrombin acts as a mitogen for smooth muscle cells and fibroblasts and stimulates the release of growth factors from endothelial cells and smooth muscle cells. Thrombin also has chemotactic activity for monocytes and inflammatory cells and influences leukocyte adhesion molecule expression by the adjacent endothelium [4,5].

Current data indicate that at least two processes are integral to the initiation of the atherogenic cascade: 1) an enhanced focal endothelial transcytosis of low-density lipoprotein that accumulates in the proteoglycan-rich subendothelial space, and 2) the preferential recruitment of blood monocytes to the intima—a process that is augmented by even, short periods of hyperlipidemia. It is, however, the dynamic balance among plasma and intimal lipoprotein concentrations, the oxidative potential of the intima, the level of intimal monocyte/macrophage recruitment, and the efficiency of the reverse cholesterol transport process that are considered key determinants for lesion progression. In lesion progression, cellular necrosis with lipid release from foam cells and lysosomal enzymes are important events because such release further modifies or injures the surrounding intimal cells

and interstitial components and induces a second cascade of inflammatory responses within the arterial intima. Evidence supports the hypothesis that progression of atherosclerotic lesions is episodic, with periods of activity followed by periods of dormancy. For example, episodes of plaque injury (splits, fissures) are often followed by repair and, perhaps, growth.

In this chapter, the normal histology of muscular and elastic arteries, early intimal lesions such as the fatty streak and diffuse intimal thickening, the raised fibrofatty plaque, and the complicated lesions are illustrated and discussed. At the appropriate places, important sequelae and complications of atherosclerotic plaques are demonstrated such as arterial luminal narrowing, plaque fissuring or rupture, and medial damage leading to arterial wall weakening, dilatation, and aneurysm formation.

NORMAL ARTERIAL HISTOLOGY

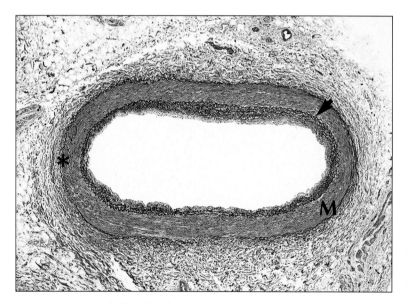

and collagenous fibers and proteoglycans; and 3) longitudinally oriented smooth muscle cells in large-caliber muscular arteries.

The interna elastic lamina (*arrow*) is a relatively thick and well-delineated band of elastic fibers, which although appears continuous on light microscopy, reveals fenestrations on electron microscopy.

The tunica media (M) is composed of approximately 40 circularly arranged smooth muscle cells, with collagenous and reticular fibers and rare fibroblasts between these layers. In large-caliber muscular arteries (*eg*, left main coronary artery), some circularly arranged elastic fibers are present between the muscle layers.

The adventitia (*asterisk*) is as thick as the media and consists of connective tissue containing varying amounts of collagenous and elastic fibers. The latter are more numerous in close proximity to the media forming the externa elastic membrane. In contrast to the interna elastica, the externa lamina is not continuous but is characteristically formed by fragmented elastic fibers arranged in a rather thick circumferential band.

There are age-related intimal and medial changes in muscular arteries, which may be focal or circumferential. The intima is thickened primarily because of increased numbers of smooth muscle cells and connective tissue matrix elaborated by these cells. The interna elastica may reveal fragmentation and reduplication. Foci of calcification at the medial aspect of the interna elastica may occur in an otherwise normal muscular artery. (Verhoeff–van Gieson elastic, original magnification, ×80.)

FIGURE 1-1. (*see* Color Plate) Normal epicardial coronary artery (minimal focal intimal thickening) from a 29-year-old woman. Small and medium-sized arteries, such as that shown, are regarded as the muscular type. Like all arteries, they have three coats or tunics with characteristically robust media. The inner coat or tunica intima has three layers: 1) the endothelium resting on a thin basal lamina; 2) the subendothelial space containing thin elastic

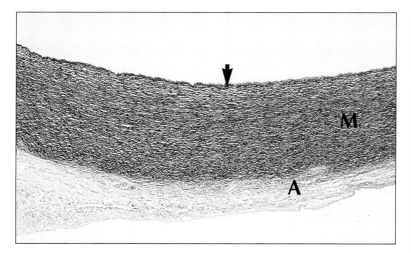

FIGURE 1-2. (*see* Color Plate) Normal aortic wall from a 2-year-old girl. Large arteries, such as the aorta (shown here), the brachiocephalic, common carotid, subclavian, and common iliac, are regarded as the elastic type. These arteries are characterized by a thin arterial wall compared with the size of their lumen. Their endothelial cells are polygonal in contrast to the elongated shape of the endothelial cells in muscular arteries. Similar to the muscular arteries, however, their subendothelial layer contains collagenous and elastic fibers, few fibroblasts, and smooth muscle cells.

Elastic arteries have no distinct interna elastica (*arrow*). Instead, they reveal longitudinal elastic fibers that merge with the elastic fibers of the media (M). The media consists of approximately 40 to 60 distinct elastic membranes arranged in a concentric way. The spaces between the elastic membranes contain smooth muscle cells (pursuing a spiral course), fibroblasts, and amorphous connective tissue matrix. The smooth muscle cells of the media are attached to the elastic membranes by short cellular processes. The adventitia (A) of elastic arteries is relatively thin, poorly organized, and merges with the surrounding connective tissue. There is no distinct externa elastica in large elastic arteries. Age-related changes in elastic arteries are characterized by elastic tissue fragmentation and medial fibrosis leading to weakening of the arterial wall and dilatation. Fibrous intimal thickening is also considered to be an age-related change, although its clinical significance or potential for subsequent development of atherosclerosis remains unclear. (Verhoeff–van Gieson elastic, original magnification, ×80.)

EARLY (PRECURSOR?) INTIMAL LESIONS: FATTY STREAK AND DIFFUSE INTIMAL THICKENING

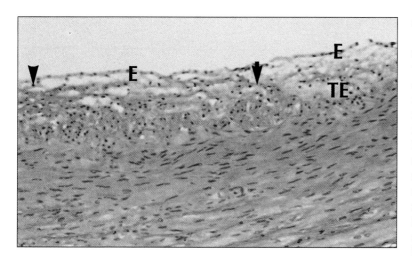

FIGURE 1-3. (*see* Color Plate) Human aorta with a flat fatty streak. The fatty streak has been considered by some as an almost physiologic event, in which the intimal macrophage system protects the arterial wall against the cytotoxic effects of the anionic OX–low-density lipoprotein. Although a number of cells are present in the subendothelial space (foamy macrophages [*arrow*] and lymphocytes [*arrowhead*]), under an intact endothelium, a modest degree of tissue spreading by what appears, under light microscopy, to be edema within the lesion, is apparent. According to recent studies in human coronary arteries, lipid deposition may occur only after an increased insudation of albumin, immunoglobulin, and fibrinogen into the intima has occurred. This finding suggests that significant changes in the endothelium and intima occur before lipid insudation becomes a factor [6]. Immunohistochemical studies of fatty streaks and atherosclerotic plaques have shown abundant protoglycan deposits in the intima of these arteries. Protoglycans most likely represent an early response to injury and are a form of provisional matrix into which cells migrate and proliferate to heal the wound. Furthermore, protoglycans play a fundamental role in self-surface anchorage for lipoprotein lipase on endothelium, in sequestration of lipoproteins in the subendothelial matrix, and presentation of lipoproteins to phagocytic intimal cells in the setting of native atherosclerosis. Thus, protoglycans have the potential to affect lesion development by regulating events such as lipid accumulation, thrombosis, and cell proliferation [7]. (Hematoxylin and eosin, original magnification, ×200.) E—endothelium; TE—tissue edema.

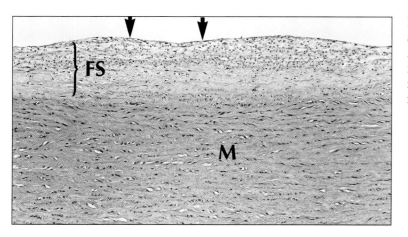

FIGURE 1-4. (*see* Color Plate) A flat fatty streak (FS) from a human aorta developed under a structurally intact endothelium (*arrows*). Although the majority of cells in the subendothelial space are foamy macrophages, several lymphocytes are also present. The media (M) is unremarkable. (Hematoxylin and eosin, original magnification, ×80.)

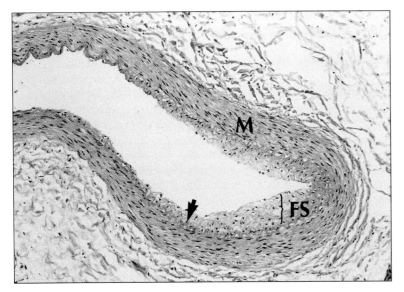

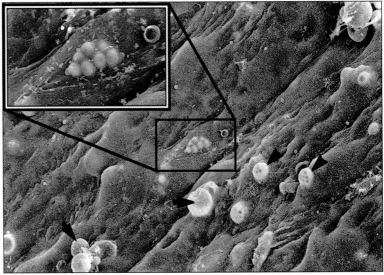

FIGURE 1-5. (*see* Color Plate) A fatty streak (FS) in an epicardial coronary artery of a 3-year-old boy. It consists of foamy macrophages, few lymphocytes, and rare smooth muscle cells. The interna elastica (*arrow*) appears intact. (Hematoxylin and eosin, original magnification, ×80.) M—media.

FIGURE 1-6. Scanning electron micrograph of coronary artery endothelium over a fatty streak. Note large blebs (*arrows*), some of which appear partially vacuolated (*arrowheads*). **Inset,** Endothelial cell lipid inclusions at higher magnification. (*Courtesy of* K. Robinson, MD, Emory University Hospital, Atlanta, GA.)

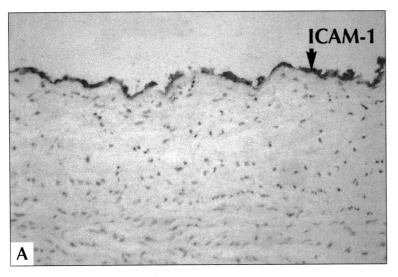

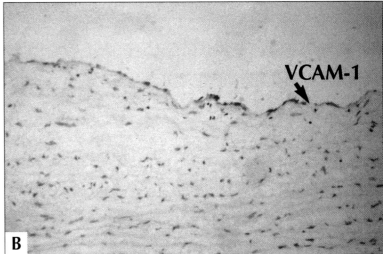

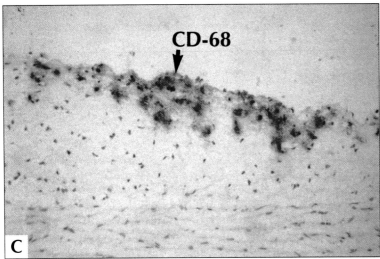

FIGURE 1-7. (*see* Color Plate) Localization of intracellular adhesion molecule (ICAM) and vascular cell adhesion molecule (VCAM) immunoreactive endothelial cells overlying human aortic fatty streaks. A human aortic fatty streak was stained using antibodies specific for ICAM-1 (**A**), VCAM-1 (**B**), and a macrophage marker, CD-68 (**C**). Original magnification, ×50. (*Courtesy of* J.N. Wilcox, MD, Emory University, Atlanta, GA.)

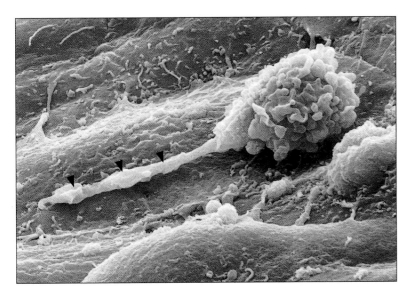

FIGURE 1-8. Scanning electron micrograph shows a monocyte with an extended pseudopod (*arrowheads*) adherent to the aortic endothelium at the site of a raised fatty streak. (*Courtesy of* K. Robinson, MD, Emory University Hospital, Atlanta, GA.)

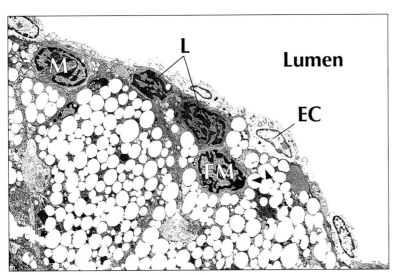

FIGURE 1-9. Transmission electron micrograph of a fatty streak in the proximal coronary artery. The endothelium is intact but shows areas of attenuation. In the subendothelium, monocytes (M), macrophage-foam cells (FM) with cytoplasmic lipid droplets (*arrowheads*) and multilamellar bodies, and lymphocytes (L) are seen (original magnification, ×5000).

The morphologic endothelial integrity in these fatty streaks (*see* Figs. 1-4 and 1-5) does not preclude a functional (activation) change of endothelial cells (EC) (*see* Fig. 1-6). An activated endothelium

produces a spectrum of cell adhesion molecules (selectins, integrins, and adhesive cytokines) (*see* Fig. 1-7) that may encourage blood-monocyte attachment (*see* Fig. 1-8). Monocyte activation occurs within the intima where they become larger and exhibit pinocytosis and phagocytosis, increased superoxide anion generation, and augmented secretion of many enzymes and growth factors. Macrophages have receptors for both native and modified low-density lipoprotein and can thus take up lipoproteins, de-esterify and re-esterify cholesterol to accumulate lipid, and become foam cells.

Fatty streaks are slightly raised, narrow, yellow lesions that are longitudinally oriented. The foam cells in the intima contain cholesterol esters and free cholesterol. The majority of the foamy cells are macrophages, although a few cells are recognized with monoclonal antibodies (α-actin) as secretory phenotypes of smooth muscle cells. However, as the lesion progresses, the smooth muscle cells become the dominant cells. In addition, varying numbers of T lymphocytes have also been demonstrated by monoclonal antibodies (Leu-22) in fatty streaks. In contrast to the fibrofatty plaque, only a minimal amount of lipid is extracellular in fatty streaks.

Fatty streaks may expand and grow by continuous chemotactic migration of additional monocytes in the intima. Migration of smooth muscle cells from the media also contributes to the growth of fatty streaks. Lipid is stored in both macrophages and smooth muscle cells and, thus, the term "foam cell" is applicable to both. Once a cell becomes heavily laden with lipid, its origin is very difficult to determine.

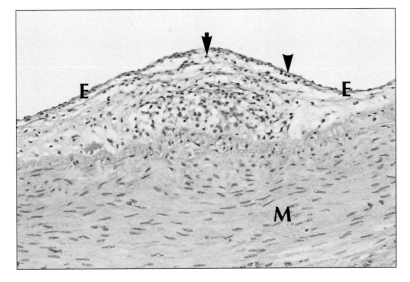

FIGURE 1-10. (*see* Color Plate) Raised fatty streak from the thoracic aorta of a 6-year-old boy. The lesion consists primarily of foamy macrophages (*arrow*) and lymphocytes (*arrowhead*) intermingled with spaces that appear to contain edema fluid, probably albumin, immunoglobulin, and fibrinogen. Note a row of mononuclear cells immediately beneath the intact endothelium (E). Those are probably monocytes or lymphocytes as seen in Figure 1-9. One of the earliest events in formation of a fatty streak is adhesion of monocytes to the endothelium. A novel vascular monocyte adhesion–associated protein (VMAP-1) has been shown to play a role in the adhesion of monocytes to activated endothelium. It is the general belief, however, that VMAP-1 is not the sole determinant of monocyte endothelial binding [8].

It is still unclear whether a fatty streak in the aorta remains harmless or even disappears. The consensus with regard to fatty streaks in coronary arteries is that they may evolve into fibrous plaques [9]. Raised fatty streaks are rare in coronary arteries before 10 years of age, increase in frequency in the second decade of life, and are almost always present beyond the age of 20 years. (Hematoxylin and eosin, original magnification, ×200.) M—media.

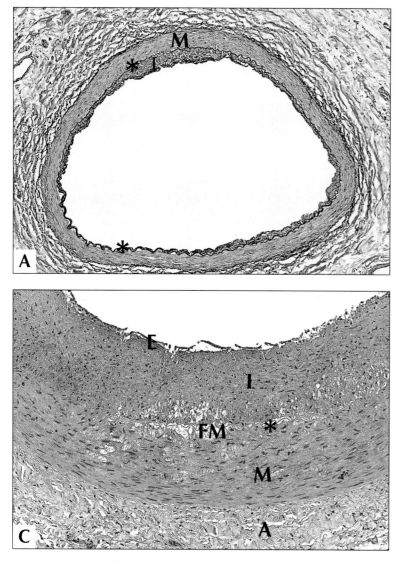

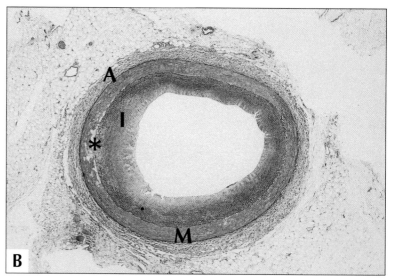

or absent. Diffuse intimal thickening is characterized by proliferation of myointimal cells (smooth muscle cells) with subsequent synthesis of collagen, elastin, and proteoglycans. An intriguing similarity exists between this vascular reaction in atherosclerosis and the lesions observed in the allograft heart, the so-called accelerated atherosclerosis, in postangioplasty restenosis, and the intimal proliferation observed in saphenous vein grafts. The underlying pathogenetic mechanisms leading to the intimal reaction in these different settings, however, are quite dissimilar, reaffirming the dictum that vascular injury—regardless of its nature or its precise localization (intima, media, or adventitia [A])—will eventually manifest as an intimal reaction. According to many investigators [10], the intimal smooth muscle masses (cushions) found near arterial branch sites are more likely to predispose to the development of atherosclerotic plaques. Thus, there is a good correlation between focal smooth muscle masses seen early in life and arteriosclerotic lesions observed later. However, lipid accumulation leads the smooth muscle cell mass to progress into an advanced atherosclerotic lesion.

According to one hypothesis, atherogenesis begins early in life as fibroblastic intimal thickening into which necrotic cores later appear. Furthermore, fibrocellular proliferation in the intima may foster lipid deposition, probably because of stimulation of smooth muscle cells by growth factors resulting in expression of additional low-density lipoprotein receptors by smooth muscle cells. With increasing age when the thick fibroproliferative intima approaches a threshold of about 150 μm, atherosclerosis occurs. The biologic threshold, therefore, appears to be determined by the product of two measured variables such as age and fibroplasia [10]. E—endothelium; FM—foamy macrophage.

FIGURE 1-11. (*see* Color Plate) Cross-sections of the left anterior descending coronary artery from a 2-year-old girl (**A**, Verhoeff–van Gieson elastic, original magnification, ×80), and from a 41-year-old man (**B**, Verhoeff–van Gieson elastic, original magnification, ×40; **C**, hematoxylin and eosin, original magnification, ×200).

Both subjects died from noncardiac causes. The photomicrographs reveal an intimal thickening that is rather limited in **A** but circumferential and of considerable thickness in **B** and **C**. The interna elastica (*asterisks*) appears to be intact except in the sections from the adult in which a focal area between the intima (I) and media (M) where foam cell infiltration is present and the interna elastica appears fragmented

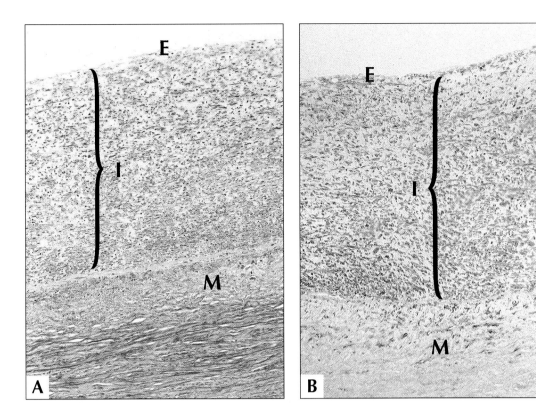

A

B

FIGURE 1-12. (*see* Color Plate) Aortic intimal myofibroblastic lesions from a 51-year-old man (**A**, Masson trichrome, original magnification, ×200; **B**, actin immunoperoxidase, original magnification, ×200). The majority of the intimal cells are of smooth muscle origin as it is depicted by the monoclonal antibody for actin immunoperoxidase stain (**B**). The absence of atheronecrosis in these sections suggests that the threshold for atheronecrosis is perhaps higher in the aorta than in coronary arteries, probably due to a relative paucity of smooth muscle cells in the latter. E—endothelium; I—intima; M—media.

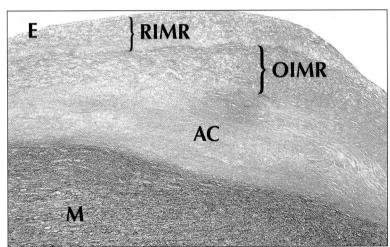

FIGURE 1-13. (*see* Color Plate) In atherogenesis, cell proliferation and extracellular matrix synthesis are neither linear nor predictable. The myofibroblastic proliferation may be episodic, *ie*, in which two distinct layers of intimal myofibroblast reactions are apparent. The upper (luminal) intimal layer of smooth muscle cells, which is the most recent, contains less connective tissue matrix and mature collagen. Plaques, such as that shown, may reveal successive cascades of intimal myoproliferative responses. (Verhoeff–van Gieson elastic, original magnification, ×80.) AC—acellular collagen; E—endothelium; M—media; OIMR—older intimal myofibroblastic reaction; RIMR—recent intimal myofibroblastic reaction.

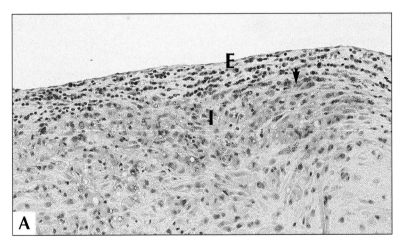

A

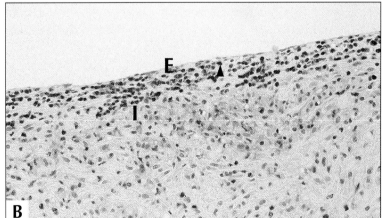

B

FIGURE 1-14. (*see* Color Plate) Diffuse intimal thickening in the aorta of a 47-year-old man. Special markers demonstrate immunocompetent cells throughout the intimal (I) lesion and, in particular, close to the luminal surface of the arterial wall. Cells identified are T lymphocytes (*arrow*) (**A**, Leu 22, original magnification, ×400) and macrophages (*arrowhead*) (**B**, Ham 56, original magnification, ×400), the presence of which strongly suggests an immune-mediated process. Because similar activated immunocompetent cells also occur in well-established atherosclerotic lesions, it may be hypothesized that diffuse intimal thickening creates a milieu for an immune-mediated response ultimately leading to the full-blown atherosclerotic lesion [11]. An understanding of the molecular mechanisms involved in the intimal cellular recruitment process may provide important information for developing therapeutic interventional strategies. E—endothelium.

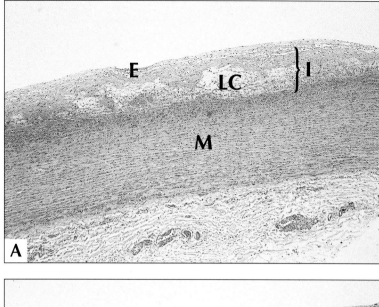

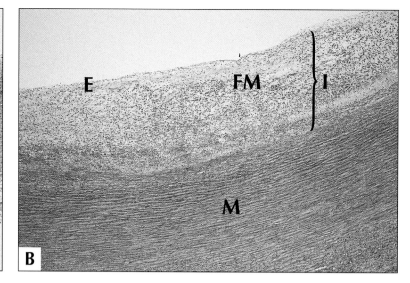

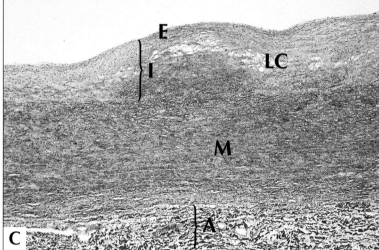

FIGURE 1-15. (*see* Color Plate) Human aortic intermediate lesions in which active replication of both smooth muscle cells and macrophages has occurred. In addition, T lymphocytes and varying amounts of connective tissue matrix are recognized. There is no distinct, well-developed fibrous cap in these lesions. Although two different phenotypes of smooth muscle cells are identified in these intermediate lesions, such as the contractile and the synthetic types, the predominant cell type is the latter. Synthetic smooth muscle cells have prominent endoplasmic reticulum and Golgi apparatus. They can synthesize extracellular matrix and contain receptors for low-density lipoprotein and, therefore, may accumulate lipid. (**A**, Hematoxylin and eosin, original magnification, ×80; **B** and **C**, Masson trichrome, original magnification, ×80.) A—adventitia; E—endothelium; FM—foamy macrophage; I—intima; LC—lipid core (intracellular and extracellular lipid); M—media.

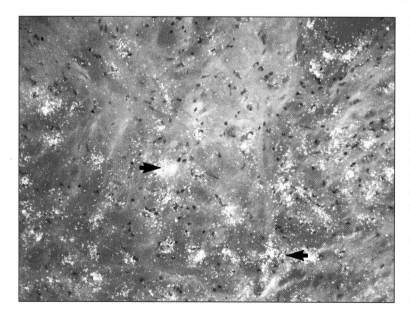

FIGURE 1-16. (*see* Color Plate) Localization of platelet-derived growth factor (PDGF) mRNA in an advanced human atherosclerotic lesion. Serial 10-μm sections of human atherosclerotic plaques were hybridized with a ^{35}S-labeled riboprobe encoding the A chain of PDGF and exposed for 8 weeks prior to development and counter-staining with hematoxylin and eosin. The presence of PDGF-A chain mRNA is indicated by the localization of silver grains in the emulsion overlying cells. This section was photographed using polarized light epiluminescence (Leitz) so that the silver grains appear white (*arrows*). PDGF-A chain mRNA was found in smooth muscle cells and mesenchymal-appearing intimal cells in the fibrous cap of this specimen apparently colocalized with PDGF-B chain and PDGF receptor mRNAs (original magnification, ×50) [12,13].

Synthetic smooth muscle cells may express genes for several growth-regulatory molecules and cytokines and may respond in an autocrine way to PDGF and other growth stimulators [14]. Smooth muscle cells also respond to many chemotactic factors and, there-fore, may migrate into the intima where replication can occur. (*Courtesy of* J.N. Wilcox, MD, Emory University, Atlanta, GA.)

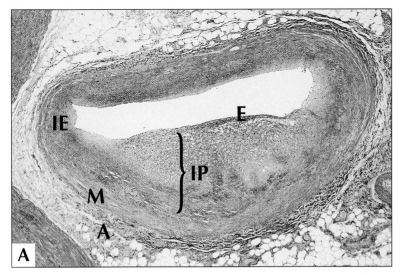

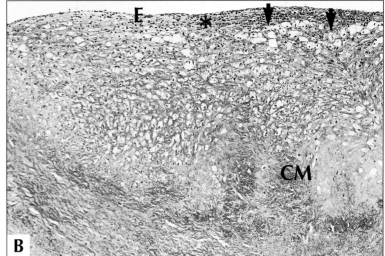

FIGURE 1-17. (*see* Color Plate) A coronary artery lesion that does not reveal a fibrous cap despite its significant thickness. Although the lesion contains a variety of cells, the predominant cell closest to the surface appears to be the foamy macrophage (*arrows*). Hypercholesterolemic monocytes are preferentially stimulated to migrate and penetrate areas of altered endothelium (E) [15].

Macrophages have receptors for both native and modified low-density lipoprotein. Their capacity to take up lipoproteins and to de- and re-esterify cholesterol is important in order to accumulate lipid and become foam cells. Furthermore, activation of the monocyte-derived macrophage may generate a variety of growth-regulatory molecules and cytokines.

Admixed with the macrophages and smooth muscle cells in this intermediate lesion are T lymphocytes (*asterisk*). Both CD4+ and CD8+, T lymphocytes, rare B lymphocytes, and natural killer cells have been identified in intermediate lesions and in fibrofatty plaques [16]. (**A**, Masson trichrome, original magnification, ×80; **B**, Masson trichrome, original magnification, ×200.) A—adventitia; CM—collagen matrix; IE—interna elastica; IP—intimal plaque; M—media.

THE FIBROFATTY PLAQUE

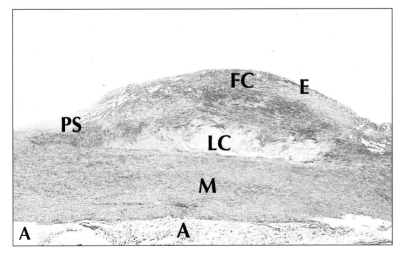

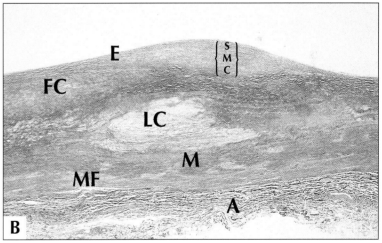

FIGURE 1-18. (*see* Color Plate) **A** and **B,** Early fibrofatty plaques in human aorta. In **B,** the media beneath the lipid core (LC) appears thin and attenuated with evidence of fibrosis. Both plaques reveal well-established fibrous caps (FC) and a moderate amount of LC.

An intermediate lesion may increase in size by continuous cell replication, focal necrosis, lipid accumulation, and connective tissue matrix formation. As these intermediate lesions progress, an FC of varying thickness forms over the lesion. The FC is usually thinner at the shoulders of the plaque where foam cells and smooth muscle cells (SMC) tend to accumulate. Fibrous tissue deposition in a plaque contributes significantly to the progression of the lesion, which appears to be regulated by growth factors acting on fibroblasts and SMC. The extracellular fibrous matrix consists of collagen (type I), elastin, proteoglycans, and glycoproteins. Whereas the latter may play a role in lipid binding, elastin may contribute to both lipid deposition and calcification [17]. One should be aware, however, that growth of an atherosclerotic plaque may also occur by outward, albuminal expansion, a remodeling process without encroachment on the arterial lumen.

Whether the two major components of a plaque—that is, atherosis (lipid deposition) and sclerosis (collagen deposition)—change proportionally as the plaque progresses with age is debated. Some investigators believe that the plaque becomes larger and softer with increasing age. Others, however, indicate that the softening of the plaque is an early event and that hard plaques represent the late sclerotic phase in the evolution of the lesion. (Masson trichrome, original magnification, ×80.) A—adventitia; E—endothelium; M—media; MF—medial fibrosis; PS—plaque shoulder.

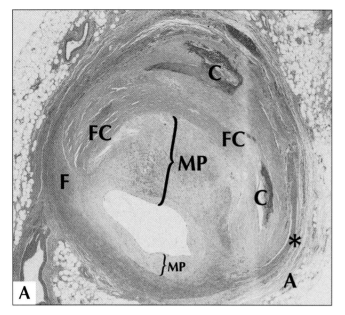

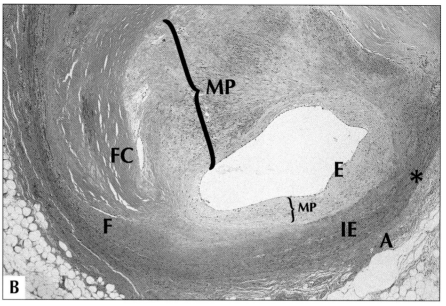

FIGURE 1-19. (*see* Color Plate) Lesion progression in a fibrofatty plaque in the left anterior descending coronary artery of a 52-year-old man who died from a cardiac ischemic episode. The eccentric fibrofatty calcified plaque occupies approximately two thirds of the arterial circumference. Luminal to the plaque, there is a concentric, relatively cellular proliferation of fibromuscular tissue that stains lighter than the underlying plaque. Similar fibromuscular tissue is also recognized extending between the fibrous cap (FC) of the original plaque and the media (*asterisks*) through an obvious fissure (F) of the FC at the shoulder region. Besides being the site of growth (recruitment of monocytes), the plaque "shoulders" also show significant neovascularization (angiogenesis). Mechanical transmural shearing forces, secondary to the cardiac cycle, are likely to be maximal at these sites, probably due to differences in compliance of the diseased versus nondiseased segment of the arterial wall. Plaques in which the lipid core is situated eccentrically are also associated with fissuring [18].

Arterial wall reaction to fissuring of a plaque may contribute to the growth of the lesion by either a neointimal proliferation or organization of a thrombus formed at the site of plaque fissuring. In the sections shown, fingerprints of a preceded thrombotic episode (hemosiderin deposition, neovascularity) are lacking. The "thrombogenic" or "encrustation" hypothesis proposes that fibrin deposition and thrombus organization on an atheromatous plaque may play a role in plaque development. Evidence that thrombus incorporation contributes to the plaque progression has been demonstrated with monoclonal antibodies, which have identified fibrin, fibrinogen, and their split products [19].

This case clearly demonstrates that the atheromatous plaque is not a static structure but is subject to either growth or dynamic modification and remodeling process (**A**, hematoxylin and eosin, original magnification, ×40; **B**, original magnification, ×80). A—adventitia; C—calcification; E—endothelium; IE—interna elastica; MP—myofibroblastic proliferation.

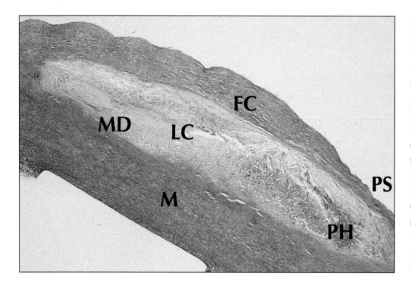

FIGURE 1-20. (*see* Color Plate) An established fibrofatty plaque in human aorta. Note that the thick fibrous cap (FC) tapers toward the right shoulder of the plaque. The large lipid core (LC) beneath the FC reveals several cholesterol clefts and foci of hemorrhage, although there is no apparent communication between the lipid pool and the lumen. Rupture of capillaries adjacent to the LC (right side of core) may be the source of the hemorrhage. The inner layers of the media (M) adjacent to the LC are focally destroyed. The mechanical strength of the FC depends on the synthesis, by smooth muscle cells, and organization of connective tissue proteins (collagen, elastin, proteoglycans). Reduction or loss of smooth muscle cells may result in degeneration and breakdown of the connective tissue. Proteolytic enzymes secreted by smooth muscle cells and macrophages may also contribute to tissue breakdown [20]. (Masson trichrome, original magnification, ×20.) MD—medial destruction; PH—plaque hemorrhage; PS—plaque shoulder.

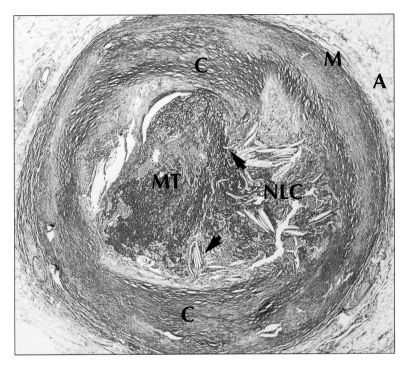

FIGURE 1-21. (*see* Color Plate) A fibrofatty eccentric coronary atherosclerotic plaque with rupture of its thin, delicate fibrous cap (*arrows*), exposure of the necrotic lipid core (NLC) to the blood stream, and subsequent luminal thrombosis precipitating an acute ischemic episode. Note that this eccentric plaque did not present a critical stenosis before rupture of its fibrous cap (estimated luminal area, 40% to 45%).

The importance of the collagenous matrix in determining plaque stability has been emphasized repeatedly in recent years. Several growth factors and cytokines have been implicated in regulating the synthesis of the interstitial forms of collagen in atherosclerotic plaque. Thus, it has been shown that whereas transforming growth factor-β and platelet-derived growth factor increase the synthesis of the precursors of the interstitial collagen types I and III, a cytokine known as interferon gamma (IFN-γ) decreases the ability of human smooth muscle cells to express the interstitial collagen genes [21]. IFN-γ is elaborated by T lymphocytes, which, with macrophages, are the predominant cells at sites of plaque disruption. Furthermore, IFN-γ may inhibit smooth muscle cell proliferation and induce their apoptotic death. However, besides impaired collagen synthesis, degradation of collagen and other extracellular matrix components by certain enzymes may also weaken the fibrous cap of a plaque and predispose it to rupture. These enzymes, known as matrix metalloproteinases (MMPs), are capable of cleaving all components of the extracellular matrix. MMPs are divided into four subfamilies: collagenases, gelatinases, stromelysins, and membrane type. Collagenases share the ability to degrade fibrillar type I, II, III, and X collagens. Collagenase-3 (MMP-13) is able to degrade gelatin in addition to fibrillar collagen. Stromelysins have a broad selection of substrates, such as proteoglycans; type IV, V, IX, and X collagens; laminin; elastin; fibronectin; and domains of procollagens I and III. Tissue inhibitors of metalloproteinases (TIMPs) bind to the active site of MMPs in a 1:1 stochiometric ratio. TIMP-3 and TIMP-4 are two of the recently cloned inhibitors. Macrophages activated by cytokines such as tumor necrosis factor, IFN-γ, interleukin-1, and macrophage colony-stimulating factor synthesize these matrix-degrading proteinases [22]. Recently, another inflammatory cell type, the mast cell, was shown to accumulate in the shoulder area of atherosclerotic plaques—the predilection site of plaque rupture [23]. Mast cells contain two neutral proteases, tryptase and chymase, which are capable of initiating matrix degradation via activation of MMPs. (Masson trichrome, original magnification, ×45.) A—adventitia; C—collagen; M—media; MT—mural thrombus.

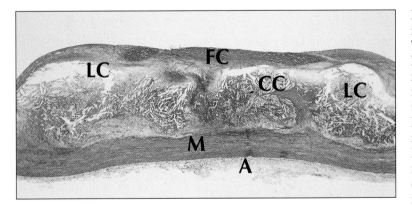

FIGURE 1-22. (*see* Color Plate) An established fibrofatty plaque from a human aorta with an excessive amount of lipid core (LC). The importance of the lipid pool in the process of plaque fissuring has been stressed in morphologic studies and has been confirmed recently by in vivo intravascular ultrasound [24]. Recent studies indicate that plaque fissuring is more common in plaques in which the lipid pool occupies more than 40% of their cross-sectional area. Furthermore, fissured plaques contain a smaller volume of smooth muscle cells and a larger volume of monocytes/macrophages and lymphocytes within the plaque cap [25]. This large array of inflammatory cells in atherosclerotic plaques clearly indicates that atherosclerosis should no longer be considered a degenerative disease; instead, it seems to be a chronic inflammatory condition. (Masson trichrome, original magnification, ×40.) A—adventitia; CC—cholesterol crystals; FC—fibrous cap; M—media.

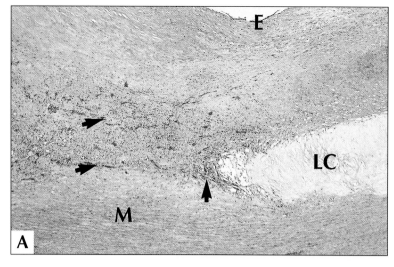

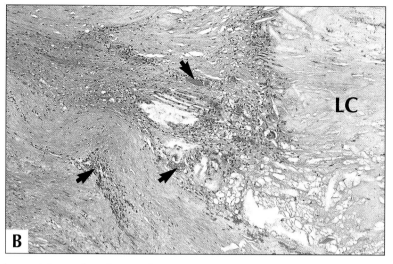

FIGURE 1-23. (*see* Color Plate) Microvessel formation (*arrows*) adjacent to the lipid core (LC) of an aortic atherosclerotic plaque. The importance of microvascular formation has been stressed with regard to the nourishment of growing plaques and as a cause of intraplaque hemorrhage. However, neither of these two hypotheses has been proven until recently [26]. Furthermore, angiogenesis is a rather complex multistep process requiring endothelial cell migration, proliferation, and, finally, morphogenesis. Recent data indicate that intimal endothelial cells, smooth muscle cells, and adventitial fibroblasts are all capable of producing angiogenic factors such as vascular endothelial growth factor (VEGF). It has also been shown that VEGF expression is upregulated by hypoxia as well as by mechanical or immune-mediated injury and that this autoregulated angiogenic process may be mediated by autocrine or paracrine mechanisms [27].

Recent investigations have shown that with increasing plaque size or greater accumulation of lipid, the intimal microvessels extend from the plaque shoulders toward the center of the plaque; their origin can be traced from the adventitia, but not from the arterial lumen. These investigators concluded that intimal vascularization is a function of intimal thickness and that when the intima is more than 50% of the overall wall thickness, vascularization occurs [26]. These findings strongly support the hypothesis that intimal microvessels nourish the growing plaques. Furthermore, newly formed vessels are usually deficient in supporting connective tissue and basement membrane and, thus, are highly permeable and fragile. It appears, therefore, that plasma components such as albumin, fibrinogen, and immunoglobulins (IgG, IgA, and IgM) may enter the atherosclerotic plaques from the intimal microvessels [26] and may contribute to the growth of the plaque. (**A,** Hematoxylin and eosin, original magnification, ×80; **B,** original magnification, ×200.) E—endothelium; M—media.

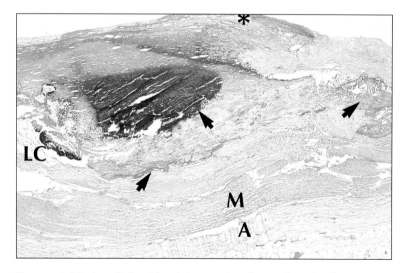

FIGURE 1-24. (*see* Color Plate) An aortic atherosclerotic plaque with extensive calcification (*arrows*). Although the plaque contains a minimal amount of lipid core (LC), the entire fibrous cap (*asterisk*) is calcified. In certain plaques, calcification is observed in the deep layers of the lesion, below the LC. In others, however, calcium deposits may occur in the fibrous cap. Although the exact reason for the mineralization of some atherosclerotic plaques is unclear or was interpreted as a form of dystrophic calcification, a recent report has emphasized the possible role of osteopontin. Osteopontin is a 44-kD phosphorylated sialoprotein that has high affinity for hydroxylapatite and, thus, it appears to have a modulating effect on the mineralization of tissues [28]. Osteopontin mRNA–expressing cells in plaques were found to be macrophages and smooth muscle cells, and such expression increased as the atherosclerotic process advanced. It has also been demonstrated that the degree of osteopontin expression is related to the degree of calcification and that osteopontin mRNA–expressing macrophages surround the atheromatous plaque crystals [29]. However, lipids may also act to nucleate the calcium mineral crystal. In addition, an oxidation product of cholesterol, namely 25-hydroxycholesterol, often found in atheromatous lesions, accelerates in vitro vascular calcification. Furthermore, in cholesterol-fed rabbits, tissues with high lipid content have a predisposition for mineralization [30]. (Hematoxylin and eosin, original magnification, ×80.) A—adventitia; M—media.

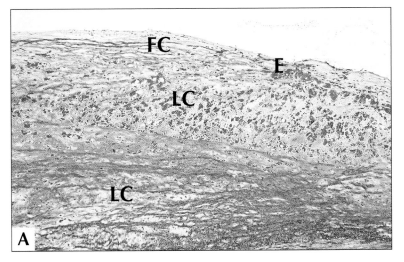

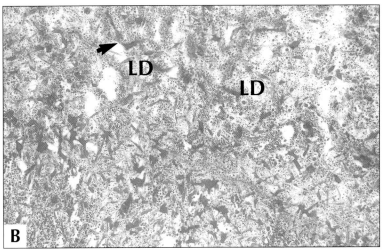

FIGURE 1-25. (see Color Plate) The lipid cores (LC) of an aortic atherosclerotic plaque in which fresh-frozen tissues were stained for lipid. A, A soft aortic atherosclerotic plaque with a poorly formed fibrous cap (FC). B, Lipid droplets (LD) very close to the endothelial lining. The lipid pool, which is avascular and almost completely acellular, contains extracellular deposits of cholesterol esters and few phospholipids. Improved electron microscopic techniques have demonstrated that small droplets of neutral lipid (profile diameter, 30 to 400 nm) and lipid vesicles with aqueous centers comprise more than 90% of the lipid-rich core region. Cholesterol clefts (arrow), LD (0.4 to 6 μm), and larger neutral lipid deposits (> 6 μm) together occupy less than 10% of the LC [31]. Furthermore, it appears that there is a stratified distribution of sequential lipid deposits that accumulates during plaque progression. The newest cholesterol deposits, consisting mainly of intracellular cholesterol ester droplets, are therefore localized beneath the intima. More inert forms of cholesterol such as cholesterol-supersaturated membranes and droplets are found deeper in the lesion. The oldest cholesterol deposit, crystalline cholesterol, is usually localized at the base of the atheroma. It has also been observed that elastic fibers are favored sites for the nucleation and growth of extracellular cholesterol droplets, probably because elastic fiber amino acid composition includes a significant proportion of hydrophobic residues [32] (A, oil red O, original magnification, ×80; B, original magnification, ×200). E—endothelium.

COMPLICATED ATHEROSCLEROTIC LESIONS

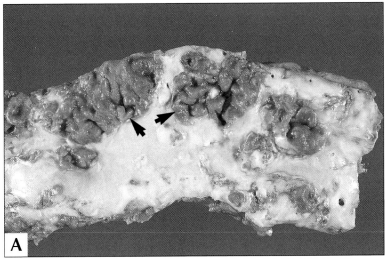

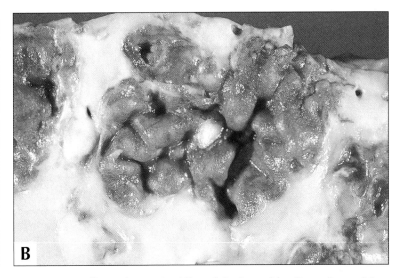

FIGURE 1-26. (see Color Plate) A to C, Gross photographs depicting multiple complicated aortic atherosclerotic lesions (arrows) characterized by ulceration or rupture of their fibrous cap and subsequent thrombosis (A and B). Plaques that fissure or rupture are advanced or of the raised fibrolipid type and have a characteristic microanatomy. Atherosclerotic lesions in such vessels as the aorta tend to develop at the entrance of branch arteries (C) and the lateral leading edges of the flow divider at the principal branches from the aorta; these are apparently sites of increased injury and continuous replacement of the endothelium. Transmission and scanning electron microscopy of these arterial sites have demonstrated alterations in the shape of endothelial cells and spaces between the endothelial cells. (continued)

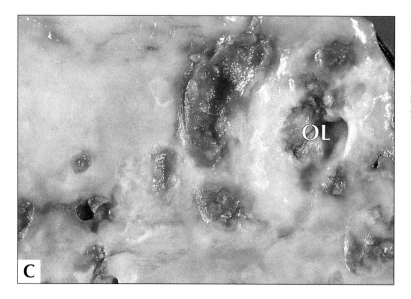

FIGURE 1-26. (*continued*) This endothelial change is apparently potentiated by factors such as hypertension, vasoactive amines, immunocomplexes, tobacco, and high fatty dietary intake [17]. However, atherosclerotic lesions may develop at sites not associated with a particular orifice, indicating that a strong correlation with specific hemodynamic forces, such as high or low shear stress, is not always present. OL—ostial lesion.

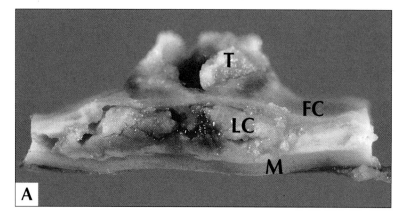

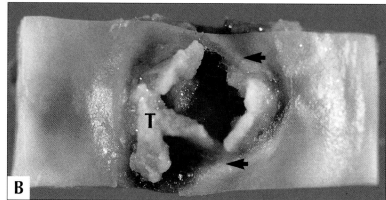

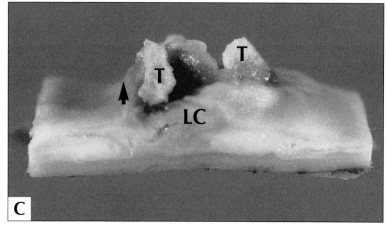

FIGURE 1-27. (*see* Color Plate) Gross photographs illustrating an aortic complicated atheromatous lesion with rupture of its fibrous cap (FC). The photographs demonstrate the overhanging ends of the ruptured FC (*arrows*) (**A**), the creation of a sizable crater, and the subsequent thrombosis at the rupture site. They also reveal the size and extent of the lipid core (LC) with a central hemorrhagic area secondary to the inrush of blood from the lumen (**B** and **C**).

These photographs also stress that plaque rupture is a deep arterial wall injury and not simply an endothelial denudation or simple ulceration. Although FCs may be five times stiffer than normal intima, their mechanical properties depend on their composition. Macrophages in the fibrous cap may synthesize and release matrix-degrading metalloproteinases, which, along with the generation of free radicals (products of lipid oxidation), may induce damage to the FC. Ruptured FCs 1) have reduced mechanical strength, 2) have increased extensibility, and 3) contain less collagen and sulfated glycosaminoglycans, more extracellular lipid, half as many smooth muscle cells, and twice as many macrophages [33]. Furthermore, plaques that undergo disruption tend to be relatively soft and have a high concentration of cholesteryl esters rather than of free cholesterol monohydrate crystals [34]. It is difficult to determine from morphology alone whether the cap 1) ruptures into the lumen or the opposite way, 2) fractures because of fatigue, 3) tears apart because of overstretching, 4) shears away secondary to hemodynamic forces, or 5) disintegrates [33]. M—media; T—thrombus.

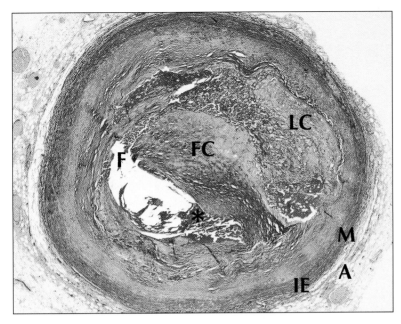

FIGURE 1-28. (*see* Color Plate) A primarily eccentric atherosclerotic plaque in the left anterior descending coronary artery of a 68-year-old woman. The fissure (F)-like rupture of the fibrous

cap (FC) appears to have occurred at the shoulder of the plaque. The lipid core (LC) is infiltrated by blood because of its communication with the lumen, which is severely stenotic and contains a recent, partially occlusive thrombus (*asterisk*). Note the medial (M) atrophy, which allows the plaque to bulge outward. This process of plaque remodeling has been clearly demonstrated by intravascular ultrasound.

Although most plaque ruptures are microscopic, some are extensive. Ruptures are more often longitudinal than transverse, and they may be single or multiple. Although the shoulder area of the plaque is more prone to rupture, the other most common site is through the center of the FC. Apparently both locations are points of high circumferential tensile stress during systole. In moderately or severely stenotic atheromatous lesions, rupture usually occurs within or proximal to the point of maximal narrowing [18]. Although collagenous tissue—often the most voluminous constituent of the plaque—is stable, a progressive extracellular lipid accumulation may destabilize the plaque by displacing and destroying the FC [35]. It has been estimated that a load of systolic wall stress seven to eight times normal may occur on the fibrous cap of a plaque. The stress is even further enhanced if the cap is thin or uneven in thickness and the stenosis not high grade [36]. (Masson trichrome, original magnification, ×40.) A—adventitia; IE—interna elastica.

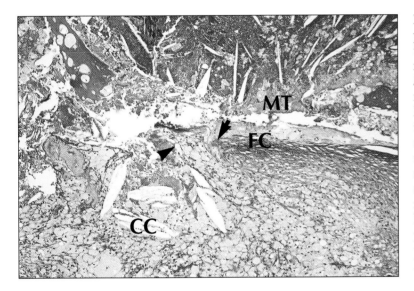

FIGURE 1-29. (*see* Color Plate) A fibrofatty coronary atherosclerotic plaque with rupture of the fibrous cap (FC; *arrow*) and luminal thrombosis. Note the extensive infiltration of the FC by foamy macrophages, several of which reach the luminal surface (*arrowhead*). The procoagulant activity of monocyte-derived macrophages after exposure to minimally oxidized low-density lipoprotein (LDL) has been documented. Macrophages express tissue factor activity upon exposure in vitro to either oxidized LDL or endotoxin (lipopolysaccharide). This activity has been associated with membrane (macrophage) vesicles that are apparently shed after procoagulant expression [37]. Furthermore, there is adequate evidence to support the hypothesis that increased macrophage density or activation, or both, may induce collagen breakdown in the FC by secreting metalloproteinases and other proteases and, thus, contribute to the plaque rupture [38]. (Masson trichrome, original magnification, ×225.) CC—cholesterol clefts; MT—mural thrombus.

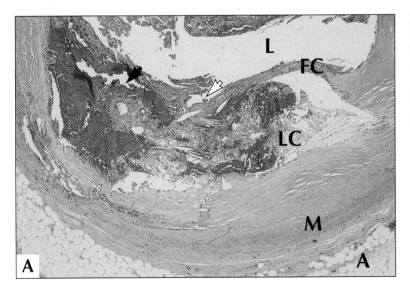

FIGURE 1-30. (*see* Color Plate) Both low (**A**, hematoxylin and eosin, original magnification, ×80) and higher (**B**, original magnification, ×200) magnification photomicrographs illustrate a soft coronary artery plaque with rupture. They also reveal a thin fibrous cap (FC) shuttered at several points and extensively infiltrated by foamy macrophages (FM). The abundant atheromatous debris appears to have extruded into the arterial lumen (L), contributing to the formation of a mural thrombus. (*continued*)

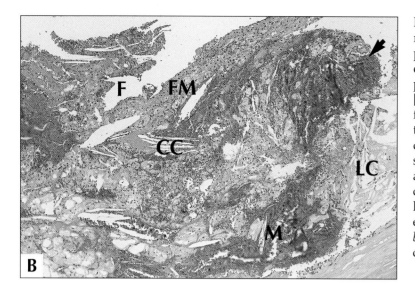

FIGURE 1-30. (*continued*) When the injury (rupture) to a plaque is mild, the thrombogenic stimulus is relatively small. However, deep plaque injury (as shown) results in exposure of collagen, lipids, and other elements of the vascular wall to blood, leading to relatively persistent thrombotic luminal occlusion and myocardial infarction [31]. It appears, therefore, that specific local factors during plaque fracture influence the degree of thrombogenicity, stability of the thrombus, and apparently the clinical symptomatology. Fluid dynamics also affect thrombus formation after plaque rupture, as seen in severely stenotic lesions in which the high local shear rate after rupture enhances platelet deposition. Moreover, evidence indicates that various systemic factors such as levels of epinephrine, levels of serum cholesterol, and impaired fibrinolysis may also enhance thrombogenicity [39]. *White arrow* indicates FC rupture; *black arrows* indicate plaque hemorrhage. A—adventitia; CC—cholesterol clefts; F—fissure; LC—lipid core; M—media.

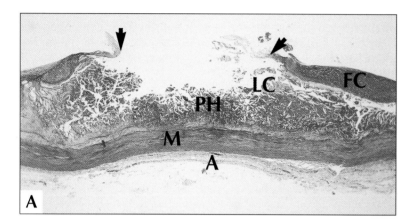

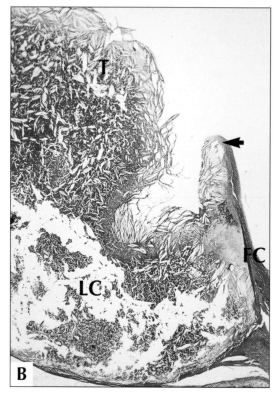

FIGURE 1-31. (*see* Color Plate) Additional examples of ruptured aortic atherosclerotic plaques with exposure of their lipid cores (LC) to blood elements and subsequent thrombosis. **A,** The ruptured ends of the fibrous cap (FC) (*arrows*) are shown to be considerably thinner than the rest of the collagenous intima over the plaque. (Masson trichrome, original magnification, ×80.) **B,** The extruded atheromatous debris is transformed into a sizable luminal thrombus (original magnification, ×200).

Although the relation between atherosclerosis and thrombosis has been recognized for more than 100 years, its importance has been downplayed. In recent years, an important link between atherosclerosis and thrombosis has been attributed to lipoprotein(a) [Lp(a)]. This lipoprotein is composed of a low-density lipoprotein particle linked by a disulfide bridge to a unique apoprotein, apo(a). Apo(a) is strikingly homologous (75% to 90%) to human plasminogen. Because of this strong homology, Lp(a) binds to fibrin, whereupon it competes with both plasminogen and tissue-type plasminogen activator (t-PA) for fibrin binding, thereby reducing the significant enhancement in t-PA's catalytic efficiency that fibrin binding facilitates [40]. Lp(a) has been demonstrated by immunohistochemistry in atheromatous lesions. By downregulating plasmin generation, Lp(a) leads to impaired activation of transforming growth factor (TGF)-β and thus may contribute to smooth muscle cell proliferation. Lp(a) may also contribute to atherogenesis by participating in the control of angiogenesis.

This latter action of Lp(a) may convert a stable plaque to an unstable plaque. Furthermore, Lp(a) may be involved in the recruitment of monocytes to the arterial wall [41]. Finally, it has been shown that patients with high levels of Lp(a) have impairment of endothelial-dependent vasodilation of epicardial arteries [42]. A—adventitia; M—media; PH—plaque hemorrhage; T—thrombus (with cholesterol clefts).

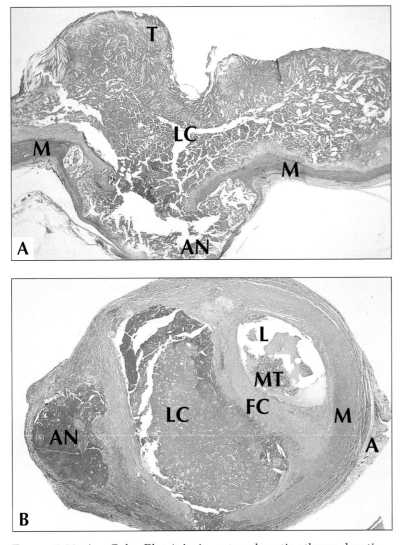

Both examples demonstrate that although the atherosclerotic process is primarily an intimal disease characterized by atherosis and sclerosis, all three layers of the arterial wall may be involved. The media (M) adjacent to the plaque may become attenuated and thin, or may even be completely destroyed. A thin media may be the result of disuse atrophy, splinting effect by the plaque, or loss of smooth muscle cells. Although advanced intimal atherosclerosis always accompanies abdominal aortic aneurysms (AAAs), structural degenerative changes of the media play a more unique role in the evolution of aneurysmal disease. Recent studies have shown that in addition to accelerated degradation of structural matrix proteins (ie, elastic, collagen), aneurysms are associated with changes in the cellular composition of the arterial wall. Vascular smooth muscle cells are the predominant cell type of the media and thereby make a major contribution to the anatomic integrity of the arterial wall through their production of collagen, elastin, and other matrix proteins. These recent studies have shown that medial smooth muscle cell (SMC) density is significantly reduced in AAA compared with normal aortas or cases of atherosclerotic occlusive disease, and that this loss of medial SMCs in aneurysms is due to SMC apoptosis [43].

With regard to atherosclerotic dilatations in the coronary arteries, discrete aneurysms (AN), which are spherical or saccular (**B**), should be separated from the fusiform coronary dilatations, which are referred to as "coronary artery ectasias." Recent evidence indicates that inflammatory cells play an important role in the pathogenesis of arterial aneurysmal disease. Tissues from human abdominal aneurysms reveal higher quantities of the chemotactic cytokines, interleukin-8 and monocyte chemoattractant protein-1 (MCP-1), than tissue from atherosclerotic aorta without aneurysms. Whereas the primary source of interleukin-8 in these tissues is the macrophage, MCP-1 is available from the macrophage and, to a lesser extent, the smooth muscle cell. The signals that regulate interleukin-8 production in the arterial wall have, however, not been identified. It appears that these two cytokines play a pivotal role in the recruitment of chronic inflammatory cells at the site of the atherosclerotic lesion, which in turn may release additional factors that contribute to the arterial wall damage and, thus, the aneurysmal dilatation [44]. A—adventitia; FC—fibrous cap; L—lumen; LC—lipid core; MT—mural thrombus; T—thrombus (with cholesterol clefts).

FIGURE 1-32. (*see* Color Plate) **A,** A ruptured aortic atherosclerotic plaque (hematoxylin and eosin, original magnification, ×80). **B,** An intact fibrofatty plaque from a coronary artery (original magnification, ×40). Both plaques reveal an additional feature of atherosclerosis—complete medial destruction at the site of the lesion with subsequent aneurysmal dilatation of the arterial wall. The atheromatous material at the aneurysm bulging is contained only by a thin strip of connective tissue of adventitial A origin.

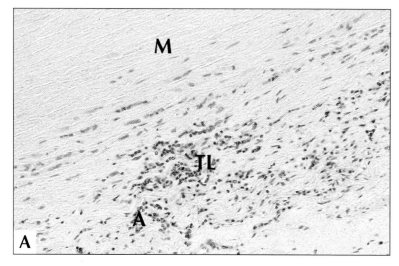

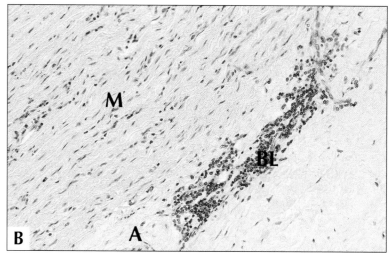

FIGURE 1-33. (*see* Color Plate) Clusters of lymphocytes at the border zone are shown between media (M) and adventitia (A) at the site of an aortic atherosclerotic lesion. Both T lymphocytes (TL; **A,** Leu 22, original magnification, ×200) and B lymphocytes (BL; **B,** L26, original magnification, ×200) are recognized with monoclonal antibodies (bright red cytoplasmic staining).

The finding of immunocompetent cells within the atheromatous plaque, including the adventitia, clearly indicates that immunologic activation is somehow associated with human atherosclerosis. The presence of immunocompetent cells does not, however, signify whether an immune response plays a primary role in atherogenesis or is merely a secondary phenomenon to antigenic stimuli arising within the plaque.

Normal aortic tissues contain few, if any, inflammatory cells in contrast to the inflammatory responses observed in atherosclerotic aortas with and without aneurysmal dilatation. It is not clear whether a specific antigen is responsible for an immune-mediated mechanism, although putative antigens such as elastic fibers or extracellularly modified lipoproteins have been suggested [45]. In atherosclerotic aortas, approximately 25% of CD3+ T lymphocytes are located in the adventitia, but the majority are within the media. CD3+ T lymphocytes may reveal several mechanisms for recruiting CD19+ B lymphocytes to the inflammatory reaction site. Interleukin-4, -5, and -6 may stimulate the growth and differentiation of CD19+ B lymphocytes, which in turn may serve as antigen-presenting cells, similar to macrophages [46]. The possible role of the immune system in atherogenesis has also been advanced after immunoglobulins and activated complement factors were identified in human atherosclerotic plaques [45].

REFERENCES

1. Wilcox JN, Harker LA: Molecular and cellular mechanisms of atherogenesis: studies of human lesions linked with animal modeling. In *Haemostasis and Thrombosis*, edn 3, vol 2. Edited by Bloom AL, Forbes CD, Thomas DP, *et al.* Edinburgh: Churchill Livingstone; 1993:1139–1152.

2. Cybulsky MI, Gimbrone MA: Endothelial expression of a mononuclear leukocyte adhesion molecule during atherogenesis. *Science* 1991, 251:788–791.

3. Celermajer DS: Endothelial dysfunction: does it matter? Is it reversible? *J Am Coll Cardiol* 1997, 30:325–333.

4. Bar Shavit R, Benezra M, Sabbah V, *et al.*: Thrombin as a multifunctional protein: induction of cell adhesion and proliferation. *Am J Respir Cell Mol Biol* 1992, 6:123–130.

5. Shultz PJ, Knauss TC, Mene P, *et al.*: Mitogenic signals for thrombin in mesangial cells: regulation of phospholipase C and PDGF genes. *Am J Physiol* 1989, 257(suppl F):366–374.

6. Zhang Y, Cliff WJ, Schoefl GI, *et al.*: Plasma protein insudation as an index of early coronary atherogenesis. *Am J Pathol* 1993, 143:496–505.

7. Evanko SP, Raines EW, Ross R, *et al.*: Proteoglycan distribution in lesions of atherosclerosis depends on lesion severity, structural characteristics, and the proximity of platelet-derived growth factor and transforming growth factor-β. *Am J Pathol* 1998, 152:533–546.

8. McEvoy LM, Sun H, Tsao PS, *et al.*: Novel vascular molecule involved in monocyte adhesion to aortic endothelium in models of atherogenesis. *J Exp Med* 1997, 185:2069–2077.

9. McGill HC Jr: Persistent problems in the pathogenesis of atherosclerosis. *Arteriosclerosis* 1984, 4:443–451.

10. Tracy RE, Kissling GE: Age and fibroplasia as preconditions for atheronecrosis in human coronary arteries. *Arch Pathol Lab Med* 1987, 111:957–963.

11. Van Der Wal AC, Das PK, Van Der Berg DB, *et al.*: Atherosclerotic lesions in humans: in situ immunophenotypic analysis suggesting an immune-mediated response. *Lab Invest* 1989, 61:166–170.

12. Wilcox JN: Analysis of local gene expression in human atherosclerotic plaques by in situ hybridization. *Trends Cardiovasc Med* 1991, 1:17–24.

13. Wilcox JN, Smith KM, Williams LT, *et al.*: Platelet derived growth factor mRNA detection in human atherosclerotic plaques by in situ hybridization. *J Clin Invest* 1988, 82:1134–1143.

14. Ross R: The pathogenesis of atherosclerosis: a perspective for the 1990's. *Nature* 1993, 362:801–809.

15. Gerrity RG, Goss JA, Soby L: Control of monocyte recruitment by chemotactic factor(s) in lesion-prone areas of swine aorta. *Atherosclerosis* 1985, 5:55–66.

16. Ross R: Atherosclerosis: a defense mechanism gone awry. *Am J Pathol* 1993, 143:987–1002.

17. Fuster V, Badimon JJ, Badimon L: Clinical-pathological correlations of coronary disease progression and regression. *Circulation* 1992, 86(suppl 6):1–11.

18. Richardson PD, Davies MS, Born GVR: Influence of plaque configuration and stress distribution on fissuring of coronary atherosclerotic plaques. *Lancet* 1989, 2:941–944.

19. Bini A, Fenoglio JJ Jr, Mesa-Tejada R, *et al.*: Identification and distribution of fibrinogen, fibrin and fibrin(ogen) degradation products in atherosclerosis: use of monoclonal antibodies. *Arteriosclerosis* 1989, 9:109–121.

20. Lendon C, Davies M, Born G, *et al.*: Atherosclerotic plaque caps are locally weakened when macrophage density is increased. *Atherosclerosis* 1991, 65:302–310.

21. Amento EP, Ehsani N, Palmer H, *et al.*: Cytokines positively and negatively regulate interstitial collagen gene expression in human vascular smooth muscle cells. *Arterioscler Thromb* 1991, 11:1223–1230.

22. Libby P: Molecular bases of the acute coronary syndromes. *Circulation* 1995, 91:2844–2850.

23. Kovanen PT, Koaartinen M, Paavonen T: Infiltrates of activated mast cells at the site of coronary atheromatous erosion or rupture in myocardial infarction. *Circulation* 1995, 92:1084–1088.

24. Nissen S, Gurley J, Booth D, *et al.*: Differences in ultrasound plaque morphology in stable and unstable patients [abstract]. *Circulation* 1991, 84:436.

25. Davies MJ, Richardson PD, Woolf N, *et al.*: Risk of thrombosis in human atherosclerotic plaques: role of extracellular lipid, macrophages and smooth muscle cell content. *Br Heart J* 1993, 69:377–381.

26. Zhang Y, Cliff WJ, Shoefl GI, *et al.*: Immunohistochemical study of intimal microvessels in coronary atherosclerosis. *Am J Pathol* 1993, 43:164–172.

27. Nicosia RF, Lin YJ, Hazelton D, *et al.*: Endogenous regulation of angiogenesis in the rat aorta model: role of vascular endothelial growth factor. *Am J Pathol* 1997, 151:1379–1386.

28. Demer LL: A skeleton in the atherosclerosis closet. *Circulation* 1995, 92:2029–2032.

29. Hirota S, Imakita M, Kohri K, *et al.*: Expression of osteopontin messenger RNA by macrophages in atherosclerotic plaques. *Am J Pathol* 1993, 143:1003–1008.

30. Demer LL: Lipid hypothesis of cardiovascular calcification. *Circulation* 1997, 95:297–298.

31. Guyton JR, Klemp KF: The lipid-rich core region of human atherosclerotic fibrous plaques: prevalence of small lipid droplets and vesicles by electron microscopy. *Am J Pathol* 1989, 134:705–717.

32. Podet EJ, Shaffer DR, Gianturco SH, *et al.*: Interaction of low density lipoproteins with human aortic elastin. *Arterioscler Thromb* 1991, 11:116–122.

33. Falk E: Why do plaques rupture? *Circulation* 1992, 86(suppl III): 30–42.

34. Theroux P, Foster V: Acute coronary syndromes: unstable angina and non-Q-wave myocardial infarction. *Circulation* 1998, 97:1195–1206.

35. Stary HC: The sequence of cell and matrix changes in atherosclerotic lesions of coronary arteries in the first forty years of life. *Eur Heart J* 1990, 11(suppl E):3–19.

36. Davies MJ: Stability and instability: two faces of coronary atherosclerosis. *Circulation* 1996, 94:2013–2020.

37. Lewis LC, Bennet-Cain AL, DeMars CS, *et al.*: Procoagulant activity after exposure of monocyte-derived macrophages to minimally oxidized low density lipoprotein. *Am J Pathol* 1995, 147:1029–1040.

38. Shah PK, Falk E, Badimon JJ, *et al.*: Human monocyte-derived macrophages induce collagen breakdown in fibrous caps of atherosclerotic plaques: potential role of matrix-degrading metalloproteinases and implication for plaque rupture. *Circulation* 1995, 92:1565–1569.

39. Badimon L, Chesebro JH, Badimon JJ: Thrombus formation on ruptured atherosclerotic plaques and rethrombosis on evolving thrombi. *Circulation* 1992, 86(suppl 6):74–85.

40. Nachman RL: Lipoprotein (alpha): molecular mischief in the microvasculature. *Circulation* 1997, 96:2485–2487.

41. Schachinger V, Halle M, Minners J, *et al.*: Lipoprotein (alpha) selectively impairs receptor-mediated endothelial vasodilator function of the human coronary circulation. *J Am Cell Cardiol* 1997, 30:927–934.

42. Lopez-Candales A, Holmes, DR, Liao S, *et al.*: Decreased vascular smooth muscle cell density in medial degeneration of human abdominal aortic aneurysms. *Am J Pathol* 1997, 150:993–1007.

43. Loscalzo J, Weinfeld M, Fless GM, *et al.*: Lipoprotein (alpha), fibrin binding, and plasminogen activation. *Arteriosclerosis* 1990, 10:240–245.

44. Koch AE, Kunkel SL, Pearce WH, *et al.*: Enhanced production of the chemotactic cytokines interleukin-8, and monocyte chemoattractant protein-1 in human abdominal aortic aneurysms. *Am J Pathol* 1993, 142:1423–1431.

45. Hanson GK, Jonasson S, Seifert PS, *et al.*: Immune mechanisms in atherosclerosis. *Arteriosclerosis* 1989, 9:567–578.

46. Koch AE, Haines K, Rizzo RJ, *et al.*: Human abdominal aortic aneurysms: immunophenotypic analysis suggesting an immune-mediated response. *Am J Pathol* 1990, 137:1199–1213.

THE ENDOTHELIUM IN ATHEROTHROMBOSIS

2

CHAPTER

Noyan Gokce and Joseph Loscalzo

Located at the interface between the vessel wall and circulating blood, the vascular endothelium plays a critical role in the homeostatic and physiologic functions of the vasculature. In response to biochemical and mechanical stimuli, endothelial cells synthesize and elaborate a number of factors that modulate vascular tone, inflammation, thrombosis, and vascular growth. Normal endothelium provides a fluid antiatherogenic environment that inhibits platelet and leukocyte adhesion, prevents vasospasm, promotes fibrinolysis, and inhibits vascular smooth muscle cell growth. Under pathologic conditions when homeostatic mechanisms are altered, the phenotypic changes that occur in endothelial cells support a vasospastic, prothrombotic, and proinflammatory milieu, and play a central role in the pathophysiology and clinical manifestations of cardiovascular disease [1].

A critical homeostatic function of normal endothelium involves control of vascular tone, determined by a dynamic balance of endothelium-derived vasoactive mediators. Dilator substances include prostacyclin, bradykinin, endothelium-derived hyperpolarizing factor (EDHF), and, importantly, nitric oxide (NO) [2]. Nitric oxide is synthesized from the conversion of the amino acid L-arginine to L-citrulline through the tightly regulated activity of the nitric oxide synthases (NOS). Nitric oxide is responsible, in part, for maintenance of basal vascular tone, and exerts a potent relaxant effect on vascular smooth muscle through activation of soluble guanylyl cyclase and the consequent increase in intracellular cGMP. NO also supports a number of additional antiatherogenic functions through inhibition of platelet aggregation, leukocyte adhesion, monocyte chemotaxis, and smooth muscle cell proliferation. Individuals with coronary risk factors or atherosclerosis demonstrate impaired NO-mediated vasomotor function and reduced NO bioactivity [3]. Vasoconstrictive substances released by the endothelium include angiotensin II, endothelium-derived constricting factor (EDCF), prostaglandin H_2, and endothelin. An imbalance favoring the predominance of constrictive agents appears to contribute to the pathophysiology of vasospasm and impaired vasomotor tone characteristic of disease states, such as hypertension, congestive heart failure, and coronary artery disease (CAD).

Another important function of the endothelium is the maintenance of thromboresistance. Intact endothelium serves as a mechanical barrier to blood elements and prevents the interaction of subendothelial matrix components, such as von Willebrand factor (vWF), fibronectin, and collagen, that initiate platelet adhesion and aggregation. When endothelial injury occurs, exposure of this highly reactive subendothelial surface triggers a cascade of events that results in platelet aggregation, coagulation, and luminal thrombosis. Under basal conditions, the endothelium maintains an homeostatic balance between thrombosis and fibrinolysis through the generation of antiplatelet mediators, such as NO and prostacyclin, and anticoagulant and fibrinolytic factors, such as thrombomodulin, heparan sulfate, and tissue-type plasminogen activator (t-PA), that inhibit local thrombosis. Disease states, such as atherosclerosis, hypercholesterolemia, and diabetes mellitus, are associated with impaired antithrombotic functions of the endothelium and increased expression of endothelium-derived prothrombotic mediators, such as plasminogen activator inhibitor-1 (PAI-1) and tissue factor, that alter this delicate balance between local fibrinolysis and thrombosis, favoring the latter [4].

Recent evidence suggests that the inflammatory response plays an important role in the development, progression, and activity of atherosclerotic lesions [5]. The endothelium normally inhibits leukocyte adhesion, lipid deposition, and smooth muscle cell proliferation. In response to injury or cytokines, activated endothelial cells upregulate adhesion molecule expression, such as intercellular adhesion molecule-1 (ICAM-1) and vascular cell adhesion molecule-1 (VCAM-1) [6], and release chemoattractants, such as monocyte chemotactic protein-1 (MCP-1), that facilitate endothelial-leukocyte interactions. Under such pathophysiologic conditions, these phenotypic changes of endothelial cells support monocyte recruitment, inflammation, foam cell formation, metalloproteinase activation, and, ultimately, plaque weakening and rupture leading to acute cardiovascular events.

"Endothelial dysfunction" represents a pathophysiologic state in which these collective homeostatic properties of normal endothelial cells are impaired or lost, thereby promoting an atherogenic milieu. Abnormalities in endothelial function are believed to play a central role in the pathophysiology of common cardiovascular syndromes, such as myocardial infarction, unstable angina, and stroke. Endothelial dysfunction is associated with a growing number of risk factors for cardiovascular disease, including smoking, diabetes mellitus, hypertension, hyperlipidemia, hyperhomocystinemia, menopause, and advanced age [3,7–9]. Importantly, in individuals with risk factors, this physiologic disturbance is detectable very early in the progression of atherosclerosis, long before the appearance of visible stenotic lesions. This association suggests a biologic link between endothelial dysfunction and vascular disease, thus making it an ideal target for primary preventive intervention.

A central feature of impaired endothelial function under pathologic conditions appears, at least in part, to relate to an abnormality in endothelium-derived NO (EDNO) bioactivity, underscoring the importance of NO in antiatherogenesis [10]. Reduced intracellular availability of L-arginine for NO synthesis, altered NO synthase activity, impaired receptor-mediated release of NO in response to stimuli, and increased inactivation of NO owing to excess vascular generation of oxidized LDL or reactive oxygen species, such as superoxide anion (O_2^{--}), are among several described mechanisms linked to reduced NO bioavailability. Increased oxidative stress, in particular, represents a mechanistic feature shared by several disease states, including hypertension, atherosclerosis, and mechanical injury and, in addition to NO inactivation, has been associated with expression of inflammatory genes and vascular smooth muscle cell proliferative responses that promote atheroma formation.

Clinical assessment of the endothelium represents a challenging task owing to its heterogeneous functions; no single test provides a comprehensive physiologic assessment of endothelial function. Several plasma measurements of endothelium-derived substances, such as PAI-1, vWF, and endothelin have been used as surrogate markers of endothelial activity and have positively correlated with adverse cardiovascular outcomes. However, most clinical studies have focused primarily on the regulation of vascular tone as a means of assessing endothelial function through interrogation of NO-mediated, endothelium-dependent vasodilator responses to specific agonists, such as acetylcholine, serotonin, or shear stress, which normally provoke vasodilation. Paradoxical constriction or attenuated dilator responses are observed in disease states associated with atherosclerosis or risk factors for coronary heart disease, reflecting impaired vasomotor function and reduced endothelial NO bioactivity.

Because abnormal endothelial physiology is implicated in the genesis and progression of vascular disease, prevention or reversal of endothelial dysfunction represents an attractive goal for therapeutic intervention. Indeed, several interventions have been consistently shown to restore endothelial vasomotor function. These include, among others, lipid-lowering therapy, angiotensin-converting enzyme (ACE) inhibitor therapy, L-arginine, tetrahydrobiopterin, folate, antioxidant and estrogen supplementation, smoking cessation, and exercise [11,12]. Interestingly, these are the very same interventions that attenuate atherosclerosis and improve morbidity and mortality outcomes from cardiovascular disease, suggesting a mechanistic link between endothelial dysfunction and atherosclerosis.

The simple presence or anatomic severity of fixed atherosclerotic lesions is not necessarily predictive of cardiac events. Instead, atherothrombotic disease is a dynamic process that relates to plaque rupture, intraluminal thrombosis, and vasospasm. The morphologic

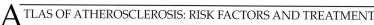

characteristics of vulnerable plaques relate to their structural and physiologic features that are largely influenced by neighboring endothelial cells. Although the precise causes of plaque rupture remain undefined, it is clear that these events reflect a dramatic loss of endothelial function and vascular homeostasis. Identification and treatment of individuals with endothelial dysfunction may lead to improvement in vascular function, attenuation of atherosclerosis progression, and a reduction in the risk of adverse cardiovascular events.

ENDOTHELIAL REGULATION OF VASOMOTOR TONE

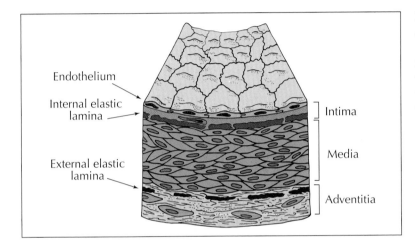

FIGURE 2-1. Structure of a normal muscular artery. The arterial wall consists of three functionally separate layers conventionally termed 1) the intima, 2) the media, and 3) the adventitia. The intimal layer is composed of a single monolayer of endothelial cells, in contact with circulating blood, that serves as a functional barrier, regulates transport and metabolism, and modulates local and systemic vascular physiologic functions. The media consists predominantly of smooth muscle cells, embedded in extracellular matrix, that regulate vascular tone in response to local and humoral stimuli. The adventitia harbors nutrient vessels (vasa vasorum), nerves, and dense fibroelastic tissue. (*Adapted from* Ross and Glomset [13].)

MAJOR ENDOTHELIAL PRODUCTS AND REGULATORY FUNCTIONS

Vasomotor tone
  Vasodilators
    Nitric oxide
    Prostacyclin
    Endothelial-derived hyperpolarizing factor
  Vasoconstrictors
    Endothelin
    Prostaglandin H_2
    Endothelium-derived constricting factor
    Angiotensin II
    Platelet-derived growth factor
    Thromboxane A_2
Fibrinolysis
  Profibrinolytic factors
    Tissue plasminogen activator
    Urokinase-type plasminogen activator
  Antifibrinolytic factor
    Plasminogen activator inhibitor-1

Thrombosis
  Anticoagulants
    Thrombomodulin
    Heparan sulfate
    Dermatan sulfate
  Platelet inhibitors
    Nitric oxide
    Prostacyclin
    Ecto-ADPase
  Procoagulant
    Tissue factor
    Fibronectin
  Platelet activator
    Von Willebrand factor

Cell growth
  Growth inhibition
    Nitric oxide
    Heparan sulfate
    Prostacyclin
  Growth promotion
    Angiotensin II
    Platelet-derived growth factor
    Endothelin
Inflammation
  Anti-inflammatory factors
    Nitric oxide
  Proinflammatory factors
    E-selectin
    Intercellular adhesion molecule-1
    Vascular cell adhesion molecule-1
    Monocyte chemotactic protein
    Interleukin-8

FIGURE 2-2. Endothelial cells regulate a number of important vascular functions, including vasomotor tone, coagulation, inflammation, and vascular growth. A dynamic balance of endothelium-derived substances that act in a paracrine-autocrine fashion largely modulates these regulatory functions. Under pathologic conditions, loss of homeostatic equilibrium owing to increased activity of proinflammatory, prothrombotic, growth promoting, and vasconstrictive factors expressed by dysfunctional endothelial cells supports the underlying pathogenesis of a given disease process. (*Adapted from* Gokce et al. [11].)

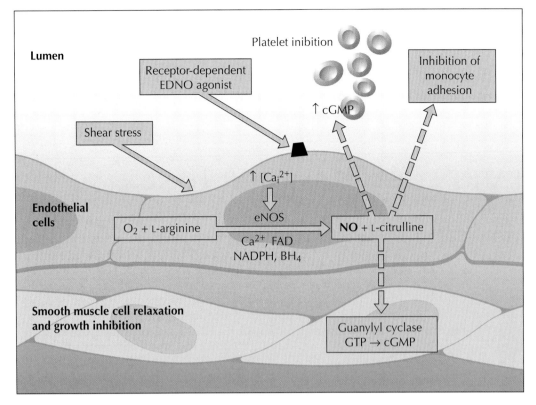

FIGURE 2-3. Endothelium-derived nitric oxide (EDNO) synthesis and action. In endothelial cells, a constitutive membrane-associated NO synthase (eNOS) catalyzes the conversion of the amino acid L-arginine to NO and L-citrulline. eNOS cofactors

include FAD (flavin adenine dinucleotide), NADPH (nicotinamide adenine dinucleotide phosphate), BH_4 (tetrahydrobiopterin), and calcium. Endothelial synthesis of NO is tightly controlled and linked to changes in ionized calcium concentration. Several agonists, including acetylcholine, bradykinin, substance P, and platelet-derived serotonin, act on specific membrane receptors that trigger cytosolic calcium release and eNOS activation. Increased shear stress from enhanced blood flow also serves as an important stimulus for NO production. NO modulates basal vascular tone, and exerts a relaxant effect on vascular smooth muscle through activation of soluble guanylyl cyclase and consequent increase in intracellular cGMP, which also mediates NO-dependent inhibition of platelet activation. Individuals with coronary risk factors or atherosclerosis demonstrate impaired shear stress– and agonist-induced endothelium-dependent vasodilation. Other actions of NO include inhibition of monocyte adhesion and smooth muscle cell proliferation. GTP—guanosine 5'-triphosphate. (*Adapted from* Gokce *et al.* [11].)

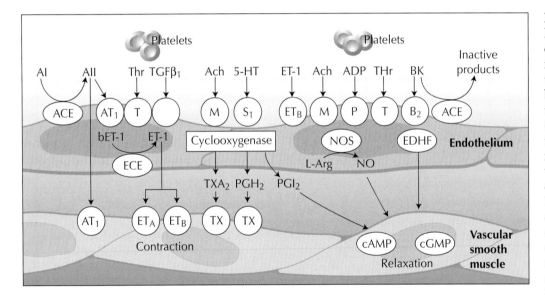

FIGURE 2-4. Endothelial vasoactive agents. Endothelial control of vascular tone is a dynamic process that involves the complex interplay of a number of vasoactive mediators, derived not only from endothelial cells but also from circulating platelets (serotonin, ADP), circulating humoral agents (epinephrine, vasopressin), and nerve terminals. The relative actions of these mediators ultimately determine effective vascular tone. ACE—angiotensin-converting enzyme; Ach—acetylcholine; BK—bradykinin; ECE—endothelin-converting enzymes; EDHF—endothelium-derived hyperpolarizing factor; ET-1—endothelin-1; 5HT—5-hydroxytryptamine (serotonin); L-arg—L-arginine; NOS—nitric oxide synthase; PGH_2—prostaglandin H_2; PGl_2—prostacyclin; $TGF\beta_1$—transforming growth-factor-β_1; Thr—thrombin; TXA_2—thromboxane A_2. *Circles* represent receptors (AT—angio-tensinergic; B—bradykinergic; M—muscarinic; P—purinergic; T—thrombin receptors.) (*Adapted from* Luscher and Noll [14].)

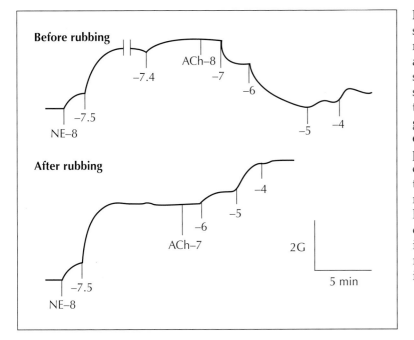

Before rubbing

After rubbing

FIGURE 2-5. A seminal observation made by Furchgott [15] underscores the critical functional importance of endothelial cells in the regulation of vascular tone. These investigators reported that acetylcholine (ACh)-mediated relaxation of isolated rabbit aorta segments was lost following "unintentional rubbing of its intimal surface against foreign substances during its preparation." In functionally normal arteries, ACh serves as an agonist for endothelial generation of NO and consequent vessel relaxation. When the endothelium is rubbed off, or rendered dysfunctional, ACh promotes "paradoxical" vasoconstriction owing to a direct constrictor effect on vascular smooth muscle cells. This highlights the potential of selective agents to evoke seemingly disparate responses depending on the functional integrity of the endothelium, and effective endothelium-derived NO release. Disease conditions associated with endothelial dysfunction are characterized by impaired agonist-mediated vascular relaxation that may result in impaired coronary blood flow and lead to myocardial ischemia. (*Adapted from* Furchgott [15].)

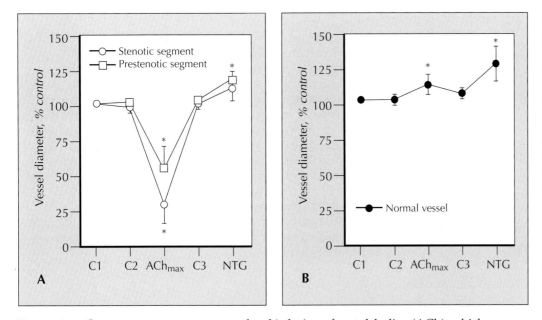

FIGURE 2-6. Coronary artery responses to local infusion of acetylcholine (ACh), which serves as an endothelium-dependent stimulus for NO release, and nitroglycerin (NTG), which

causes vasodilation through a direct (endothelium-independent) effect on vascular smooth muscle cells. **A,** Coronary ACh infusion results in pathologic constriction at sites of minimal or advanced coronary atherosclerotic lesions, arguing for impaired local endothelium-derived NO release in these regions. **B,** In contrast, normal coronary arteries demonstrate intact vasodilator responses to both ACh and NTG. This "paradoxical" constriction of atherosclerotic coronary artery segments provides evidence for endothelial dysfunction not only in vessels with advanced lesions but also in arteries with minimal, nonobstructive atherosclerosis early in the course of the disease process. Impaired vasomotor function may contribute to flow disturbances and clinical symptoms in vessels that do not appear to have flow-limiting obstructive lesions. *Asterisks* indicate $P < 0.05$ C—control. (*Adapted from* Ludmer *et al.* [16].)

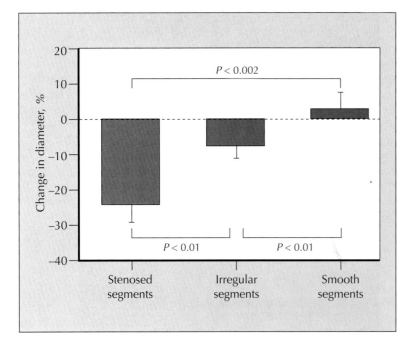

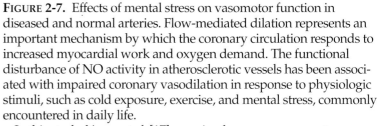

FIGURE 2-7. Effects of mental stress on vasomotor function in diseased and normal arteries. Flow-mediated dilation represents an important mechanism by which the coronary circulation responds to increased myocardial work and oxygen demand. The functional disturbance of NO activity in atherosclerotic vessels has been associated with impaired coronary vasodilation in response to physiologic stimuli, such as cold exposure, exercise, and mental stress, commonly encountered in daily life.

In this study, Yeung *et al.* [17] examined coronary vasomotor responses to mental stress testing by intentionally frustrating willing participants who were asked to perform rapid mathematical calculations during cardiac catheterization. Diseased vessels developed up to 24% constriction in the setting of mental stress testing, in contrast to normal vessels with preserved dilator responses. Impaired vasomotor function may evoke myocardial ischemia in individuals with fixed coronary stenoses and aggravate a supply-demand mismatch. In addition, clinical stimuli such as cold exposure and mental stress are associated with increased circulating catecholamines, and individuals with endothelial dysfunction exhibit a greater sensitivity to the constrictor effects of catecholamines [18] that may further augment the functional severity of fixed lesions. (*Adapted from* Yeung *et al.* [17].)

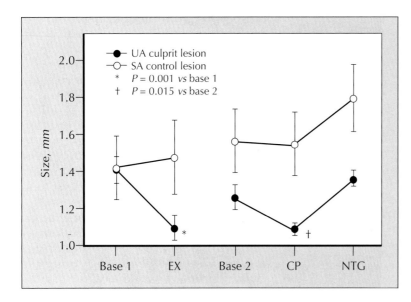

FIGURE 2-8. Abnormal vasoreactivity is also involved in the pathogenesis of acute coronary syndromes. This figure demonstrates changes in luminal diameter of the culprit coronary artery lesion in unstable angina (UA) compared with a control lesion in stable angina (SA) at baseline, with exercise (EX), with the cold pressor test (CP), and following exposure to nitroglycerin (NTG). The culprit lesion involved in unstable angina exhibits a greater degree of vasoconstriction in comparison to stable lesions. Loss of flow-mediated dilation and increased coronary vasoconstriction may in turn lead to elevated shear stress at the site of an atherosclerotic lesion and increase the likelihood of plaque rupture and thrombosis. In the face of ineffective endothelium-derived NO release, local generation of platelet-derived products, including serotonin and thrombin, may further induce vasoconstriction and result in severe flow limitation superimposed on mechanical obstruction and vascular thrombosis. (*Adapted from* Bogaty *et al.* [19].)

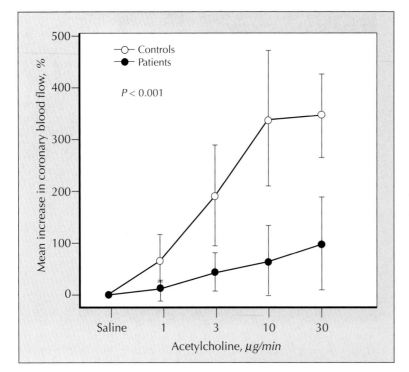

FIGURE 2-9. Endothelial dysfunction and microvascular angina. Endothelial dysfunction may predominantly involve coronary resistance vessels in the absence of detectable obstructive epicardial coronary artery disease. Impaired endothelium-dependent microvascular dilation has been demonstrated in individuals with syndrome X, a clinical entity characterized by anginal chest pain, elevated coronary sinus lactate concentrations, and angiographically normal epicardial coronary arteries. Impaired vasomotor regulation in resistance vessels may represent one mechanism underlying the pathophysiology of myocardial ischemia in these individuals with altered microvascular physiology and otherwise "normal" coronary angiograms. Deficient NO activity has also been demonstrated in arteries of patients with vasospastic angina, who otherwise also have angiographically smooth vessels. (*Adapted from* Egashira *et al.* [20].)

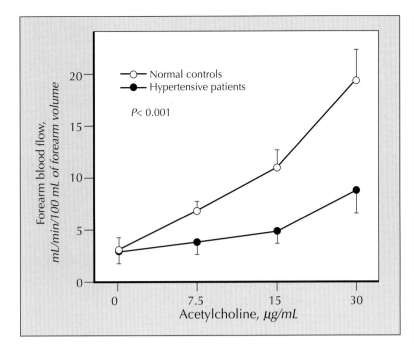

FIGURE 2-10. Hypertension is among several risk factors for coronary artery disease , including diabetes mellitus, hypercholesterolemia, and tobacco use, that are characterized by impaired endothelium-derived nitric oxide (EDNO) bioactivity. Hypertensive individuals display impaired epicardial and resistance vessel dilation in response to EDNO agonists in both the peripheral and coronary circulations. Whether loss of EDNO action is a consequence of chronically elevated blood pressure or, instead, is involved in the pathogenesis of hypertension itself, is unclear. Normotensive offspring of individuals with essential hypertension have impaired vasodilator responses to acetylcholine [21], which suggests a primary abnormality and genetic basis for a defect involving NO activity in some forms of hypertension. Excess production of endogenous vasconstrictors, such as angiotensin-II and endothelin, decreased availability of the NO precursor L-arginine, defects in G-protein–dependent intracellular signaling pathways, and NO inactivation owing to excess generation of reactive oxygen species are mechanisms implicated in the pathophysiology of hypertension. (*Adapted from* Panza *et al.* [22].)

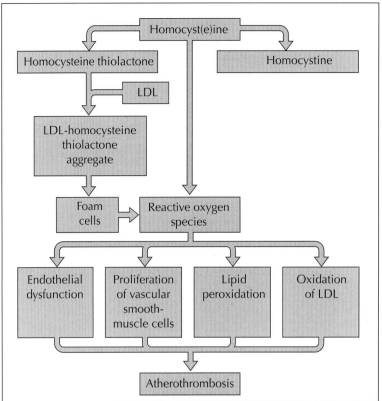

FIGURE 2-11. Hyperhomocystinemia has recently emerged as a modifiable independent risk factor for atherosclerosis and atherothrombosis involving the coronary and peripheral circulations. Elevations in plasma homocysteine are generally caused by enzymatic defects or cofactor/vitamin deficiencies (B_{12}, folate) involved in pathways of homocysteine metabolism. The atherogenic propensity associated with hyperhomocystinemia has been linked to impaired endothelial function at several levels, including reduced NO synthesis, altered endothelial antithrombotic activity, enhanced oxidative vascular injury, and increased vascular smooth muscle cell proliferation [23]. LDL—low-density lipoprotein. (*Adapted from* Welch and Loscalzo [24].)

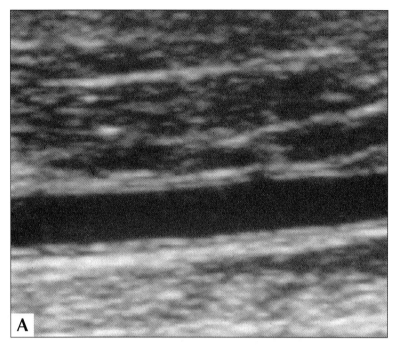
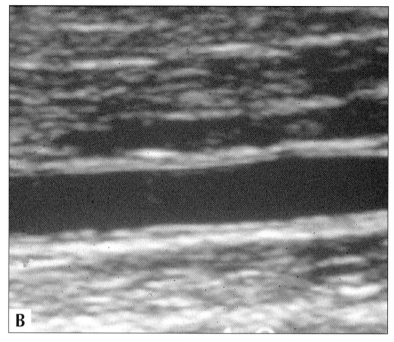
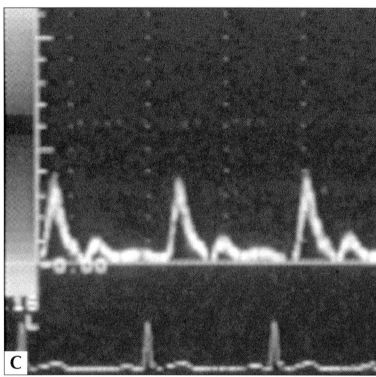
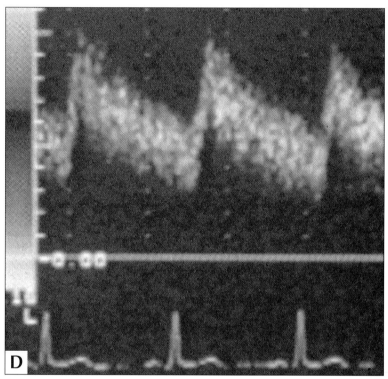

FIGURE 2-12. Clinical studies of in vivo endothelial NO action have generally required the use of invasive catheter techniques for local intra-arterial delivery of NO agonists to interrogate coronary and peripheral physiologic responses. The need for invasive techniques has limited the number of subjects who can be studied and the number of studies that can be repeated in each individual. This limitation has recently led to the development of noninvasive tools to examine vasomotor function with the use of high-resolution vascular ultrasound. This figure shows flow-mediated, endothelium-dependent brachial artery dilation in a healthy individual. Two-dimensional (**A** and **B**) and Doppler (**C** and **D**) images were obtained using an ultrasound system with a 7.5-MHz linear array probe. Images were obtained at baseline (**A** and **C**) and after induction of hyperemia (**B** and **D**) that mediates shear stress-induced endothelium-derived nitric oxide (EDNO) release produced by deflating a forearm cuff following a 5-minute flow occlusion period. In normal individuals, greater than 10% vasodilation of the brachial artery is typically observed, whereas in individuals with coronary artery disease or risk factors for coronary artery disease, the dilator response is blunted or absent. A close correlation has been demonstrated between the presence of endothelial dysfunction in the brachial artery and dysfunction in the coronary circulation [25]. Interventions that reduce cardiovascular risk and improve coronary EDNO action also have similar effects in the brachial circulation. Thus, examination of brachial artery vasomotor function may provide noninvasive information potentially applicable to vascular physiology in the coronary and, possibly, cerebrovascular beds [25,26].

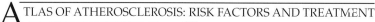

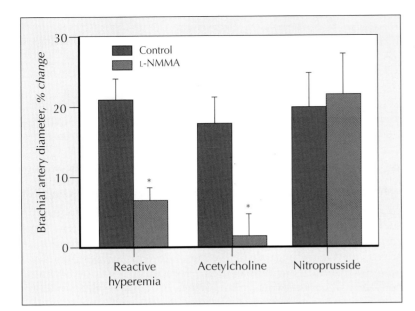

FIGURE 2-13. The dilator response to reactive hyperemia in the forearm circulation is largely NO-dependent. In this figure, brachial artery diameter was measured in response to hyperemia, during intra-arterial acetylcholine infusion, and during infusion of the endothelium-independent vasodilator nitroprusside. Extent of vasodilation is expressed as a percent change from baseline. After infusion of the NO synthase antagonist, NG-monomethyl-L-arginine (L-NMMA), the dilator responses to hyperemia and acetylcholine are significantly reduced, providing evidence for the dependence of these responses on endothelium-derived NO action. L-NMMA has no effect on endothelium-independent relaxation to nitroprusside. (*Adapted from* Lieberman *et al.* [27].)

POSSIBLE MECHANISMS OF REDUCED EDNO ACTIVITY IN CARDIOVASCULAR DISEASE

Reduced availability of substrate
  Arginine deficiency
  Reduced activity/expression of cationic amino acid transporter
  Increased activity/expression of arginase
  Reduced activity of argininosuccinate synthetase
Antagonism of NOS
  Overproduction of ADMA
  Decreased activity/expression of DDAH
  Inhibition by endogenous NO
  Inhibition by exogenous NO donors
Alterations in NOS
  Reduced expression
  Reduced dimerization
  Aberrant palmitoylation, myristoylation, or phosphorylation
Degradation of NO
  Increased generation of O_2^-
Reduced availability of cofactors
  Folate deficiency
  Reduced generation of tetrahydrobiopterin

FIGURE 2-14. A central mechanistic feature of impaired endothelial function under pathologic conditions relates, at least in part, to abnormalities in NO bioactivity. Derangements in the NO pathway have been linked to the pathophysiology of a number of cardiovascular disorders including atherosclerotic coronary artery disease, systemic and pulmonary hypertension, congestive heart failure, vasospasm, microvascular angina, and ischemia-reperfusion injury. Possible mechanisms of reduced endothelium-derived NO bioactivity include decreased availability of substrate or cofactors for NO synthesis, impaired NO synthase (NOS) activity, endogenous inhibition of NOS (by ADMA), and increased NO degradation. ADMA—asymmetric dimethylarginine; DDAH—dimethylarginine dimethylaminohydrolase. (*Adapted from* Cooke and Dzau [28].)

$$NO \cdot \xrightarrow{\;O_2^{-\cdot}\;} OONO^- \xrightarrow[\text{SOD, Fe}^{2+}]{\;H^+\;} NO_2^+ + OH^-$$

$$NO \cdot \xrightarrow[\;H_2O\;]{\;O_2\;} NO_2^- + H^+ \xrightarrow[\;O_2\;]{\;H^+\;} NO_3^- + H^+$$

FIGURE 2-15. Ample evidence suggests that increased vascular oxidative stress plays an important role in reduced endothelium-derived nitric oxide (EDNO) bioactivity. Oxidative stress describes a pathophysiologic state in which endothelial cells are exposed to excessive levels of reactive oxygen species (ROS). ROS are products of normal cellular metabolism whereby oxygen undergoes a series of univalent reductions, producing a number of highly reactive intermediates, including superoxide anion ($O_2^{-\cdot}$), which directly inactivates NO and produces peroxynitrite anion ($OONO^-$). Peroxynitrite anion is capable of causing lipid peroxidation and promoting the formation of other oxidants, including hydroxyl radical ($\cdot OH$), hypochlorous acid (HOCl), reactive aldehydes, and nitrogen oxides. Major enzymatic sources of ROS are linked to the activity of cyclooxygenases, the mitochondrial electron transport chain, eNOS, and membrane-bound NADH/NADPH oxidases that are expressed by endothelial and vascular smooth muscle cells and fibroblasts. NADH/NADPH oxidase activity is enhanced by angiotensin-II (AT-II) in animal models of hypertension [29]. Excessive production of superoxide is a common feature of several disease states, including hypertension, hypercholesterolemia, atherosclerosis, diabetes mellitus, and congestive heart failure, providing evidence for increased NO inactivation in these pathologic conditions. Fe^{2+}—ferrous iron; NADH—nicotinamide adenine dinucleotide phosphate; NADPH—reduced nicotinamide adenine dinucleotide phosphate; NO_2^-—nitrite; NO_3^-— nitrate; SOD—superoxide dismutase. (*Adapted from* Cohen [30].)

ENDOTHELIAL DYSFUNCTION AND INFLAMMATION

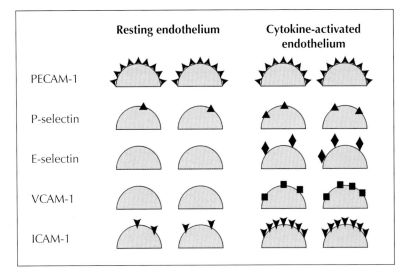

FIGURE 2-16. The inflammatory response plays an important role in the development, progression, and activity of atherosclerotic lesions. Monocyte adhesion to the endothelial surface represents one of the earliest stages in atherosclerotic lesion formation. Cell-surface integrins and adhesion molecules facilitate endothelial-leukocyte interactions, and play an important role in modulating cellular transmigration and signal transduction. Upregulation of surface ligands becomes manifest under pathologic conditions, such as atherosclerosis, supporting the inflammatory process. As a correlate, plasma concentrations of soluble adhesions molecules are elevated in individuals with coronary artery and peripheral vascular disease, providing evidence for a mechanistic association between inflammation and atherosclerosis; ICAM-1—intracellular adhesion molecule-1; VCAM-1—vascular cell adhesion molecule-1. PECAM-1—platelet-endothelial cell adhesion molecule-1. (*Adapted from* Stein *et al.* [31].)

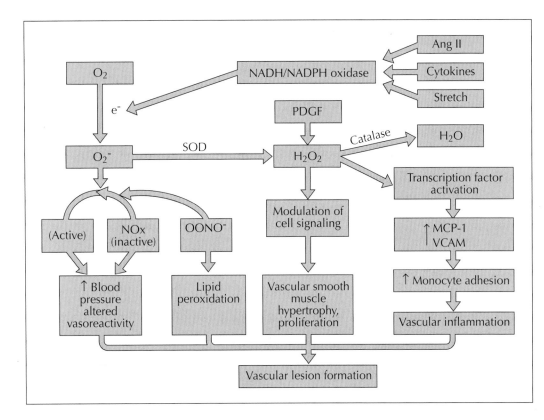

FIGURE 2-17. In the setting of increased oxidative stress, endothelial cells lose their protective phenotype and express proinflammatory, vasoconstrictive, and growth promoting factors that support atherogenesis. These processes appear to be, in part, mediated by excess vascular superoxide formation that stimulates surface adhesion molecule expression, inactivates NO, alters cell signaling, and promotes lipid peroxidation. Expression of many adhesion molecules is controlled by the transcriptional regulatory protein nuclear factor-κ regulated by intracellular signal pathways sensitive to the intracellular redox state [32]. H_2O_2— hydrogen peroxide; AngII—angiotensin II; PDGF—platelet-derived growth factor; SoD—superoxide dismutase; MCP-1—monocyte chemotactic protein-1; VCAM-1—vascular cell adhesion molecule-1. (*Adapted from* Kojda and Harrison [33].)

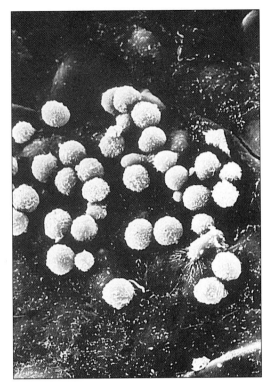

FIGURE 2-18. Electron micrograph demonstrating leukocytes adherent to vascular endothelium. Accumulation of monocytes on the endothelial surface and subsequent transformation into lipid-laden foam cells leads to "fatty streak" formation, representing the earliest visible lesion in atherosclerosis. Fatty streaks along the vascular wall are detectable as early as adolescence, with the potential to develop into complex lesions depending on the presence of atherogenic stimuli. (*From* Ross [34]; with permission.)

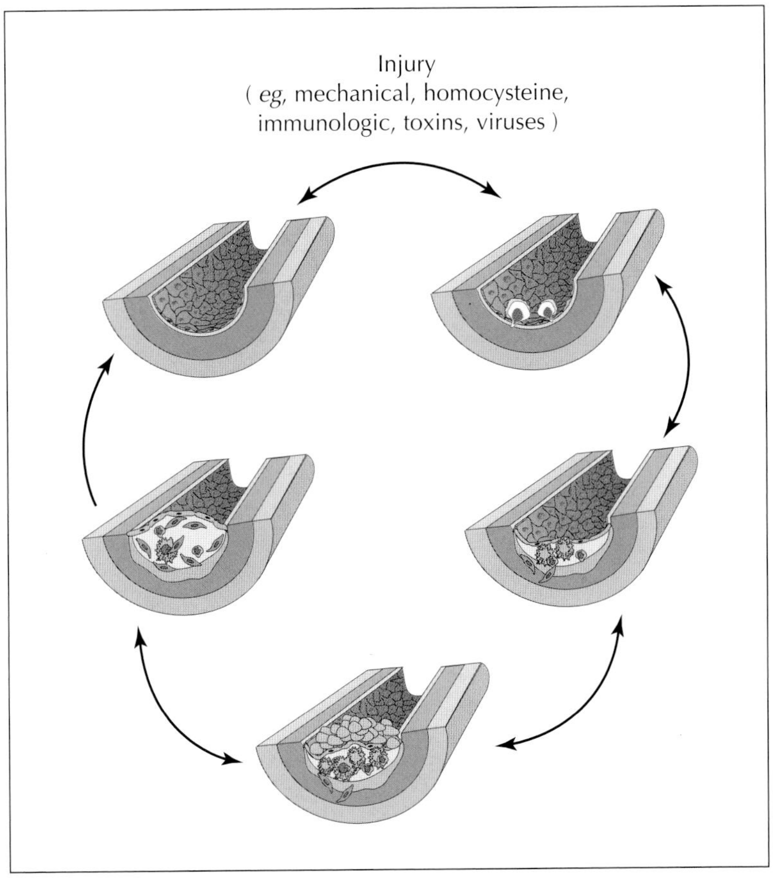

Injury
(*eg*, mechanical, homocysteine,
immunologic, toxins, viruses)

FIGURE 2-19. The response-to-injury hypothesis of atherosclerosis. In response to mechanical injury or exposure to atherogenic stimuli, such as hypercholesterolemia, diabetes mellitus, hyperhomocysteinemia, and cigarette smoking, endothelial cells express adhesion molecules and elaborate growth factors that lead to recruitment of leukocytes in an inflammatory response to injury. Leukocytes adhere and migrate into the vessel wall, localize subendothelially, and develop into lipid-laden macrophages (foam cells). Foam cells, in turn, release growth factors and cytokines that promote recruitment of smooth muscle cells and stimulate neointimal proliferation, continue to accumulate lipid, and support endothelial cell dysfunction. Collectively, these events promote the development of a lipid-rich atheromatous lesion. Subsequent denudation of the endothelium exposes circulating platelets and coagulants to the underlying matrix, thereby initiating thrombosis, and triggering a cascade of events leading to a fibroproliferative lesion and luminal narrowing. (*Adapted from* Ross [35].)

PLASMA MARKERS OF ENDOTHELIAL CELL FUNCTION

Markers for which clinical data are available
  Fibrinolytic substances
    Plasminogen activators
    Plasminogen activator inhibitor-1
  Procoagulant substances
    Von Willebrand factor
    Fibronectin
  Antiplatelet substances
    Nitric oxide
    Prostacyclin
  Metabolic substances
    Lipoprotein lipase
Potential markers
  Activated protein C
  Antithrombin II
  Angiotensin-converting enzyme
  Heparan sulfate
  Laminin
  Protease nexin
  Thrombospondin
  Tissue factor
  Vitronectin

FIGURE 2-20. In addition to the regulation of vascular tone and inflammation, the endothelium plays an important role in the maintenance of thromboresistance. Endothelial cells are capable of synthesizing a number of antithrombotic, fibrinolytic, and procoagulant factors that are biochemically detectable in plasma. The antithrombotic/procoagulant balance is tightly regulated, and depends on dynamic shifts in the localized vascular milieu that are disturbed in pathologic disease conditions. (*Adapted from* Mendelsohn and Loscalzo [36].)

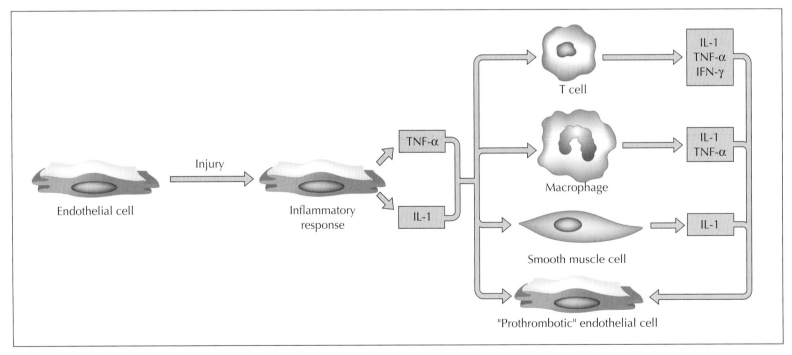

FIGURE 2-21. The role of cytokines in atherothrombosis. Endothelial injury, or exposure to atherogenic stimuli, triggers endothelial cell inflammatory responses leading to recruitment of leukocytes and release of cytokines, including tumor necrosis factor-α (TNF-α), interleukin-1 (IL-1), and interferon gamma (IFN-γ). These cytokines, in addition to amplifying the immune response, alter endothelial cell function towards a prothrombotic phenotype, characterized by increased production of plasminogen activator inhibitor-1, tissue factor expression (and activation of the extrinsic coagulation pathway), and release of platelet-derived growth factors (PDGF). (*Adapted from* Dobroski *et al.* [37].)

NORMAL VERSUS. DYSFUNCTIONAL ENDOTHELIAL CELLS

NORMAL ENDOTHELIAL CELL	DYSFUNCTIONAL ENDOTHELIAL CELLS
PGI_2 production	Decreased PGI_2 production
EDRF release	Decreased EDRF release
t-PA production	Increased thromboplastin production
Ecto-ADPase activity	Inhibition of endothelial cell-dependent protein C activation
Facilitation of vascular uptake and degradation of prothrombotic amines	Decreased resistance to platelet adhesion
Thrombin-binding and inactivation	Increased PAI-1 release
Thrombomodulin expression	Impaired thrombomodulin expression
Glycosaminoglycan expression	Tissue factor expression

FIGURE 2-22. Thromboresistant properties of normal endothelial cells are impaired in pathologic conditions associated with disease states such as hypertension, diabetes mellitus, smoking, hypercholesterolemia, and hyperhomocysteinemia. Altered antithrombotic functions of diseased endothelium may be one mechanism linked to increased propensity for atherothrombosis associated with these disease states. EDRF—endothelium-derived relaxing factor; PAI-1—platelet activator inhibitor-1; PGI_2—prostacyclin; t-PA—tissue plasminogen activator. (*Adapted from* Dobroski *et al.* [37].)

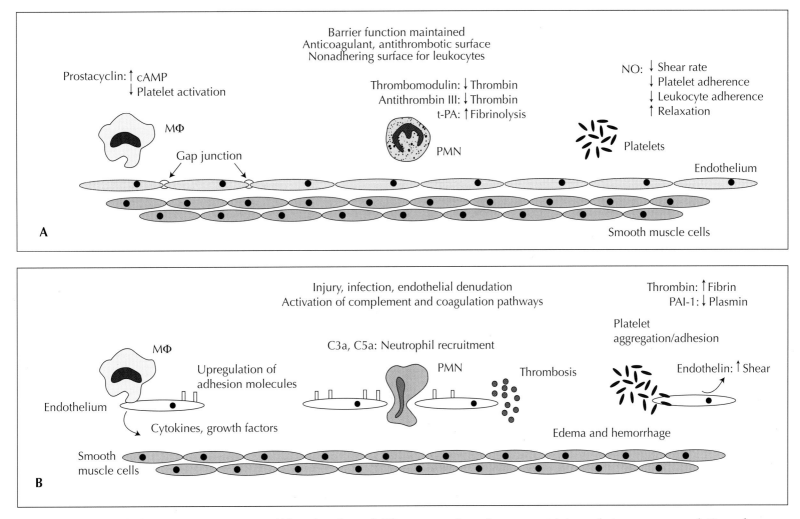

FIGURE 2-23. Metabolic events in quiescent (**A**) and activated (**B**) endothelium. In response to injury or exposure to atherogenic stimuli, the phenotypic alterations that occur in "activated" endothelial cells impose a loss on normal homeostatic functions, and promote atherogenesis and thrombosis. Characteristics of activated endothelium include impaired NO release, increased generation of vasoconstrictor substances, upregulation of inflammatory mediators and leukocyte recruitment, increased expression of prothrombotic factors, and loss of mechanical barrier function. MΦ—macrophage; PAI-1—platelet activator inhibitor-1; PMN—polymorphonuclear leukocyte; t-PA—tissue plasminogen activator. (*Adapted from* Makrides and Ryan [38].)

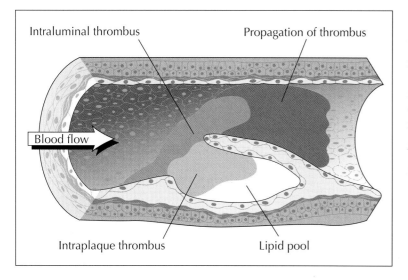

Intraluminal thrombus Propagation of thrombus

Blood flow

Intraplaque thrombus Lipid pool

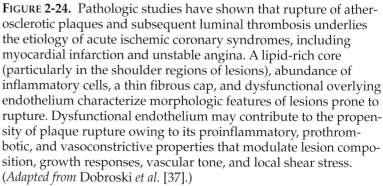

FIGURE 2-24. Pathologic studies have shown that rupture of atherosclerotic plaques and subsequent luminal thrombosis underlies the etiology of acute ischemic coronary syndromes, including myocardial infarction and unstable angina. A lipid-rich core (particularly in the shoulder regions of lesions), abundance of inflammatory cells, a thin fibrous cap, and dysfunctional overlying endothelium characterize morphologic features of lesions prone to rupture. Dysfunctional endothelium may contribute to the propensity of plaque rupture owing to its proinflammatory, prothrombotic, and vasoconstrictive properties that modulate lesion composition, growth responses, vascular tone, and local shear stress. (*Adapted from* Dobroski *et al.* [37].)

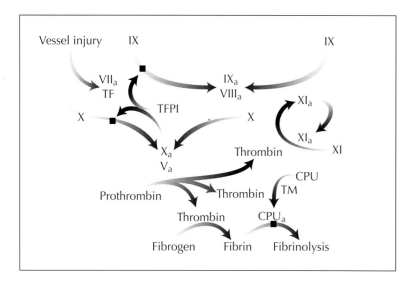

FIGURE 2-25. Intimal injury and exposure of circulating blood to subendothelial matrix components triggers a series of thrombotic events that result in luminal occlusion. Initial events include platelet adhesion and aggregation at the site of localized injury, followed by tissue factor-mediated activation of the coagulation cascade leading to thrombin formation, and rapid generation of fibrin intermeshed with aggregating platelets to form a thrombus. Dysfunctional endothelium may potentiate the extent of localized thrombosis and flow occlusion through enhanced expression of prothrombotic factors, such as plasminogen activator inhibitor-1, tissue factor, and factor V; impaired effective release of antiplatelet factors, including NO and prostacyclin; and increased generation of vasoconstrictor substances. CPU—carboxypeptidase-U; TF—tissue factor; TFPI—tissue factor pathway inhibitor; TM—thrombomodulin. (*Adapted from* Broze [39].)

POTENTIAL THERAPIES TO IMPROVE ENDOTHELIAL FUNCTION

POTENTIAL INTERVENTIONS TO IMPROVE ENDOTHELIAL FUNCTION

Lipid-lowering therapy
Angiotensin-converting enzyme inhibitors
Estrogen replacement therapy
Exercise
α-Tocopherol
Probucol
Ascorbic acid
Glutathione repletion
Pyrrolidine dithiocarbamate
Deferoxamine
L-Arginine
Tetrahydrobiopterin
Smoking cessation
? glucose control
? blood pressure control
Folate

FIGURE 2-26. Because endothelial dysfunction is believed to play a role in atherogenesis and the development of acute cardiovascular clinical syndromes, guided therapy toward restoring endothelial function represents an attractive therapeutic goal. Indeed, several acute and chronic interventions have been convincingly shown to improve endothelium-dependent vasomotor function. These include, among others, lipid-lowering therapy, angiotensin-converting enzyme inhibitor therapy, L-arginine, antioxidant and estrogen supplementation, smoking cessation, and exercise. Interestingly, these are the same primary and secondary interventions that have been associated with reduced morbidity and mortality from cardiovascular disease, suggesting a link between amelioration of endothelial function and improved clinical outcomes from vascular disease. (*Adapted from* Gokce *et al.* [11].)

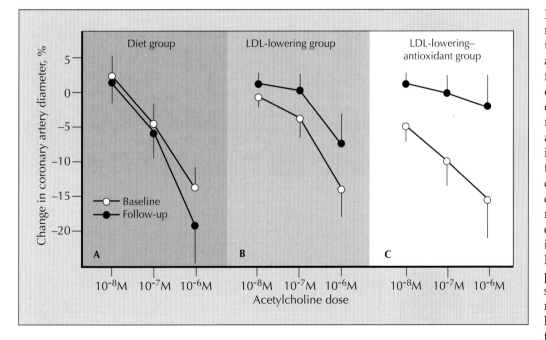

A

B

C

FIGURE 2-27. Endothelium-dependent coronary artery vasomotion in hypercholesterolemic subjects in response to intracoronary acetylcholine infusion at baseline and following 1-year treatment with **A**, diet; **B**, diet + lovastatin and cholestyramine; and **C**, diet + lovastatin and probucol. The medical regimens that consisted of lipid-lowering and antioxidant therapy resulted in greater improvement in endothelial vasomotor function as compared to diet alone. Although cholesterol-lowering therapy clearly reduces cardiovascular events, the mechanism for this reduction does not appear to be regression of existing atherosclerotic lesions [40]. Rather, improved endothelial function and effective NO release, altered lesion composition, and plaque stabilization with a reduced propensity toward lesion ulceration or rupture may represent alternative beneficial effects of lipid-lowering therapy. LDL—low-density lipoprotein. (*Adapted from* Anderson *et al.* [41].)

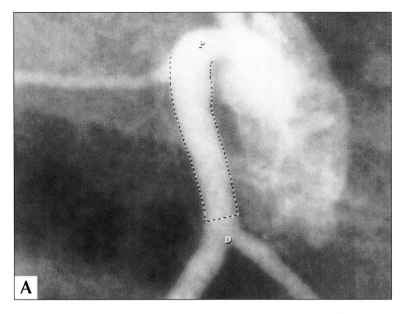

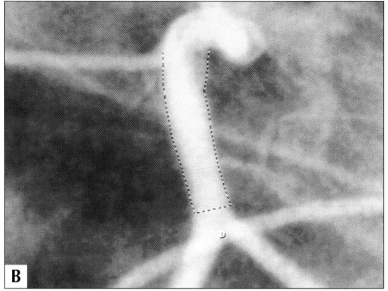

FIGURE 2-28. Coronary angiogram demonstrating improved NO-dependent dilator responses to acetylcholine at baseline (**A**) and following 6 months of treatment with quinapril (**B**). Angiotensin-converting enzyme (ACE) inhibitor therapy has been shown to improve dilator responses in both the coronary and peripheral (forearm) circulations following short-term (1 month) or prolonged therapy. There are a number of potential mechanisms by which ACE inhibitors might improve effective endothelium-derived NO action.

ACE inhibitors reduce production of angiotensin II (AT-II) and prevent ACE-mediated breakdown of the NO-agonist bradykinin. Reduction of AT-II formation may have other effects with regard to endothelial function, including reduction of endothelin-1 synthesis, inhibition of AT-II–induced stimulation of NADH/NADPH oxidases that generate superoxide and degrade NO, reduction in plasminogen activator inhibitor-1 expression, and reduction in vascular smooth muscle cell growth. (*From* Mancini *et al.* [42]; with permission.)

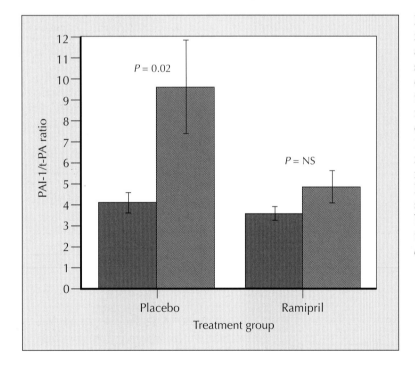

FIGURE 2-29. Although most therapeutic clinical studies have focused primarily on the regulation of NO-dependent vasodilation as a means of assessing endothelial function, there is evidence to suggest that beneficial effects of some interventions extend to other aspects of endothelial function. This point is illustrated by the effect of the angiotensin-converting enzyme (ACE) inhibitor ramipril on vascular fibrinolytic activity in subjects with acute coronary syndromes. In individuals with myocardial infarction, a 14-day treatment with ramipril was associated with a significant reduction in plasminogen activator inhibitor-1 (PAI-1)/tissue plasminogen activator (t-PA) ratios as compared to placebo. Elevated PAI-1 levels have correlated with increased risk of cardiovascular syndromes, and therapeutic manipulation of endothelial antithrombotic activity may represent another salutary effect of ACE inhibitor therapy. Baseline is indicated by *light bars*; day 14 is indicated by *dark bars*. (*Adapted from* Vaughan *et al.* [43].)

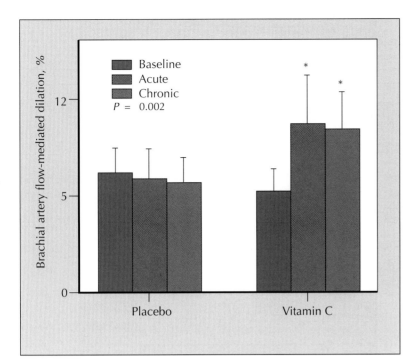

FIGURE 2-30. Considering the relevance of increased oxidative stress as a mechanism of endothelial dysfunction in several disease states, including atherosclerosis, hypertension, diabetes mellitus, hyperhomocysteinemia, and smoking, therapy with antioxidant supplementation has been an attractive therapeutic goal. In individuals with documented coronary disease, ascorbic acid (vitamin C) has been shown to improve endothelium-dependent vasodilation following acute (2 hour) and chronic (1 month) therapy. Similar benefits, in several disease states and different vascular beds, have also been reported with other antioxidants including α-tocopherol (vitamin E), probucol, glutathione, and flavonoid compounds, among others. Potential mechanisms of benefit have included scavenging of superoxide anion, inhibition of low-density lipoprotein oxidation, modulation of intracellular redox state, regulation of inflammatory gene expression, prevention of leukocyte adhesion, and alteration of endothelial NO synthase activity. Vitamin C therapy has also been shown to reduce blood pressure in hypertensive individuals [44]. (*Adapted from* Gokce *et al.* [45].)

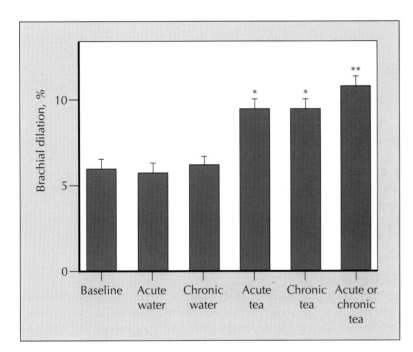

FIGURE 2-31. Epidemiologic data suggest an inverse relationship between tea consumption and cardiovascular disease, an effect that has been attributed to the antioxidant actions of flavonoid compounds. In this study, patients with coronary artery disease were randomly assigned to consume brewed black tea or water in a crossover design. Endothelium-dependent vasodilation improved acutely 2 hours following 450 mL of black tea consumption, and this effect was sustained after 1 month of daily use. Potential beneficial cardiovascular actions of flavonoid compounds including scavenging of reactive oxygen species, inhibition of lipid peroxidation through chelation of transition metal ions, reduction in low-density lipoprotein susceptibility to oxidation, and increased NO bioactivity. Other sources of flavonoids, such as purple grape juice and red wine, have also been shown to improve endothelial function. Some have suggested that high flavonoid intake may serve as a potential explanation for the "French paradox." (*Adapted from* Duffy *et al.* [46].)

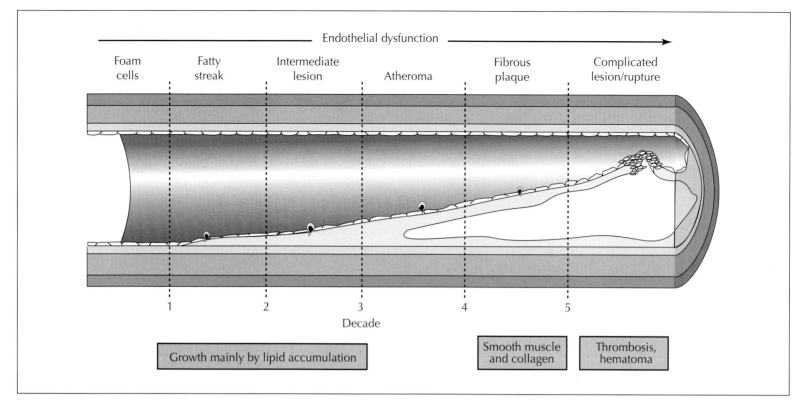

Endothelial dysfunction ──────────────────────────────────────▶

Foam cells | Fatty streak | Intermediate lesion | Atheroma | Fibrous plaque | Complicated lesion/rupture

1   2   3   4   5
Decade

Growth mainly by lipid accumulation

Smooth muscle and collagen | Thrombosis, hematoma

FIGURE 2-32. Atherosclerosis timeline. Physiologic disturbances associated with endothelial dysfunction are detectable very early in the progression of atherosclerosis, long before the appearance of visible obstructive lesions. This suggests a patho-physiologic link between endothelial dysfunction and vascular disease, underscoring the importance of early identification and treatment of risk factors for coronary heart disease. (*Adapted from* Pepine [47].)

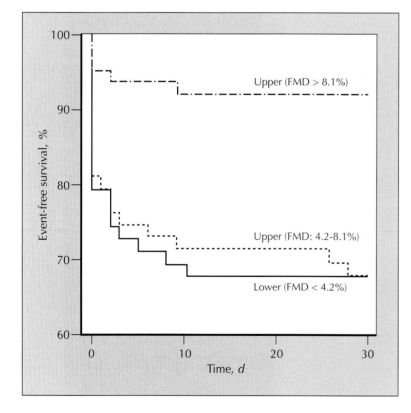

Upper (FMD > 8.1%)

Upper (FMD: 4.2–8.1%)

Lower (FMD < 4.2%)

Event-free survival, %

Time, *d*

FIGURE 2-33. Kaplan-Meier event-free survival curves according to tertile of brachial flow-mediated dilation. The pathophysiologic link between endothelial dysfunction and cardiovascular disease activity is strengthened by recent coronary angiographic studies demonstrating that individuals with impaired endothelial function are at increased risk for future cardiovascular events, independent of coronary lesion severity and traditional cardiac risk factors [48,49]. Ultrasound assessment of brachial artery flow-mediated dilation (FMD) has emerged as a broadly applicable noninvasive method of examining endothelial function, and has shown close correlation with responses in the coronary circulation. To examine the predictive value of brachial artery reactivity testing for future cardiovascular events in patients with atherosclerosis, 187 subjects undergoing elective vascular surgery underwent preoperative brachial ultrasonography and were followed 30 days postoperatively for adverse events, such as myocardial infarction, stroke, unstable angina, or death. This figure demonstrates that individuals with preserved endothelium-dependent vascular dilation had significantly fewer events compared with patients with lower dilator responses. Multivariate analysis identified impaired brachial flow-mediated dilation as a strong independent predictor of adverse postoperative complications (OR 3.7, 1.6–9.3; $P = 0.007$). Thus, endothelial dysfunction in the brachial artery may reflect the integrated effects of systemic risk factors on the entire vasculature, and thus may prove useful in assessing cardiovascular risk noninvasively. Normalization of vascular endothelial function may become a useful target for coronary risk reduction in the future. (*Adapted from* Gokce *et al.* [50].)

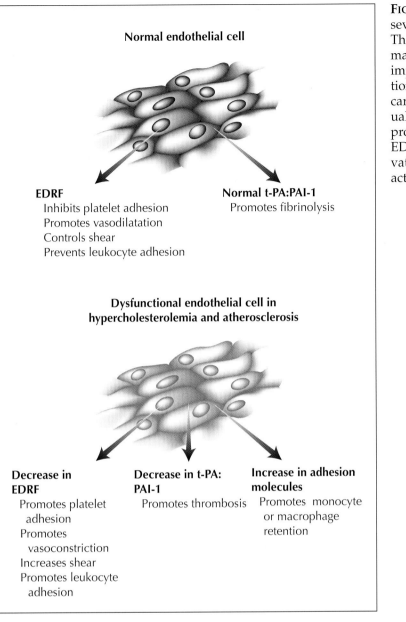

Normal endothelial cell

EDRF
Inhibits platelet adhesion
Promotes vasodilatation
Controls shear
Prevents leukocyte adhesion

Normal t-PA:PAI-1
Promotes fibrinolysis

Dysfunctional endothelial cell in hypercholesterolemia and atherosclerosis

Decrease in EDRF
Promotes platelet adhesion
Promotes vasoconstriction
Increases shear
Promotes leukocyte adhesion

Decrease in t-PA: PAI-1
Promotes thrombosis

Increase in adhesion molecules
Promotes monocyte or macrophage retention

FIGURE 2-34. In summary, endothelial function is a feature of several vascular disease states associated with atherothrombosis. There is strong evidence that phenotypic changes that become manifest in dysfunctional endothelial cells characterized by impaired vasodilator, antithrombotic, and anti-inflammatory functions contribute to the pathogenesis of vascular disease and acute cardiovascular syndromes. Identification and treatment of individuals with endothelial dysfunction may attenuate atherosclerosis progression, and reduce the risk of adverse cardiovascular events. EDRF—endothelium-derived relaxing factor; PAI-1—platelet activator inhibitor-1; PGI$_2$—prostacyclin; t-PA—tissue plasminogen activator. (*Adapted from* Levine *et al.* [40].)

REFERENCES

1. Levine GN, Keaney JF, Jr, Vita JA: Cholesterol reduction in cardiovascular disease: clinical benefits and possible mechanisms. *N Engl J Med* 1995, 332:512–521.

2. Moncada S, Higgs A: The L-arginine nitric oxide pathway. *N Engl J Med* 1993, 329:2002–2012.

3. Vita JA, Treasure CB, Nabel EG, *et al.*: Coronary vasomotor response to acetylcholine relates to risk factors for coronary artery disease. *Circulation* 1990, 81:491–497.

4. Vaughan DE, Schafer AI, Loscalzo J: Normal mechanisms of hemostasis and fibrinolysis. In *Vascular Medicine: A Textbook of Vascular Biology and Diseases*. Edited by Loscalzo J, Creager MA, Dzau VJ: Boston: Little, Brown and Company; 1996: 207–216.

5. Ross R: Atherosclerosis: an inflammatory disease [review]. *N Engl J Med* 1999, 340:115–126.

6. Allen S, Khan S, Al-Mohanna F, *et al.*: Native low density lipoprotein–induced calcium transients trigger VCAM-1 and E-selectin expression in cultured human vascular endothelial cells. *J Clin Invest* 1998, 101:1064–1075.

7. Celermajer DS, Sorensen KE, Georgakopoulos D, *et al.*: Cigarette smoking is associated with dose-related and potentially reversible impairment of endothelium-dependent dilation in healthy young adults. *Circulation* 1993, 88:2149–2155.

8. Johnstone MT, Creager SJ, Scales KM, *et al.*: Impaired endothelium-dependent vasodilation in patients with insulin-dependent diabetes mellitus. *Circulation* 1993, 88:2510–2516.

9. Bellamy MF, McDowell IFW, Ramsey MW, *et al.*: Hyperhomocystinemia after an oral methionine load acutely impairs endothelial function in healthy adults. *Circulation* 1998, 98:1848–1852.

10. Keaney JF, Jr, Vita JA: Atherosclerosis, oxidative stress, and antioxidant protection in endothelium-derived relaxing factor action. *Prog Cardiovasc Dis* 1995, 38:129–154.

11. Gokce N, Keaney JF, Jr, Vita JA: Endotheliopathies: clinical manifestations of endothelial dysfunction. In *Thrombosis and Hemorrhage*, edn 2. Edited by Loscalzo J, Schafer AI. Philadelphia: Lippincott Williams & Wilkins; 1998: 901–924.

12. Stroes ES, van Faasen EE, Yo M, *et al.*: Folic acid reverts dysfunction of endothelial nitric oxide synthase. *Circ Res* 2000, 86:1129–1134.

13. Ross R, Glomset JA: The pathogenesis of atherosclerosis (part 1). *N Engl J Med* 1976, 295:369–377.

14. Luscher T, Noll G: Coronary blood flow and myocardial ischemia. In *Heart Disease*. Edited by Braunwald E. Philadelphia: WB Saunders; 1997:1161–1184.

15. Furchgott R: Role of endothelium in responses of vascular smooth muscle. *Circ Res* 1983, 53:557–573.

16. Ludmer PL, Selwyn AP, Shook TL, *et al.*: Paradoxical vasoconstriction induced by acetylcholine in atherosclerotic coronary arteries. *N Engl J Med* 1986, 315:1046–1051.

17. Yeung AC, Vekshtein VI, Krantz DS, *et al.*: The effect of atherosclerosis on the vasomotor response of coronary arteries to mental stress. *N Engl J Med* 1991, 325:1551–1556.

18. Vita JA, Treasure CB, Yeung AC, *et al.*: Patients with evidence of coronary endothelial dysfunction as assessed by acetylcholine infusion demonstrate marked increase in sensitivity to constrictor effects of catecholamines. *Circulation* 1992, 85:1390–1397.

19. Bogaty P, Hackett D, Davies G, Maseri A: Vasoreactivity of the culprit lesion in unstable angina. *Circulation* 1994, 90:5–11.

20. Egashira K, Inou T, Hirooka Y, *et al.*: Evidence of impaired endothelium-dependent coronary vasodilatation in patients with angina pectoris and normal coronary angiograms. *N Engl J Med* 1993, 328:1659–1664.

21. Taddei S, Virdis A, Mattei P, *et al.*: Defective L-arginine-nitric oxide pathway in offspring of essential hypertensive patients. *Circulation* 1996, 94:1298–1303.

22. Panza JA, Quyyumi AA, Brush JE, Epstein SE: Abnormal endothelium-dependent vascular relaxation in patients with essential hypertension. *N Engl J Med* 1990, 323:22–27.

23. Eberhardt RT, Forgione MA, Cap A, *et al.*: Endothelial dysfunction in a murine model of mild hyperhomocyst(e)inemia. *J Clin Invest* 2000, 106:483–491.

24. Welch GN, Loscalzo J: Homocysteine and atherothrombosis. *N Engl J Med* 1998, 338:1042–1050.

25. Anderson TJ, Uehata A, Gerhard MD, *et al.*: Close relation of endothelial function in the human coronary and peripheral circulations. *J Am Coll Cardiol* 1995, 26:1235–1241.

26. Vita JA, Keaney JF, Jr: Ultrasound assessment of endothelial vasomotor function. In *Diagnostics of Vascular Diseases: Principals and Technology*. Edited by Lanzer P, Lipton M: Berlin: Springer; 1996: 249–259.

27. Lieberman EH, Gerhard MD, Uehata A, *et al.*: Flow-induced vasodilation of the human brachial artery is impaired in patients < 40 years of age with coronary artery disease. *Am J Cardiol* 1996, 78:1210–1214.

28. Cooke JP, Dzau JV: Derangements of the nitric oxide synthase pathway, L-arginine, and cardiovascular disease. *Circulation* 1997, 96: 379–382.

29. Rajagopalan S, Kurz S, Munzel T, *et al.*: Angiotensin II-mediated hypertension in the rat increases vascular superoxide production via membrane NADH/NADPH oxidase activation. *J Clin Invest* 1996, 97:1916–1923.

30. Cohen RA: Endothelium-derived vasoactive factors. In *Thrombosis and Hemorrhage*. Edited by Loscalzo J, Schafer AI. Philadelphia: Lippincott Williams & Wilkins; 1998:387–404.

31. Stein B, Khew-Goodall, Gamble J, Vadas MA: Transmigration of leukocytes. In *The Endothelium in Clinical Practice: Source and Target of Novel Therapies*. Edited by Rubanyi GM, Dzau JV. New York: Marcel Dekker; 1997:149–202.

32. Mihm S, Galter M, Droge W: Modulation of transcription factor NF kappa B activity by intracellular glutathione levels and by variations of the extracellular cysteine supply. *FASEB J* 1995, 9:246–252.

33. Kojda G, Harrison DG: Interactions between NO and reactive oxygen species: pathophysiologic importance in atherosclerosis, hypertension, diabetes, and heart failure. *Cardiovasc Res* 1999, 43:562–571.

34. Ross R: The pathogenesis of atherosclerosis. In *Heart Disease: A Textbook of Cardiovascular Disease*. Edited by Braunwald E. Philadelphia: WB Saunders; 1997:1105–1125.

35. Ross R: The pathogenesis of atherosclerosis: a perspective for the 1990s. *Nature* 1993, 362:801–809.

36. Mendelsohn ME, Loscalzo J: The endotheliopathies. In *Vascular Medicine*. Edited by Loscalzo J, Creager MA, Dzau J. London: Little, Brown and Company; 1992:279–305.

37. Dobroski DR, Rabbani LE, Loscalzo J: The relationship between thrombosis and atherosclerosis. In *Thrombosis and Hemorrhage*. Edited by Loscalzo J, Schafer AI. Philadelphia: Lippincott Williams & Wilkins; 1998:837–861.

38. Makrides SC, Ryan US: Overview of the endothelium. In *Thrombosis and Hemorrhage*. Edited by Loscalzo J, Schafer AI. Philadelphia: Lippincott Williams & Wilkins; 1998:295–306.

39. Broze GJ: The tissue factor pathway of coagulation. In *Thrombosis and Hemorrhage*. Edited by Loscalzo J, Schafer AI. Philadelphia: Lippincott Williams & Wilkins; 1998:77–104.

40. Levine GN, Keaney JF, Jr, Vita JA: Cholesterol reduction in cardiovascular disease: clinical benefits and possible mechanisms. *N Engl J Med* 1995, 332:512–521.

41. Anderson TJ, Meredith IT, Yeung AC, *et al.*: The effect of cholesterol lowering and antioxidant therapy on endothelium-dependent coronary vasomotion. *N Engl J Med* 1995, 332:488–493.

42. Mancini GB, Henry GC, Macaya C, *et al.*: Angiotensin-converting enzyme inhibition with quinapril improves endothelial vasomotor dysfunction in patients with coronary artery disease. The TREND (Trial on Reversing ENdothelial Dysfunction) Study. *Circulation* 1996, 94:258–265.

43. Vaughan DE, Rouleau J, Ridker PM, *et al.*: Effects of ramipril on plasma fibrinolytic balance in patients with acute anterior myocardial infarction. *Circulation* 1997, 96:442–447.

44. Duffy SJ, Gokce N, Holbrook M, *et al.*: Treatment of hypertension with ascorbic acid. *Lancet* 1999, 354:2048–2049.

45. Gokce N, Keaney JF, Jr, Frei B, *et al.*: Long-term ascorbic acid administration reverses endothelial vasomotor dysfunction in patients with coronary artery disease. *Circulation* 1999, 99:3234–3240.

46. Duffy SJ, Keaney JR, J, Holbrook M, *et al.*: Short- and long-term black tea consumption reverses endothelial dysfunction in patients with coronary artery disease. *Circulation* 2000, 104:151–156.

47. Pepine CJ: The effects of angiotensin-converting enzyme inhibition on endothelial dysfunction: potential role in myocardial ischemia. *Am J Cardiol* 1998, 82(10[A]):235–275.

48. Al Suwaidi J, Hamasaki S, Higano S, *et al.*: Long-term follow-up of patients with mild coronary artery disease and endothelial dysfunction. *Circulation* 2000, 101:948–954.

49. Schachinger V, Britten MB, Zeiher AM: Prognostic impact of coronary vasodilator dysfunction on adverse long-term outcome in coronary artery disease. *Circulation* 2000, 101:1899–1906.

50. Gokce N, Keaney JF, Jr, Hunter LM, *et al.*: Risk stratification for postoperative cardiovascular events via non-invasive assessment of endothelial function: a prospective study. *Circulation* 2002, 105: 1567–1572.

THE MACROPHAGE AND THE ATHEROSCLEROTIC PROCESS

3

CHAPTER

Peter Libby

Data from pathologic studies and clinical trials over the past decade have led to a reassessment of the pathogenesis and treatment of atherosclerotic disease. Angiography performed at the time of acute myocardial infarction demonstrated that culprit lesions frequently caused only mild to moderate stenoses, not high-grade lesions that nearly obstructed the coronary arteries. Arteriographic regression trials that used lipid interventions to lower low-density lipoprotein (LDL) cholesterol frequently demonstrated only mild changes in the angiographic appearance of stenotic lesions identified at the baseline catheterization, but participants in these trials enjoyed a consistent reduction in clinical events [1–3].

Pathologic studies have shown on many occasions that growth of an atherosclerotic plaque occurs by expansion outward from the lumen. Obstructive plaques typically pass through a subclinical phase that may last years, accompanied by remodeling, without luminal encroachment. When the plaque burden nears approximately half of the luminal area, the plaque often becomes visible on an angiogram and can impair blood flow. Clinical and pathologic studies currently focus attention on the pathophysiology of the acute coronary syndromes, emphasizing the signaling between the cellular components and the dynamics of the plaque itself, not simply considering events that occur within the lumen [4].

Arterial plaques develop insidiously over years, eventually leading to the development of lesions with a lipid-rich core in the central portion of the eccentrically thickened intima. This central core contains many lipid-rich macrophage foam cells derived from circulating monocytes [5]. Once monocytes have passed through the arterial wall and become lipid-rich macrophages, the latter produce large amounts of tissue factor, a potent procoagulant when it comes into contact with blood. A strong fibrous cap favors stability of an atherosclerotic plaque and protects tissue factor and other matrix elements in the core from contacting the lumen and promoting thrombus formation [6].

Serologic studies over the past several years have renewed interest in the role of infectious agents in the causation of atherosclerotic disease. Among a variety of agents, *Helicobacter pylori*, cytomegalovirus, and *Chlamydia pneumoniae* have received the greatest attention. Direct and indirect effects of infectious agents on the vascular wall may modulate atherogenesis. For instance, microbial agents can infect and, in the case of viruses, transform vascular wall cells. Infected cells may survive but display deleterious functions that may promote arterial lesion formation. Additionally, infections may affect the signaling processes between the endothelial and smooth muscle cells. The indirect effects may particularly affect leukocytes already present in evolving atheroma, leading to dysregulated function and signaling, fostering lesion development [7].

Cytokines, protein mediators of inflammation and immunity, are important in the pathogenesis of atherosclerotic disease. Interferon gamma (IFN-γ), elaborated by T lymphocytes, decreases the ability of human smooth muscle cells to express interstitial collagen genes in the basal state and after exposure to transforming growth factor-beta (TGF-β), the most potent stimulus for interstitial collagen gene expression for these cells. Sites of plaque rupture have increased numbers of T cells and macrophages, and high levels of a transplantation antigen (HLA-DRα). Results from a variety of investigations reveal chronic immune stimulation within atheroma, favoring elaboration of IFN-γ from T cells and inhibition of collagen synthesis in the fibrous cap, favoring the development of a vulnerable cap. IFN-γ can also inhibit smooth muscle cell proliferation and contribute to apoptosis in human vascular smooth muscle cells [3,6].

Once collagen smooth muscle cells form, they can be degraded by a variety of matrix metalloproteinases (MMPs) that act extracellularly. These proteolytic enzymes require activation and can be inhibited by tissue inhibitors of metalloproteinase (TIMPs) under normal circumstances. Exposure to inflammatory cytokines such as interleukin-1 (IL-1), tumor necrosis factor (TNF), or CD-40 ligand can induce smooth muscle cells to express interstitial collagenase, a form of gelatinase not normally expressed, and stromelysin. Whereas nonatherosclerotic arteries in humans contain TIMPs 1 and 2 and gelatinase A, in atherosclerotic plaques, smooth muscle cells, T cells, and macrophages can express interstitial collagenases, gelatinase B, and stromelysin. In addition, endothelial cells overlying atheroma contain interstitial collagenases. This MMP may facilitate new capillary through the dense extracellular matrix of complicated plaques [8]. Atheroma overexpress all three kindred human interstitial collagenases: MMP-1, -8, and -13 [9].

Monocytes and macrophages play important roles at all phases of the atherosclerotic process. Monocytes herald the development of the early lesions as they adhere to the vascular endothelial surface, pass through this barrier, and insinuate themselves in the subendothelial space. There these phagocytic cells participate in subsequent steps of atherogenesis, characterized by the development of lipid-laden macrophages and the elaboration of extracellular matrix. Finally, macrophages contribute to the development and remodeling of more mature plaques. Greater numbers of macrophages exist in culprit plaques that are responsible for unstable coronary syndromes than in those with chronic stable angina [6,9].

LESION FORMATION

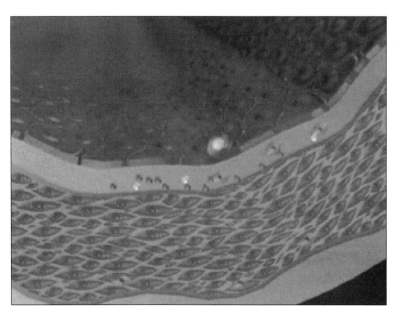

FIGURE 3-1. Endothelial dysfunction in atherosclerosis involves a series of early changes that precede lesion formation. The changes include greater permeability of lipoproteins, upregulation of leukocyte and endothelial adhesion molecules, and migration of leukocytes into the artery wall. This figure shows a cross-section of a portion of an artery with a leukocyte adherent to activated endothelial cells overlying an intima that contains low-density lipoprotein particles both native (*light areas*) and modified (*dark areas*) [10–12].

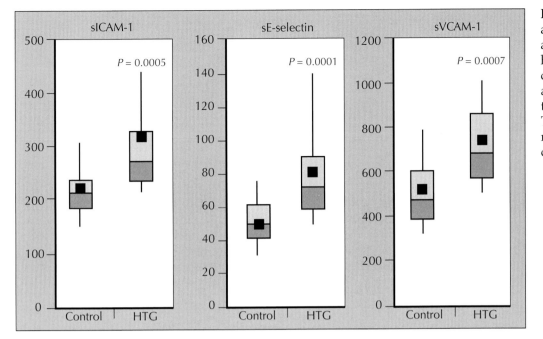

FIGURE 3-2. Concentrations of cellular adhesion molecules sICAM-1, sE-selectin, and sVCAM-1 were higher in the serum of hypertriglyceridemic (HTG) patients compared with 20 normal controls. The top and bottom of the whisker correspond to the 90th and 10th percentiles, respectively. The *small dark squares* indicate the arithmetic mean. *P values* are compared with normal controls. (*Adapted from* Abe *et al.* [13].)

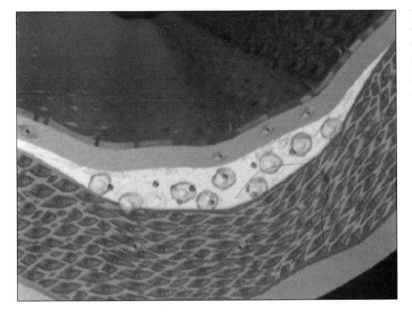

FIGURE 3-3. Fatty-streak formation in atherosclerosis occurs early with filtration by lipid-laden monocytes and macrophages along with T lymphocytes. Later lesions include smooth muscle cells. A complicated series of steps is involved, including smooth muscle migration, T-cell activation, foam cell formation, and platelet adherence and aggregation.

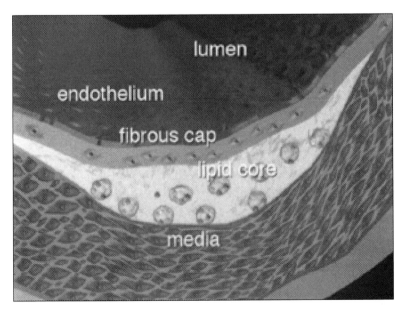

FIGURE 3-4. Formation of advanced, complicated lesions in atherosclerosis includes development of a fibrous cap that creates a barrier between the lesion and the lumen. Leukocytes, lipid, and debris localize under the cap and a necrotic core may form. Lesions expand at the shoulders by continued leukocyte adhesion.

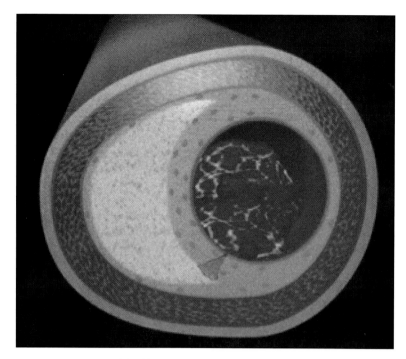

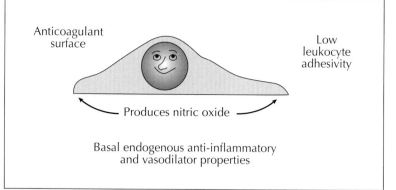

FIGURE 3-6. A normal endothelial wall is characterized by a surface that has anticoagulant properties and has low leukocyte adhesivity. Such a cell produces nitric oxide and has normal endogenous anti-inflammatory and vasodilator properties.

FIGURE 3-5. Unstable fibrous plaques in atherosclerosis can rupture and ulcerate, followed by rapid development of thrombi. Rupture usually occurs at sites of thinning and is associated with regions where there is greater influx and activation of macrophages, accompanied by release of metalloproteinases.

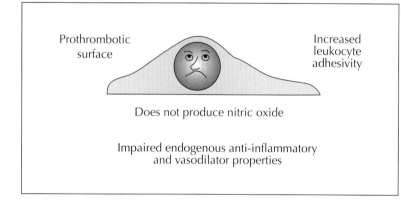

FIGURE 3-7. An "activated" endothelial cell has a prothrombotic surface and increased leukocyte adhesivity. This cell has impaired endogenous anti-inflammatory and vasodilator properties.

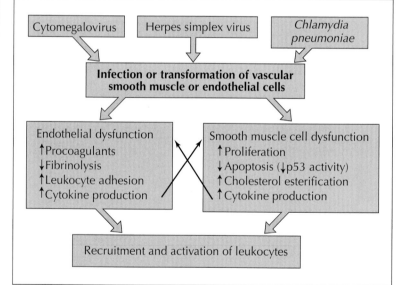

FIGURE 3-8. Microbial agents can infect and, in the case of viruses, transform vascular wall cells. Lethal lytic damage may result (not shown). Alternatively, the infected cells may survive but display deleterious functions such as those listed that could promote arterial lesion formation. Note potential cross talk between intrinsic vascular wall cells (endothelium and smooth muscle) and among vascular cells and leukocytes. (*Adapted from* Libby *et al.* [7].)

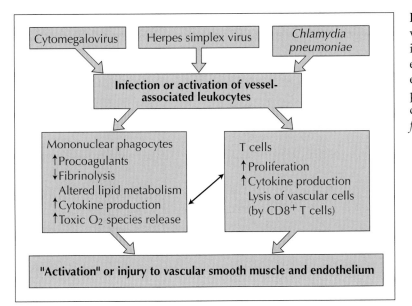

FIGURE 3-9. Indirect effects of infectious agents on intrinsic vascular wall cells. Microbial agents may infect leukocytes, including macrophages and lymphocytes, already present in the evolving atheroma. Infected leukocytes may be activated to express maladaptive functions such as those depicted, which may promote lesion evolution. Note potential cross-talk between leukocytes and intrinsic endothelium and smooth muscle cells. (*Adapted from* Libby *et al.* [7].)

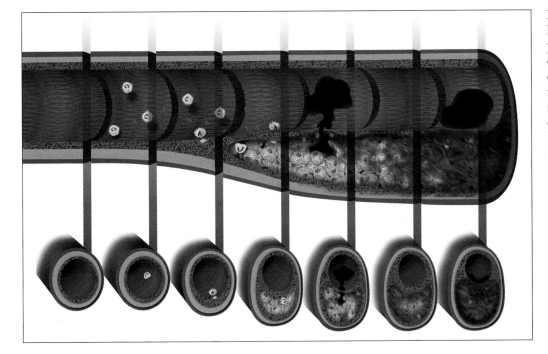

FIGURE 3-10. Schematic time course of human atherogenesis that progresses over years from "no symptoms" to symptomatic disease (from left to right). Thrombosis can occur in macrophage-rich lesions that do not necessarily cause critical stenosis. Late sequelae include ischemic heart disease, cerebrovascular disease, and peripheral vascular disease. (*From* Herman *et al.* [11]; with permission.)

MACROPHAGE INFILTRATION

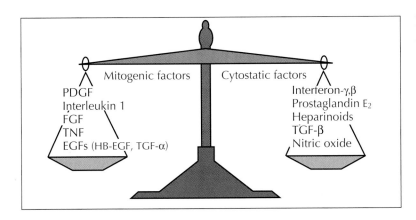

FIGURE 3-11. The balance between mitogenic and cytostatic factors helps to determine the progression of smooth muscle growth. The mitogenic factors include platelet-derived growth factor (PDGF), interleukin-1, fibroblast growth factors (FGF), tumor necrosis factor (TNF), endothelial growth factors (EGF), and transforming growth factor-α (TGF-α). Counterweighting these factors are the cytostatic influences of interferon (IFN) β and γ, prostaglandin E_2, heparinoids, transforming growth factor β (TGF-β), and nitric oxide.

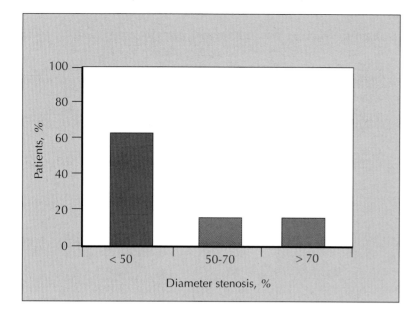

FIGURE 3-12. Severity of coronary artery stenosis before acute myocardial infarction (MI). This composite, derived from the experience of four studies, shows that stenosis of a coronary artery prior to an acute myocardial infarction is often less severe than previously thought. Approximately 60% to 70% of patients who develop an MI have lesions that occlude less than 50% of an artery's diameter. (*Adapted from* Smith [2].)

CHARACTERISTICS OF PLAQUES PRONE TO RUPTURE

Thin fibrous caps
Lipid, macrophage-rich
Smooth muscle poor

FIGURE 3-13. Characteristics of plaques that are prone to rupture include the presence of a thin fibrous cap, a core that is rich in lipids and macrophages, and a relative paucity of smooth muscle cells [13].

STRUCTURAL INTEGRITY OF THE PLAQUES'S FIBROUS CAP

Depends on interstitial collagen fibrils (types I and II) synthesized by smooth muscle cells

FIGURE 3-14. The structural integrity of the plaque's fibrous cap depends on the interstitial collagen fibrils (types I and III) synthesized by smooth muscle cells [14].

FIGURE 3-15. Smooth muscle cells produce the arterial extracellular matrix, and the components include collagens, elastin, and proteoglycans.

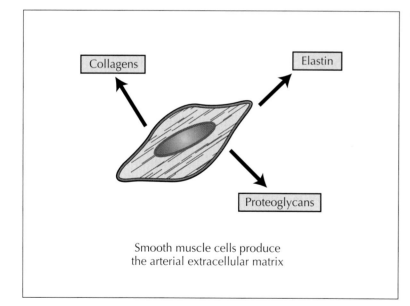

Smooth muscle cells produce
the arterial extracellular matrix

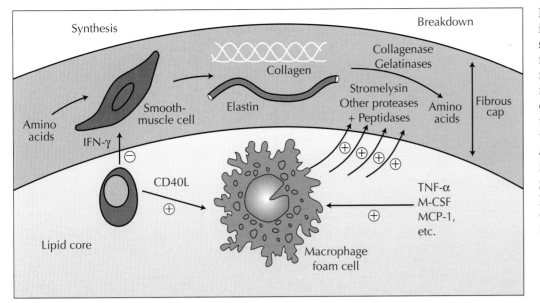

FIGURE 3-16. Matrix metabolism and integrity depends on the balance of synthesis and breakdown products in the fibrous cap, especially at the shoulder regions. T lymphocytes provide signals via interferon gamma, (IFN-γ), leading to decreased collagen formation. Aggravating these effects is the action of interleukin-1, tumor necrosis factor-α (TNF-α), MCP-1, and M-CSF on macrophages, leading to increased production of collagenases, gelatinases, stromelysin, and other proteases and peptidases that break down and limit accretion of collagen in the fibrous cap [3]. (*Adapted from* Libby [3].)

EXTRACELLULAR MATRIX DEGRADATION MECHANISMS

TYPE	EXAMPLES	LOCATION	EXAMPLES OF SUBSTRATES
Serine protease	Plasmin, urokinase, cathepsin G, TPA	Pericellular/extracellular	Fibrin, fibronectin, laminin, some proteoglycans
Cysteine protease	Cathepsins B, D, H, L, N, K, S	Usually cytosol/lysosomal	Wide range, including collagen, proteoglycans, and elastin
Matrix metalloproteinases	Interstitial collagenases (MMP-1,-8,-13)	Extracellular	Collagens I, III, III, VII, X
	Gelatinase A (MMP-2)	Extracellular	Collagens IV, V, VII, X
	Stromelysin-1 (MMP-3)	Extracellular	Collagens III, IV, V, IX; laminin, fibronectin, elastin, proteoglycans
	PUMP-1 (MMP-7)	Extracellular	Gelatin, fibronectin, laminin, collagen type IV, procollagenase, and proteoglycan core protein
	Neutrophil collagenase (MMP-8)	Extracellular	Collagens I, II, III, and proteoglycans
	Gelatinase B (MMP-9)	Extracellular	Collagens IV, V, VII, X, elastin
	Stromelysin-2 (MMP-10)	Extracellular	Similar to stromelysin-1
	Stromelysin-3 (MMP-11)	Extracellular	Gelatin, fibronectin, and proteoglycans
	Metalloelastase (MMP-12)	Extracellular	Elastin
	MT-MMP (MMP-14)	Cell surface	Collagen IV, gelatin, and progelatinase A

FIGURE 3-17. Several matrix metalloproteinases (MMPs), with their location and examples of their substrates. They typically act to degrade specific types of collagen, elastins, and proteoglycans. (*Adapted from* Lee and Libby [4].)

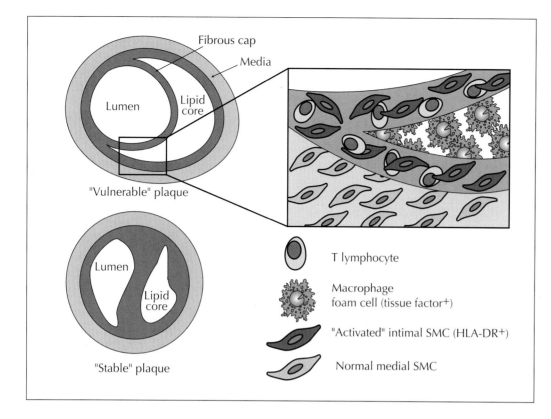

FIGURE 3-18. Vulnerable plaques typically have thin fibrous caps, a core rich in lipid and macrophages, and less evidence of smooth muscle proliferation, as shown in this schema. SMC—smooth muscle cell. (*Adapted from* Libby [3].)

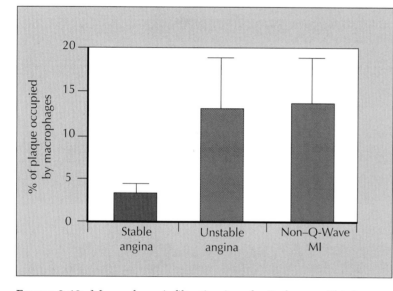

FIGURE 3-19. Macrophage infiltration in culprit plaques. This bar graph shows significantly more macrophage infiltration in culprit plaques responsible for unstable coronary syndromes (*n* = 18) than in those responsible for chronic stable angina (*n* = 8). Macrophages were identified by immunohistochemical technique, using a specific monoclonal antibody against macrophages (PG-M1 from Dako). MI—myocardial infarction. (*Adapted from* Falk *et al.* [6].)

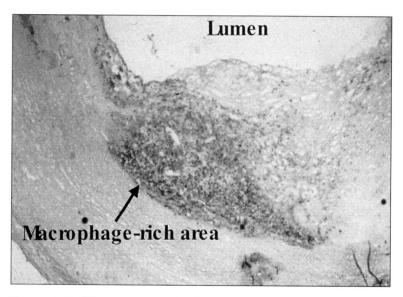

FIGURE 3-20. Photomicrograph of a shoulder region of an athero-sclerotic plaque with evidence of a macrophage-rich area at the site.

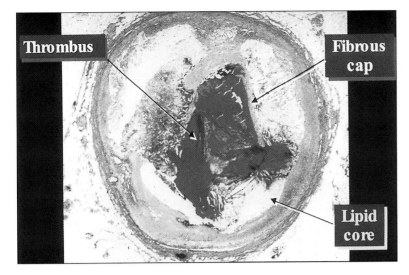

FIGURE 3-21. Photomicrograph of a ruptured plaque with thrombosis.

REFERENCES

1. Libby P, Schoenbeck U, Mach F, *et al.*: Current concepts in cardio-vascular pathology: the role of LDL cholesterol in plaque rupture and stabilization. *Am J Med* 1998, 104:14S–18S.

2. Smith SC, Jr.: Risk-reduction therapy: the challenge to change. *Circulation* 1996, 93:2205–2211.

3. Libby P: Molecular bases of the acute coronary syndromes. *Circulation* 1995, 91:2844–2850.

4. Lee RT, Libby P: The unstable atheroma. *Arterioscler Thromb Vasc Biol* 1997, 17:1859–1867.

5. Ross R: Atherosclerosis: an inflammatory disease. *N Engl J Med* 1999, 340:115–126.

6. Falk E, Shah PK, Fuster V: Coronary plaque disruption. *Circulation* 1995, 92:657–671.

7. Libby P, Egan D, Skarlatos S: Roles of infectious agents in athero-sclerosis and restenosis: an assessment of the evidence and need for future research. *Circulation* 1997, 96:4095–4103.

8. Libby P, Schonbeck U: Drilling for oxygen: angiogenesis involves proteolysis of the extracellular matrix. *Circ Res* 2001, 89:195–197.

9. Galis ZS, Sukhova GK, Lark MW, Libby P: Increased expression of matrix metalloproteinases and matrix degrading activity in vulner-able regions of human atherosclerotic plaques. *J Clin Invest* 1994, 94:2493–2503.

10. Sukhona GK, Schonbeck U, Rabkin E, *et al.*: Evidence for increased collagenolysis by interstitial collagenases-1 and -3 in vulnerable human atheromatous plaques. *Circulation* 1999, 99:2503–2509.

11. Herman MP, Sukhova GK, Libby P, *et al.*: Expression of neutrophil collagenase (matrix metalloproteinase-8) in human atheroma: a novel collagenolytic pathway suggested by transcriptional profiling. *Circulation* 2001, 104:1899–1904.

12. Moreno PR, Falk E, Palacios IF, *et al.*: Macrophage infiltration in acute coronary syndromes: implications for plaque rupture. *Circulation* 1994, 90:775–778.

13. Abe Y, El Masri B, Kimball KT, *et al.*: Soluble cell adhesion mole-cules in hypertriglyceridemia and potential significance on mono-cyte adhesion. *Arterioscler Thromb Vasc Biol* 1998,18:723–731.

14. Davies MJ, Richardson PD, Woolf N, *et al.*: Risk of thrombosis in human atherosclerotic plaques: role of extracellular lipid, macrophage, and smooth muscle cell content. *Br Heart J* 1993, 69:377–381.

STRUCTURE OF THE PLASMA LIPOPROTEINS

4

CHAPTER

G.M. Anantharamaiah, David W. Garber, and Jere P. Segrest

Lipoproteins are subcellular-sized particles composed of lipids and proteins held together by noncovalent forces. Their general structure is that of an oil droplet formed from an outer layer of phospholipids, unesterified cholesterol, and proteins, with a core of neutral lipids, predominantly cholesterol ester and triglycerides [1]. Their main function is to transport lipids and lipid-soluble material throughout the body.

Although the oil droplet is the basic structural motif of the different lipoprotein classes, these classes differ in the relative proportion of lipids, in the protein:lipid ratio, and in the protein species present, resulting in differences in size, density, and electrophoretic mobility [2]. Although lipoproteins were classified originally by their electrophoretic mobility, they are now most commonly classified by density. Each lipoprotein class also can be subdivided both structurally and metabolically into several subclasses.

Proteins associated with lipoproteins are referred to as *apolipoproteins* (apos). Apos are amphipathic in nature in that they have both hydrophobic and hydrophilic regions [3] and can therefore interact both with the lipids of the lipoprotein and with the aqueous environment. Because of the nature of these amphipathic regions, termed *amphipathic α helixes*, most apos act as detergents and have a major role in determining and stabilizing the size and structure of the lipoprotein particle [4]. In addition, apos act as mediators of metabolism, either as ligands for cellular receptors [5,6] or as cofactors for enzymes involved in lipoprotein metabolism [7,8].

Triglyceride-rich lipoproteins follow two parallel metabolic courses, the exogenous and endogenous pathways [2]. The exogenous pathway deals with dietary lipids and begins with intestinal absorption of those lipids and their secretion into the blood by the intestine as chylomicrons. In the blood, chylomicrons are acted upon by the enzyme lipoprotein lipase, which catabolizes triglycerides to free fatty acids and glycerol. The chylomicron particle diameter decreases as a result of triglyceride depletion through the action of lipoprotein lipase. Excess surface material, such as apos and lipids, leave the particle and enter the high-density lipoprotein (HDL) class. The chylomicron remnant is cleared rapidly from the blood through receptor-mediated uptake by the liver.

The endogenous pathway is similar to the exogenous pathway, except that it involves lipids already present in the body. The liver synthesizes and secretes very low-density lipoprotein (VLDL). Again, lipoprotein lipase catabolizes the triglyceride in VLDL to produce VLDL remnants called intermediate-density lipoprotein (IDL), with production of excess surface material; these surface remnants are taken up by HDL.

In humans, 20% to 60% of the VLDL is ultimately converted to low-density lipoprotein (LDL), with the rest being cleared from the blood. The catabolic cascade depletes most of the triglyceride from the particle; thus the LDL is a cholesterol-rich particle. From epidemiologic evidence, the level of LDL cholesterol is known to correlate strongly with the incidence of atherosclerosis [9]. Triglyceride levels and IDL cholesterol may also be important risk factors for atherosclerosis in some persons.

A variant lipoprotein, lipoprotein (a) [Lp(a)], is present in varying concentrations depending on the genetic composition of an individual; *eg*, African-Americans have higher levels on average than Americans of European extraction. Shown to be an independent risk factor for atherosclerosis [10], Lp(a) represents an LDL particle to which an extra apo, apo(a), is attached. Apo(a) is highly homologous to plasminogen, and its role in the atherogenic process may partly be related to this relationship.

Like LDL, HDL is a cholesterol-rich particle and is distinct from the other lipoprotein classes in that it does not contain apo B. HDL levels are inversely correlated with risk for atherosclerosis. Nascent HDL particles are produced by direct synthesis and by generation of surface components of phospholipid and apos from chylomicrons and VLDL produced during the action of lipoprotein lipase and hepatic triglyceride lipase. HDL appears to be involved in the delivery of cholesterol to steroidogenic tissues (adrenal, ovary, and testis), as well as in the removal and the excretion from the system of excess cholesterol from peripheral tissues [11]. Although apos present in HDL are cleared by the liver, the reverse cholesterol transport pathway has never been directly demonstrated.

Apos can be grouped into two general classes, the nonexchangeable apos (apo B-100 and apo B-48) and the exchangeable apos (all others). The B apos, present in chylomicrons, VLDL, IDL, LDL, and Lp(a), are highly insoluble in aqueous solutions and thus remain with the lipoprotein particle throughout its metabolism. Because of their size and insoluble nature, it has been difficult to deduce the structural motif(s) responsible for the lipid-associating properties of B apos [12]. The exchangeable apos are, however, soluble in water and have been studied extensively to determine the structural motif responsible for their lipid association. The common structural motif in exchangeable apos that provides amphipathicity is the amphipathic α helix. This motif is not only responsible for lipid association but is also an innate part of many biologic functions mediated by apos.

DEFINITION AND CLASSIFICATION

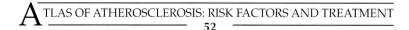

B. TYPES OF HYPERLIPOPROTEINEMIA DEFINED BY INCREASES IN LIPOPROTEIN FRACTIONS

TYPE	INCREASED LIPOPROTEIN FRACTION(S)
I	Chylomicrons
IIA	LDL
IIB	LDL and VLDL
III	β-VLDL
IV	VLDL
V	VLDL and chylomicrons

FIGURE 4-1. Classification of lipoproteins and hyperlipoproteinemias. **A,** Lipoproteins can be separated by agarose gel or paper electrophoresis. When plasma is subjected to these procedures and stained for lipids, three major bands are obtained. The band moving farthest toward the cathode, called α-migrating lipoprotein, represents high-density lipoprotein (HDL). The least-migrating band is called β-migrating lipoprotein and represents low-density lipoprotein (LDL); pre–β-migrating lipoproteins are intermediate to α and β in migration distance and usually represent very low-density lipoprotein (VLDL). Sometimes, especially after a fatty meal, a lipid-staining band is found that does not move from the origin; this usually represents chylomicrons.

B, Electrophoresis can be used to classify hyperlipoproteinemias using the Fredrickson nomenclature [13]; six patterns can be defined by increases in one or two lipoprotein fractions. (*Adapted from* Grundy [14].)

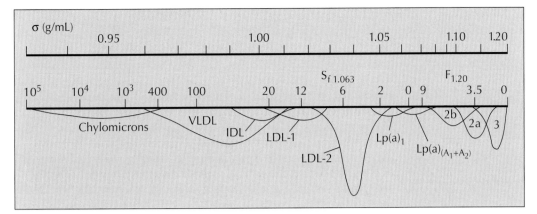

FIGURE 4-2. A summary of lipoprotein components subfractionated and characterized by analytic ultracentrifugation. The determination of both lipoprotein flotation coefficient distribution and refractometric concentration can be achieved by analytic ultracentrifugation. The lipoprotein (a) [Lp(a)] generally occurs at relatively low concentrations and normally is not resolved. IDL—intermediate-density lipoprotein; LDL—low-density lipoprotein; VLDL—very low-density lipoprotein. (*Adapted from* Lindgren [15].)

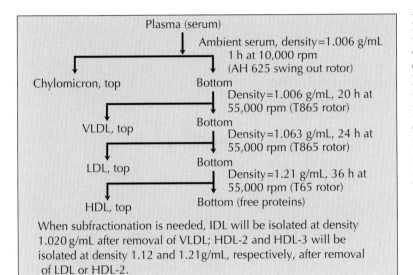

FIGURE 4-3. Sequential flotation ultracentrifugation separates lipoproteins on the basis of equilibrium density and can be adapted for preparing large quantities of individual lipoprotein classes. Commonly separated classes are called very low-density lipoproteins (VLDLs; density below 1.006), low-density lipoproteins (LDLs; density between 1.019 and 1.06), and high-density lipoproteins (HDLs; density between 1.06 and 1.21). When present, chylomicrons can be separated in a high-speed centrifuge. Other minor subclasses can also be separated, including intermediate-density lipoproteins (IDLs; density between 1.006 and 1.019), and subfractions of HDL, termed *HDL-2* and *HDL-3*. HDL-1 is a buoyant subclass not normally found in humans.

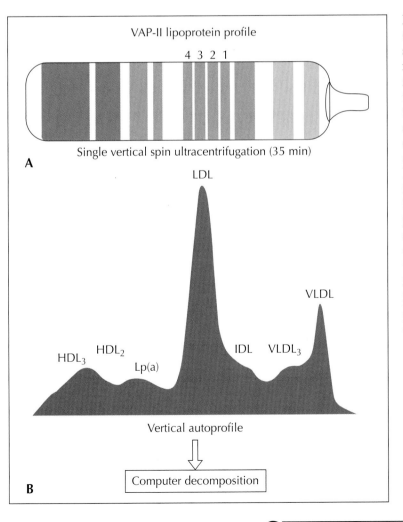

FIGURE 4-4. Single vertical spin density gradient ultracentrifugation (vertical auto lipoprotein profile). This figure illustrates single vertical spin inverted rate-zonal density gradient ultracentrifugation. If necessary, chylomicrons are removed from the sample by centrifugation of plasma. After adjusting the sample density and loading the sample to be separated in a centrifuge tube, a two-layer discontinuous salt density gradient is made by overlayering the density-adjusted plasma with a salt solution of lower density. Tubes are centrifuged with vertical rotors using slow acceleration and deceleration speed in a Beckman L8-80 ultracentrifuge (Beckman Instruments, Inc., Fullerton, CA). The tubes are then drained and fractions collected. **A,** An ultracentrifuge tube after centrifugation in which a lipid-specific stain (Sudan black) was added to the plasma. After centrifugation, the tube is placed in a fractionator apparatus and drained from the bottom into a continuous flow cholesterol analyer (Atherotech.com, Birmingham, AL), where the tube eluent is mixed with an enzymatic cholesterol reagent. **B,** The resulting cholesterol profile is decomposed mathematically into individual lipoprotein species by computer. HDL—high-density lipoprotein; IDL—intermediate-density lipoprotein; Lp(a)—lipoprotein (a); VLDL—very low-density lipoprotein.

BASIC STRUCTURE

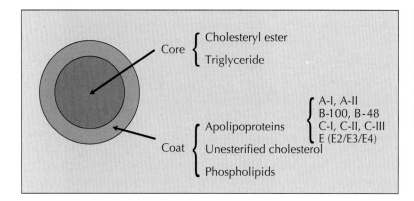

FIGURE 4-5. A lipoprotein particle structure and its components. Lipoproteins are composed of an outer layer containing apolipoproteins, phospholipids, and unesterified cholesterol; the core contains cholesteryl ester and triglycerides. The size and density of lipoproteins differ with different amounts and species of cholesterol and cholesteryl ester, individual apolipoproteins, and phospholipids; generally, the larger the particle, the less dense the lipoprotein.

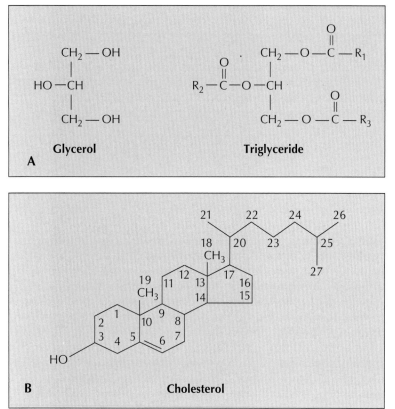

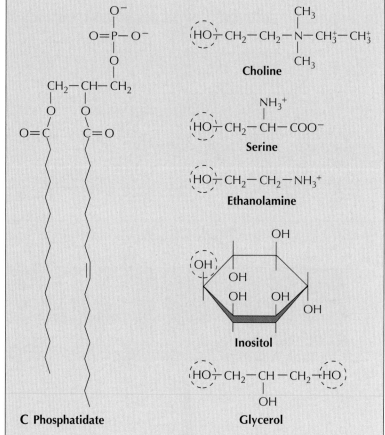

FIGURE 4-6. General chemical structures of the lipids present in lipoprotein species. The lipids present in essentially all lipoprotein species are cholesterol, cholesteryl ester, phospholipids, and triglycerides. **A,** R1, R2, and R3 represent fatty acyl chains attached to the glycerol backbone to form triglyceride. **B,** Structure of cholesterol. Cholesteryl esters can be formed by attachment of a fatty acid to the hydroxyl group on carbon 3. **C,** The general structure of phospholipids, in which various head groups can combine with the phosphatidate; variation in the polar head groups of phospholipids results in neutral, acidic, or basic functional groups. (*Adapted from* Schreiber [16].)

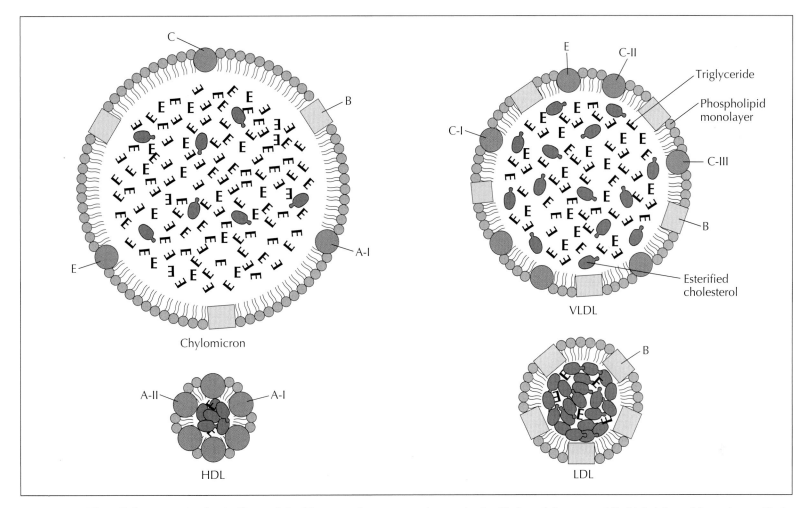

FIGURE 4-7. The oil-drop or mixed micelle model of lipoprotein structure for chylomicron, very low-density lipoprotein (VLDL), low-density lipoprotein (LDL), and high-density lipoprotein (HDL). Apolipoproteins in the outer phospholipid membrane are designated by letters. The major differences between the different lipoproteins are in the 1) size of the neutral lipid (triglyceride and esterified cholesterol, reverse cholesterol transport) core; 2) lipid composition in the core; and 3) apolipoprotein composition. Although not shown, unesterified cholesterol is found predominantly in the phospholipid monolayer. (*Adapted from* Oberman *et al.* [17].)

FIGURE 4-8. Molecular weights and putative functions for the most common apolipoproteins (apos). (*Adapted from* Segrest *et al.* [4].)

MOLECULAR WEIGHTS AND FUNCTIONS OF MAJOR APOS

APO	MOLECULAR WEIGHT, D*	PUTATIVE FUNCTION
B-100	550,000	Structural; ligand for low-density lipoprotein (B/E) receptor
B-48	264,000	Structural
E	33,000	Ligand for various receptors
C-I	6630	Inhibition of interaction with hepatic receptors
C-II	8900	Activation of lipoprotein lipase
C-III	8800	Inhibition of interaction with hepatic receptors; inhibition of lipoprotein lipase
A-I	28,000	Activation of lecithin:cholesterol acyl transferase
A-II	17,400	Structural
A-IV	44,500	Surface activity buffer

*Molecular weights shown are for human apos; the weight for apo A-II is for the dimer.

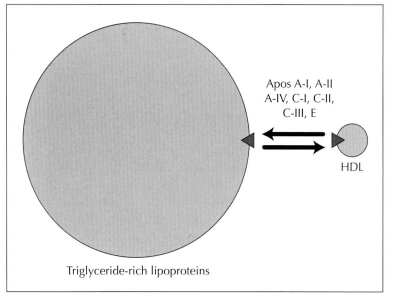

FIGURE 4-9. Exchangeable apolipoproteins (apos) readily shuttle from triglyceride-rich lipoprotein particles to high-density lipoprotein (HDL) and back again.

Apos A-I, A-II
A-IV, C-I, C-II,
C-III, E

HDL

Triglyceride-rich lipoproteins

NATURE OF THE BOND FORMED BETWEEN APOLIPOPROTEINS AND LIPIDS

Phase	Molecular shape
Bilayer	Cylindric
Micellar	Inverted cone
Hexagonal (H$_{II}$)	Cone

FIGURE 4-10. Detergent micelles, membrane bilayers, and inverted nonbilayers. The tendency of phospholipids to form various types of aggregated structures is determined by the relative cross-sectional areas of the head groups versus the fatty acyl chains and, to a lesser extent, the length of the fatty acyl chains. Cone-shaped phospholipids, such as lysophospholipids and many detergents (wedge-shaped in cross-section), contain a relatively large polar head group and a single fatty acyl chain and favor a positive surface curvature and the micellar phase (*ie*, a spheroidal particle). A lipoprotein particle is an example of a micelle formed from several different lipids and proteins. Cylindric-shaped phospholipids (*eg*, phosphatidylcholine) are those whose head groups and fatty acyl chains have approximately equal cross-sectional areas and favor a flat surface, the membrane bilayer phase. Inverted cone-shaped phospholipids (inverted wedge-shaped in cross-section) include phosphatidylethanolamine; these contain relatively large acyl chain cross-sectional areas favoring a negative surface curvature and inverted nonbilayer phases.

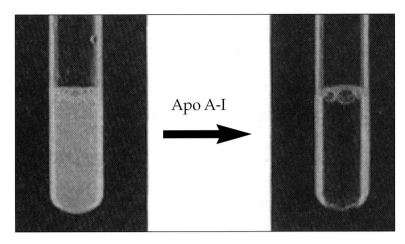

Apo A-I

DMPC

Lipoprotein
complex

FIGURE 4-11. Apolipoproteins (apos) solubilize phospholipid dispersions. Phospholipids (dimyristoyl phosphatidylcholine; DMPC) suspended in water and vortexed form large particles containing concentric (onion-skin) layers of membrane bilayer called *multilamellar liposomes*. Because of their large size, these liposomes scatter light and produce a cloudy suspension. Addition of certain apos, such as apo A-I, have the dramatic effect of completely clarifying the cloudy suspension. Thus, certain apos act as protein detergents by associating with the lipid to convert multilamellar liposomes to smaller particles that do not scatter light. (*From* Anantharamaiah *et al.* [18]; with permission.)

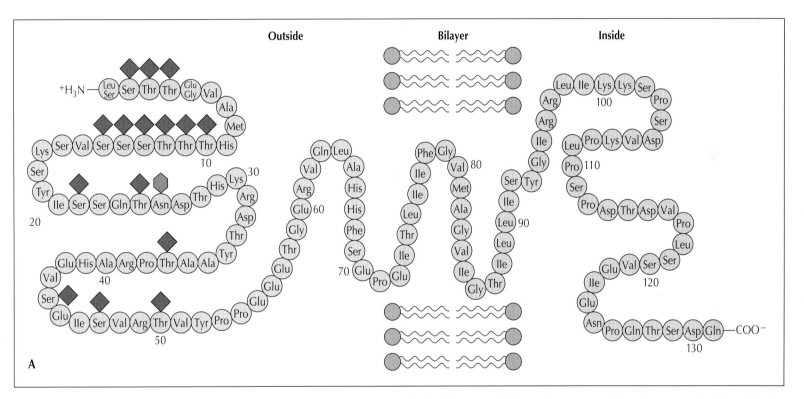

FIGURE 4-12. What is there about exchangeable apolipoproteins (apos) that allows them to associate with lipid and act as protein detergents? Although the exchangeable apos and membrane-spanning proteins both have high lipid affinity, they differ in that the latter associate irreversibly with lipid. **A,** A single transmembrane α helical domain of the erythrocyte surface glycoprotein, glycophorin, was the first lipid-associating structure described [3]; this structural motif, made up of a domain of hydrophobic amino acid residues 20 to 23 long, is repeated in many membrane-spanning proteins. (*continued*)

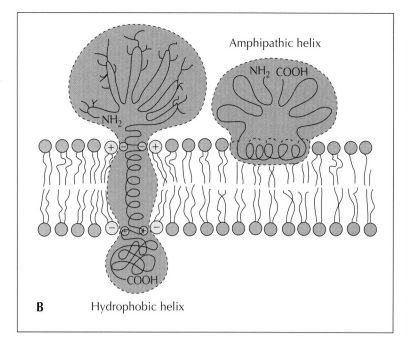

B Hydrophobic helix

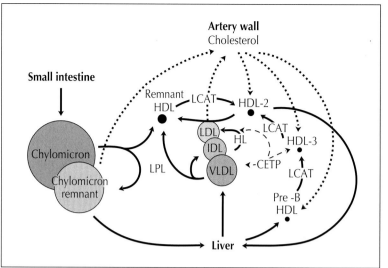

FIGURE 4-13. Metabolic interrelationships of lipoproteins. *Solid lines* represent interconversion of particles; *dotted lines* represent movement of cholesterol; and *dashed lines* represent transfer of lipids mediated by cholesteryl ester transfer protein (CETP). HDL—high-density lipoprotein; HL—hepatic lipase; IDL—intermediate-density lipoprotein; LCAT—lecithin:cholesterol acyl transferase; LPL—lipoprotein lipase; VLDL—very low-density lipoprotein. (*Adapted from* Segrest *et al.* [4].)

FIGURE 4-12. (*continued*) **B,** The exchangeable apos have no such domain. Rather, they contain helical domains composed of both hydrophobic and hydrophilic amino acids. These amino acid residues are arranged such that when the sequence is folded as a helix, it forms opposing polar and nonpolar faces. These structures, named *amphipathic helixes*, differ from the membrane-spanning structures in that they limit their interactions to the surface of the membrane rather than penetrating completely through it. (Part A *adapted from* Stryer [19].)

STRUCTURE OF INDIVIDUAL LIPOPROTEIN CLASSES AND SUBCLASSES

DISCOIDAL HIGH-DENSITY LIPOPROTEIN

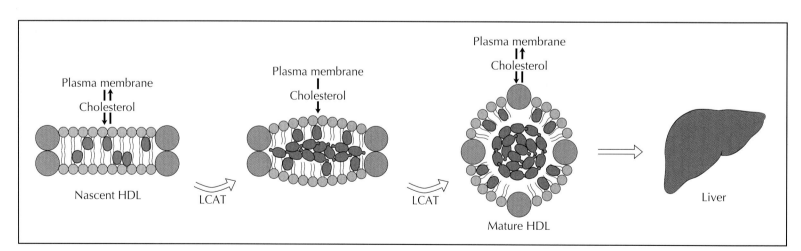

FIGURE 4-14. Discoidal high-density lipoprotein (HDL) conversion to spheroidal HDL. In the lymph, HDL is present in the form of discoidal particles. Upon conversion of cholesterol to cholesteryl ester by the enzyme lecithin:cholesterol acyl transferase (LCAT), the cholesteryl ester enters the core of the HDL, converting the discoidal into spherical HDL. Discoidal HDL particles are not found in circulating blood, except in subjects lacking LCAT activity and in those with severe liver dysfunction. Discoidal HDL has, however, been demonstrated in lymph.

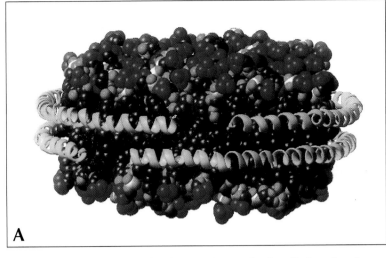

A

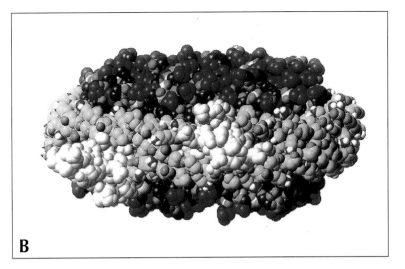

B

FIGURE 4-15. (*see* Color Plate) Two views of a detailed molecular belt model for the discoidal form of high-density lipoprotein (HDL) developed by mapping three self-evident conformational constraints—amphipathic helix, planar discoidal (nascent) HDL geometry, and helix curvature dictated by the dielectrical boundary between lipid and solvent—onto the linear sequence of apolipoprotein (apo) A-I [20]. **A,** Apo A-I shown as an α-helical ribbon. **B,** Both lipid and apo A-I shown as space-filling molecules. (*From* Segrest *et al.* [20]; with permission.)

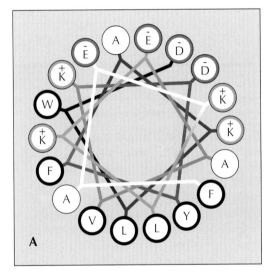

A

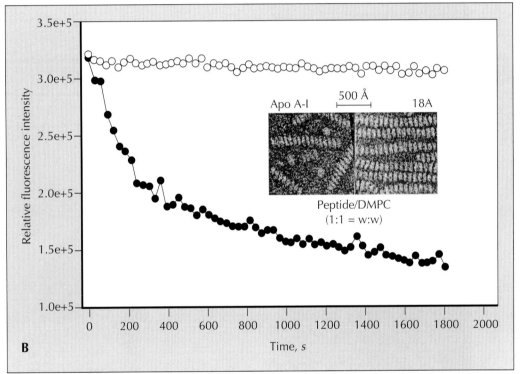

B

FIGURE 4-16. Synthetic discoidal high-density lipoprotein (HDL). **A,** Based on the concept that apolipoprotein (apo) A-I possesses several tandem repeats of amphipathic helical domains, a peptide was designed with 18 amino acid residues and the sequence Ac-Asp-Trp-Leu-Lys-Ala-Phe-Tyr-Asp-Lys-Val-Ala-Glu-Lys-Leu-Lys-Glu-Ala-Phe-NH$_2$. This sequence possesses no primary sequence homology to any of the naturally occurring apo sequences. However, when folded as an α-helix, it forms a helix that possesses a polar face and nonpolar face. The charged residues are arranged similarly to an archtypical apo amphipathic helical domains in that the positively charged residues reside at the polar-nonpolar interface and negatively charged residues reside at the center of the polar face. This type of structure is termed *class A amphipathic helix* [21].

B, When mixed with multilamellar vesicles of lipid, similarly to apo A-I, the peptide is also capable of clearing phospholipids as determined by the decrease of light scattering intensity (inset). When the solution produced by this peptide–lipid mixture is compared with the solution of apo A-I–lipid mixture by the negative stain electron microscopy, the discoidal complexes are similar in size. Thus, the research on "synthetic discoidal HDL" was initiated [21]. (*continued*)

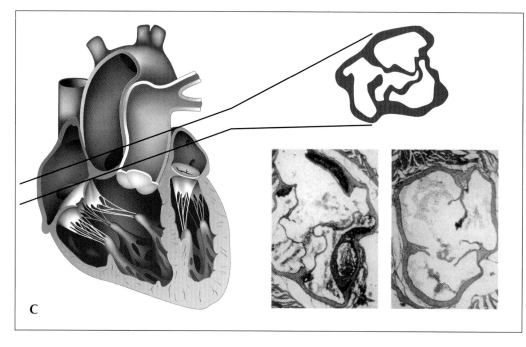

of the proximal aortic sinus. The *left image* represents an aortic sinus cross-section of a C57BL/6J control mouse administered an atherogenic diet for 16 weeks. The *right image* represents a similar cross-section from peptide 5F-administered (20 µg/d) mice. The cross-sections are stained with oil red O and counterstained with hematoxylin. Lipid accumulation can be seen in control mice (n=14, mean cross-sectional lesion area=22.12 ± 3.3 × 10^3 µm^2), almost no lesion was observed in the peptide-administered mice (n=15, mean cross-sectional area=9.34 ± 1.55 × 10^3 µm^2). The protection in atherosclerosis was observed despite no changes in the levels of plasma cholesterol levels. Further investigations have revealed that the peptide, similar to human apo A-I, was able to clear "seeding molecules" from the surface of low-density lipoprotein, rendering them nonatherogenic [23]. (*Adapted from* Anantharamaiah *et al.* [18].)

FIGURE 4-16. (*continued*) C, Recently, it has been shown that daily intraperitoneal administration of an analogue of this peptide, referred to as 5F, inhibits diet-induced atherosclerosis in mice that are sensitive to atherosclerosis [22]. This figure is a cross-section

CIRCULATING HIGH-DENSITY LIPOPROTEIN STRUCTURE

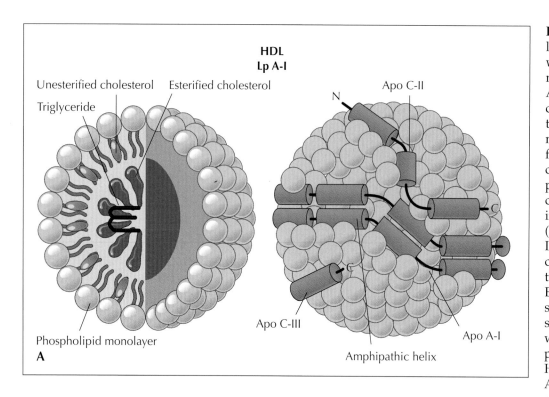

FIGURE 4-17. Structure of high-density lipoprotein (HDL). More than 50% of HDL weight is from apolipoproteins (apos), more than 90% of which are apos A-I and A-II. The core of HDL consists mostly of cholesteryl ester and small amounts of triglycerides, and the surface contains mostly phosphatidylcholine and unesterified cholesterol (*see* Fig. 4-7). Despite these common features, HDL is heterogenous in particle size or density, as well as apo composition. Not only is apo heterogeneity in the form of particles containing apo A-I (Lp A-I) and those containing both apos A-I and A-II (Lp A-I/A-II), but HDL also contains small amounts of the remainder of the exchangeable apos, apos C-I, C-II, C-III, E, and A-IV. These general features are schematically illustrated here. The relative size and density of HDL can be compared with other lipoproteins (*see* Fig. 4-19A); the presence of multiple subpopulations of HDL is also seen. **A,** The Lp A-I particle. Apo C-II, C-I, and C-III are likely to be associated predominantly with this particle. (*continued*)

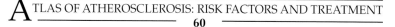

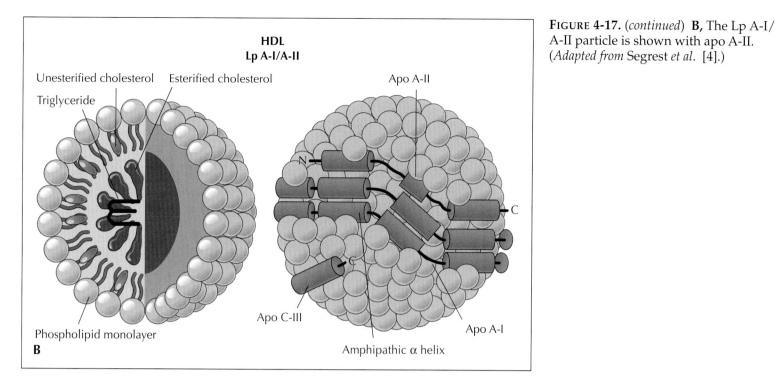

HDL
Lp A-I/A-II

Unesterified cholesterol   Esterified cholesterol

Triglyceride

Apo A-II

N

C

Apo C-III

Phospholipid monolayer

B

Apo A-I

Amphipathic α helix

FIGURE 4-17. *(continued)* **B,** The Lp A-I/A-II particle is shown with apo A-II. *(Adapted from* Segrest *et al.* [4].)

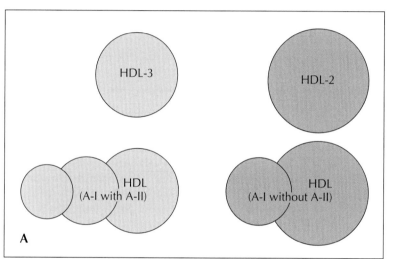

HDL-3

HDL-2

HDL (A-I with A-II)

HDL (A-I without A-II)

A

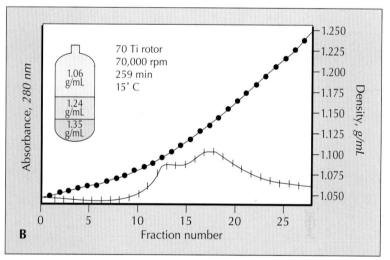

FIGURE 4-18. High-density lipoprotein (HDL) subspecies. HDL can be separated into several subclasses on the basis of size, density, and apolipoprotein (apo) composition. **A,** HDL has been separated schematically into HDL-3 (smaller and more dense) and HDL-2 (larger and less dense) by size or density alone. Many studies have suggested that HDL-2 is the HDL fraction that is most protective against the development of coronary heart disease. Another way of separating HDL subspecies is to divide HDL into HDL particles that contain apo A-I without apo A-II (Lp A-I) and those that contain both apo A-I and apo A-II (Lp A-I/A-II). Lp A-I contains at least two distinct types of particles, one in the HDL-3 subclass and another in the HDL-2 subclass. Lp A-I/A-II contains at least three distinct types of particles: one lies in the HDL-3 subclass, another in the HDL-2 subclass, and the third lies intermediate between the two. Using this classification, Lp A-I has been suggested to be antiatherogenic and Lp A-I/A-II either neutral or actually atherogenic.

B, Bottom densities of 1.30 g/mL with an overlay with physiologic saline provide optimal separation of HDL from the other lipoproteins using a 70-Ti angled head rotor and a single 4-h spin. The HDL profile shown here demonstrates two HDL subspecies, HDL-3 and HDL-2. *(continued)*

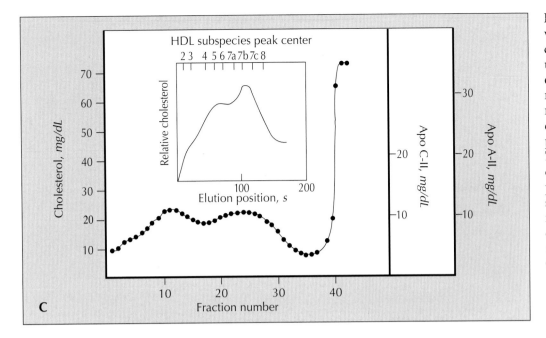

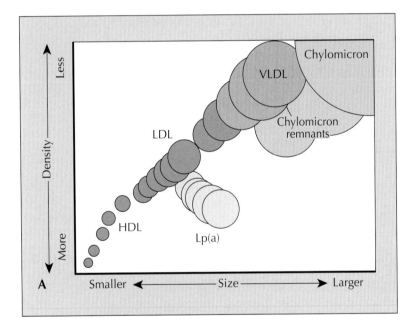

FIGURE 4-18. (*continued*) **C (inset),** HDL–vertical auto profile density gradient ultracentrifugation separation of HDL subspecies uses a bottom density of 1.21 g/mL and an overlay of 1.06 g/mL and a VTi80 vertical rotor centrifuged at 80,000 rpm for 90 minutes; the analysis of cholesterol is by a continuous flow method [21]. The resulting profile is superior to that obtained with a 70-Ti angled head rotor; three to five peaks can be identified. HDL single vertical spin preparative fractionation of HDL subspecies from the same plasma sample used in the *inset* is shown in **C.** The resolution is comparable with, or superior to, that shown in the inset. (Part C *adapted from* Cheung *et al.* [22].)

CIRCULATING VERY LOW-DENSITY LIPOPROTEIN

FIGURE 4-19. A, Although lipoproteins are similar in their basic structure, they differ in size and density. **B,** Very low-density lipoprotein (VLDL) structure. VLDL is a triglyceride-rich lipoprotein secreted directly by the liver. It possesses high levels of triglycerides and some esterified cholesterol in its core; its surface lipids are predominantly phosphatidylcholine and unesterified cholesterol. There are many apolipoproteins (apos) on the surface, including apos B-100, E, C-I, C-II, and C-III. The carboxy-terminal G amphipathic helix is the domain of apo C-II that activated lipoprotein lipase; lipoprotein lipase hydrolyzes triglycerides to produce VLDL remnants called *intermediate-density lipoprotein* (IDL, *see* Fig. 4-19). Further metabolism produces low-density lipoprotein (LDL) (*see* Fig. 4-22). During this process, excess surface remnants are removed by apo A-I–containing high-density lipoprotein (HDL) particles to produce remnant HDL particles that contain the apos C-I, C-II, and C-III. The schematic model for VLDL shown here is simplified to contain only one copy of apos C-I, C-II, C-III, and E; there may be up to 20 molecules of apo E per VLDL particle, for example. Apo B-100 is shown in a more extended conformation than that shown for LDL. (*Adapted from* Segrest *et al.* [4].)

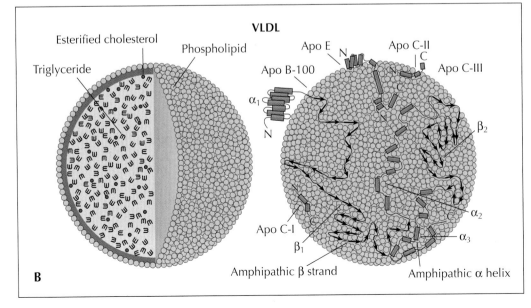

INTERMEDIATE-DENSITY LIPOPROTEIN

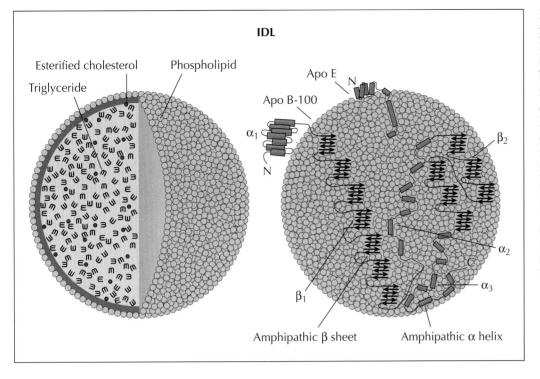

IDL

Esterified cholesterol

Triglyceride

Phospholipid

Apo E

Apo B-100

α_1

β_2

N

α_2

α_3

β_1

Amphipathic β sheet

Amphipathic α helix

FIGURE 4-20. Intermediate-density lipoprotein (IDL) structure. This particle is a remnant of very low-density lipoprotein (VLDL) and differs from its parent particle by 1) having a lower triglyceride to esterified cholesterol ratio; 2) containing less apolipoprotein (apo) C but still significant levels of apo E; and 3) having a smaller diameter. The presence of excess apo C-III may inhibit the metabolism of this particle, whereas an abundance of apo E appears to speed its uptake and metabolism by cells such as in the liver. Apo B-100, as the result of smaller particle size, is shown with a somewhat more condensed structure in the β_1 and β_2 amphipathic β sheet domains than in the model for VLDL. (*Adapted from* Segrest *et al.* [4].)

CIRCULATING LOW-DENSITY LIPOPROTEIN

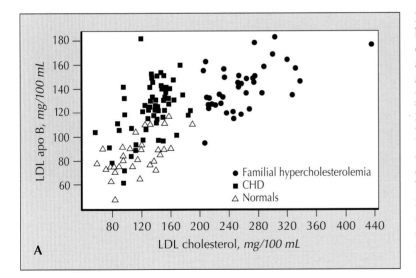

LDL apo B, mg/100 mL

- Familial hypercholesterolemia
- CHD
- Normals

LDL cholesterol, *mg/100 mL*

A

FIGURE 4-21. Low-density lipoprotein (LDL) subspecies. LDL can be separated into several subclasses on the basis of size or density. Unlike high-density lipoprotein, however, the apolipoprotein (apo) composition of the different LDL subspecies appears to be invariant; apo B-100 is essentially the only apo present in circulating LDL. The smaller, denser forms of LDL have been shown to be associated with a greater risk for coronary heart disease (CHD) than a comparable level (based on cholesterol) of the larger, more buoyant forms of LDL. This has been demonstrated in two ways. The ratio of apo B-100 mass to LDL cholesterol is greater for small, dense LDL than for larger, more buoyant LDL (when the number of such particles in plasma is increased, the term *hyperapobetalipoproteinemia* is used; this is associated with an increased risk of CHD). **A,** Scatter plot comparing LDL apo B with LDL cholesterol in subjects with familial hypercholesterolemia, CHD, and normals. (*continued*)

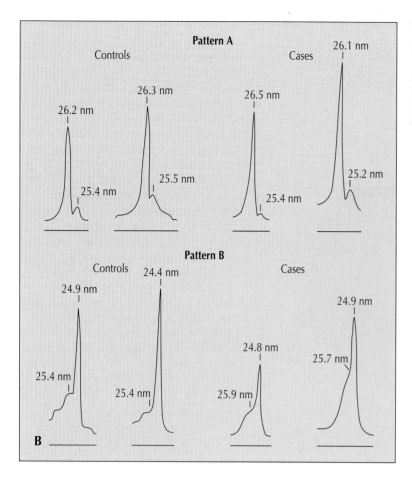

Pattern A

Controls — 26.2 nm, 25.4 nm; 26.3 nm, 25.5 nm

Cases — 26.5 nm, 25.4 nm; 26.1 nm, 25.2 nm

Pattern B

Controls — 24.9 nm, 25.4 nm; 24.4 nm, 25.4 nm

Cases — 24.8 nm, 25.9 nm; 24.9 nm, 25.7 nm

B

FIGURE 4-21. (*continued*) **B,** Using nondenaturing gradient gel electrophoresis, at least six different LDL subclasses have been demonstrated. This approach has been used to divide the population into two LDL phenotypes, namely, pattern A (larger, more buoyant LDL) and pattern B (smaller, more dense LDL). Pattern B represents up to 40% of the adult population and carries an increased risk for CHD. (Part A *adapted from* Teng *et al.* [24]; part B *adapted from* Austin *et al.* [25].)

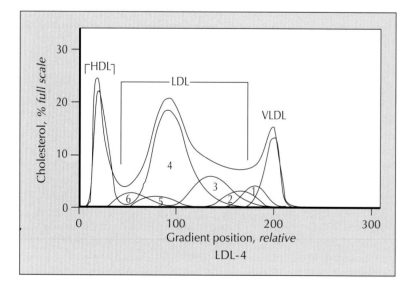

LDL-4

FIGURE 4-22. Low-density lipoprotein (LDL)–vertical auto profile (VAP) density gradient ultracentrifugation separation of LDL subspecies. A rapid, reproducible way to quantify the distribution of LDL subclasses in individuals is the LDL-VAP procedure. This procedure uses a bottom density of 1.08 g/mL, an overlay of 1.041 g/mL, and a VTi80 vertical rotor centrifuged at 80,000 rpm for 150 minutes; as with the high-density lipoprotein (HDL)-VAP, the analysis of cholesterol in the LDL-VAP is by a continuous flow method [21]. At least six subspecies of LDL having distinct densities can be demonstrated by this procedure. VLDL—very low-density lipoprotein.

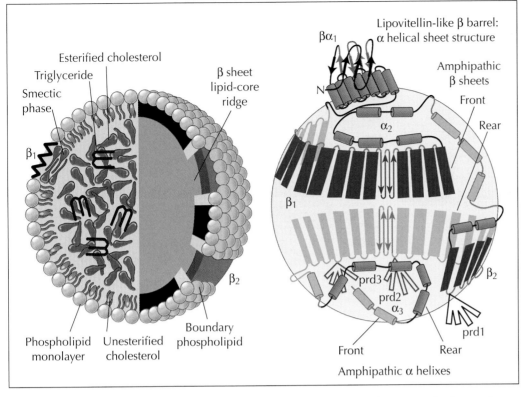

Labels on figure (left panel): Esterified cholesterol; Triglyceride; Smectic phase; β_1; Phospholipid monolayer; Unesterified cholesterol; Boundary phospholipid; β_2; β sheet lipid-core ridge

Labels on figure (right panel): Lipovitellin-like β barrel: α helical sheet structure; $\beta\alpha_1$; N; Amphipathic β sheets; Front; Rear; α_2; β_1; β_2; prd3; prd2; α_3; prd1; Front; Rear; Amphipathic α helixes

Figure 4-23. Low-density lipoprotein (LDL) structure. This is the major cholesterol-carrying particle in humans and some other species, with a core consisting primarily of

cholesteryl ester and little triglyceride and a surface of phosphatidylcholine and unesterified cholesterol. Apolipoprotein (apo) B-100, essentially the sole apo on the surface, is one of the largest proteins known with 4565 amino acid residues. Apo B serves as a ligand for the LDL receptor that mediates LDL uptake by cells. Apo B-100, shown here, is associated with the surface of LDL via two clusters of amphipathic helices located in the middle and at the carboxy-terminal end of the protein; this feature of apo B-100 structure is based on both experimental and molecular modeling studies from several laboratories. Other modeling studies suggest that the gap regions on both sides of the middle cluster of amphipathic helices are also lipid-associating but through an amphipathic β-strand motif. The amino terminal end of apo B-100 also contains amphipathic helices but they are predominantly of the non–lipid-associating G class. Apo B-100, as the result of small LDL particle size, is shown with a fully condensed structure in the β_1 and β_2 amphipathic β sheet domains. (*Adapted from* Segrest *et al.* [4].)

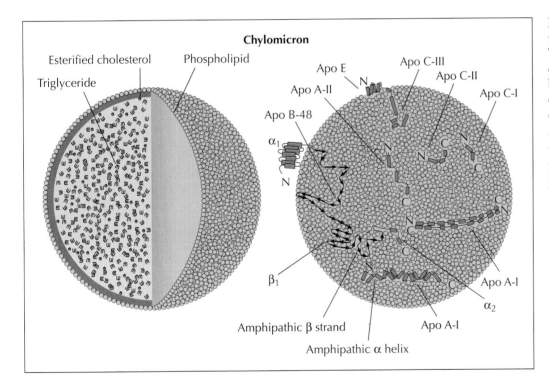

Chylomicron

Labels on figure: Esterified cholesterol; Triglyceride; Phospholipid; Apo E; Apo A-II; Apo B-48; α_1; N; N; β_1; Apo C-III; Apo C-II; Apo C-I; N; C; N; C; N; C; C; C; N; C; N; C; Apo A-I; α_2; Apo A-I; Amphipathic β strand; Amphipathic α helix

Figure 4-24. Chylomicrons are secreted by the intestine in response to fat in the diet. They have some similarities to very low-density lipoprotein (VLDL) but differ by being larger, containing a higher triglyceride:unesterified cholesterol ratio, and containing apolipoproteins (apos) A-I and A-IV and a truncated form of apo B-100, apo B-48, that contains intact α_1 and β_1 amphipathic domains and a small fragment of the α_2 domain. (*Adapted from* Segrest *et al.* [4].)

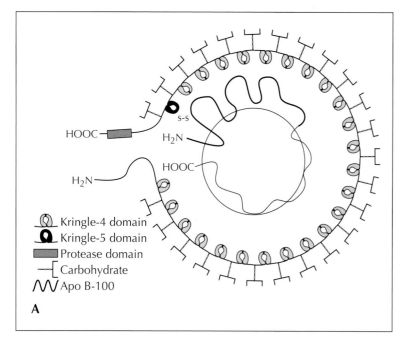

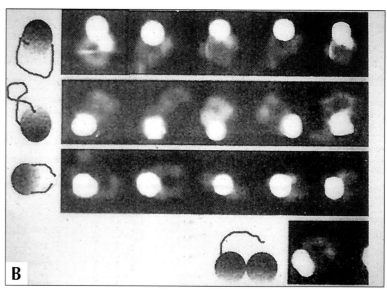

FIGURE 4-25. Lipoprotein (a) or [Lp(a)]. This variant lipoprotein particle is present in varying levels in different ethnic populations. **A,** Lp(a) consists of low-density lipoprotein particles with an extra protein called apo (a) apparently covalently associated with apo B-100. Apo(a) contains repeated structural regions, called kringles, homologous to those contained in the fibrinolytic enzyme plasminogen. In several studies, Lp(a) has been associated with a greater risk of coronary heart disease, and also with accelerated restenosis of coronary artery bypass grafts. Conflicting data, however, also exist. The relationship to atherosclerosis is complex and only partly related to the levels of Lp(a), which appear to be largely genetically determined. Diet and most medications have little effect on circulating levels of Lp(a). The mechanism for the atherogenicity of Lp(a) may be related to its homology to plasminogen and involve an aberration in the thrombotic system. **B,** Images of Lp(a) obtained by scanning tunneling electron microscopy. (Part B *from* Xu [26]; with permission.)

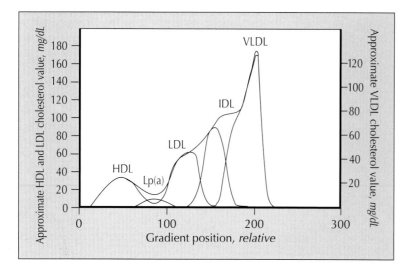

FIGURE 4-26. β-very low-density lipoprotein (β-VLDL) is found in subjects with reduced clearance of VLDL, such as those with type III dysbetalipidemia. Subjects with type III dysbetalipidemia have an abnormal vertical auto profile, with greater intermediate-density lipoprotein (IDL) than low-density lipoprotein (LDL). HDL—high-density lipoprotein; Lp(a)—lipoprotein (a); VLDL—very low-density lipoprotein.

REFERENCES

1. Scanu AM, Landsberger FR, eds: Lipoprotein structure. *Ann N Y Acad Sci* 1980, 348:1–436.

2. Gotto AM, Pownall HJ, Havel RJ: Introduction to the plasma lipoproteins. *Methods Enzymol* 1986, 128:3–41.

3. Segrest JP, Jackson RL, Morrisett JD, *et al.*: A molecular theory of lipid-protein interactions in the plasma lipoproteins. *FEBS Lett* 1974, 38:247–253.

4. Segrest JP, Garber DW, Brouillette CG, *et al.*: The amphipathic α helix: a multifunctional structural motif in plasma lipoproteins. *Adv Protein Chem* 1994, 45:303–369.

5. Brown MS, Kovanen PT, Goldstein JL: Receptor mediated uptake of lipoprotein-cholesterol and its utilization for steroid synthesis in the adrenal cortex. *Recent Prog Horm Res* 1979, 35:215–231.

6. Windler E, Chao YS, Havel RJ: Determinants of hepatic uptake of triglyceride-rich lipoproteins and their remnants in the rat. *J Biol Chem* 1980, 255:5475–5480.

7. Glomset JA: The plasma lecithin:cholesterol acyltransferase reaction. *J Lipid Res* 1968, 9:155–167.

8. Hahn PF: Abolishment of alimentary lipemia following injection of heparin. *Science* 1943, 98:19.

9. The Expert Panel: Report of the National Cholesterol Education Program Expert Panel on detection, evolution, and treatment of high cholesterol in adults. *Arch Intern Med* 1988, 148:36–69.

10. Scanu AM: Lipoprotein (a) and coronary artery disease. In *Plasma, Lipoproteins, and Coronary Artery Disease*. Edited by Kriesberg RA, Segrest JP. Cambridge, MA: Blackwell Scientific; 1992:175–199.

11. Eisenberg S: High density lipoprotein metabolism. *J Lipid Res* 1984, 25:1146–1152.

12. Segrest JP, Jones MK, Mishra VK, *et al.*: Apolipoprotein B-100 has a pentapartite structure composed of three amphipathic α helical domains alternating with two amphipathic β strand domains: detection by the computer program LOCATE. *Arterioscler Thromb* 1994, 14:1674–1685.

13. Fredrickson DS, Levy RI, Lees RS: Fat transport in lipoproteins: an integrated approach to mechanisms and disorders. *N Engl J Med* 1967, 276:148–156.

14. Grundy SM: *Cholesterol and Atherosclerosis: Diagnosis and Treatment.* New York: Gower Medical Publishing; 1990:2.1–2.25.

15. Lindgren FT: The plasma lipoproteins: historical developments and nomenclature. *Ann N Y Acad Sci* 1980, 348:1–15.

16. Schreiber WE: *Medical Aspects of Biochemistry.* Boston: Little, Brown & Company; 1984:57–90.

17. Oberman A, Kreisberg RA, Henkin Y, eds: *Principles and Management of Lipid Disorders.* Baltimore: Williams & Wilkins; 1992:87–105.

18. Anantharamaiah GM, Datta G, Garber DW: Toward the design of peptide mimics of antiatherogenic apolipoproteins A-I and E. *Current Science* 2001, 81:53–65.

19. Stryer L: *Biochemistry*, edn 3. New York: WH Freeman; 1988:283–312 .

20. Segrest JP, Jones MK, Klon AE, *et al.*: A detailed molecular belt model for apolipoprotein A-I in discoidal high density lipoprotein *J Biol Chem* 1999, 274:31755–31758.

21. Kulkarni KR, Garber DW, Marcovina SM, *et al.*: Quantification of cholesterol in all lipoprotein classes by the VAP-II method. *J Lipid Res* 1994, 35:159–168.

22. Cheung MC, Segrest JP, Albers JJ, *et al.*: Characterization of high density lipoprotein subspecies: structural studies by single vertical spin ultracentrifugation. *J Lipid Res* 1987, 28:913–929.

23. Garber D, Datta G, Chaddha M, *et al.*: A new class A amphipathic helical peptide analog protects mice from diet-induced atherosclerosis. *J Lipid Res* 2001, 42:545–552.

24. Teng B, Thompson GR, Sniderman AD, *et al.*: Composition and distribution of low density lipoprotein fractions in hyperapobeta-lipoproteinemia, normolipidemia, and familial hypercholesterolemia. *Proc Natl Acad Sci U S A* 1983, 80:6662–6666.

25. Austin MA, Breslow JL, Hennekens CH, *et al.*: Low-density lipoprotein subclass patterns and risk of myocardial infarction. *JAMA* 1988, 260:1917–1921.

26. Xu S: Apolipoprotein (A) binds to low-density lipoprotein at two distinct sites in lipoprotein(a). *Biochemistry* 1998, 37:9284–9294.

TRIGLYCERIDE-RICH LIPOPROTEINS

5

CHAPTER

Ngoc-Anh Le and
W. Virgil Brown

Elevated plasma triglycerides (TG) are an indicator of increased risk of arteriosclerotic vascular disease. However, the relationship between atherogenesis and increased levels of specific TG-carrying lipoproteins is complex and convoluted. Several primary and secondary disorders cause plasma triglyceride elevations. An increase in the risk of arteriosclerotic disease is observed in some of these disorders. Risk appears more strongly associated with concomitant alterations in high-density lipoprotein (HDL) and low-density lipoprotein (LDL) metabolism and with the accumulation of partially digested TG-rich lipoproteins, commonly referred to as "remnant" lipoproteins. In addition, the association of hypertriglyceridemia with other risk factors, such as diabetes mellitus and high blood pressure, causes linkage to atherosclerosis in epidemiologic studies to be less clear-cut.

Triglycerides and their components, the fatty acids, provide for an efficient mechanism of energy transport and storage in the body. The high energy content of TG (9.4 kcal/g) allows the 68-kg person with 20% body fat to store over 120,000 kcal. An equal amount of available energy from glycogen, or protein, would require a body weight of almost 182 kg, because storage of a gram of these nutrients requires 3 to 4 g of water and electrolytes. The intestine and liver are the sources of plasma TGs. These are contained in the inner core of chylomicrons and very low-density lipoproteins (VLDL). In addition, smaller amounts of triglyceride are carried in intermediate-density lipoproteins (IDL), LDL, and HDL. Total TG transport in these lipoproteins may be 100 to 500 g daily, depending on body size, dietary composition, and energy expenditure.

To understand the relationship between TGs and atherosclerosis, it is useful to review the absorption of dietary fats by the intestine, their synthesis into chylomicrons, and the clearance of chylomicrons from the plasma into various tissues. The liver plays a central role receiving excess energy in the form of free fatty acids from adipose tissue as well as carbohydrates, protein, and fat from the diet. Energy balance in the liver is maintained through the synthesis of TGs and their secretion in VLDL. Increased TGs may be associated with high ratios of LDL synthesis, which are then converted to LDL leading to a higher risk of vascular disease. The catabolism of VLDL and their conversion to LDL also involves an important set of interactions with HDL.

At the arterial wall, remnant lipoproteins of both VLDL and chylomicron may interact with endothelial cells, causing changes that may enhance transendothelial passage of the remnants and circulating monocytes into the intima. Monocyte-derived macrophages take up and store remnant lipoproteins and LDL. The low HDL cholesterol levels associated with hypertriglyceridemia may impair the normal system maintaining an efflux of cholesterol from arterial cells. The combination of these mechanisms may explain the apparent acceleration in atherogenesis in patients with some hypertriglyceridemic syndromes.

As these TG-rich lipoproteins of hepatic and intestinal origin undergo catabolism in the circulation, the composition of these lipoprotein particles determines the rate at which they are metabolized in vivo as well as the fate of these particles. Two key apolipoproteins that can modulate these processes are apo C-III and apo E. While a proportion of the TG-rich lipoproteins can be removed directly from the circulation, the majority of these particles are converted to the atherogenic LDL. The relative contents of these two apolipoproteins may affect the catabolic rate and metabolic fate of the particles. Of these, the gene of apo C-III contains a number of regulatory response elements, some of which have been suggested to indicate susceptibility for the development of hypertriglyceridemia. The efficacy of some management programs such as fibrates and insulin has been directly linked to these regulatory response elements. Additional evidence has been accumulated on the potential association between the apo E isoform and the interactions of TG-rich lipoproteins with cell-surface receptors.

When elevated triglyceride levels are found, the physician is often confronted with a high-risk patient. The coexistence of other risk factors, however, must be fully defined before the most effective treatment plan can be devised. To reduce vascular disease risk successfully, treatment must address all deranged lipoproteins, particularly elevated LDL and low HDL. Diet and drug therapy are available for this purpose.

PLASMA TRIGLYCERIDES AND RISK OF CARDIOVASCULAR DISEASE

TRIGLYCERIDE VALUES IN AMERICANS

| AGE, Y | PLASMA TRIGLYCERIDE LEVEL, *mg/dL* | | |
	10TH PERCENTILE	50TH PERCENTILE	90TH PERCENTILE
Males			
10	37	60	100
20	50	85	160
30	55	100	210
40	65	120	245
50	65	125	250
60	65	120	235
Females			
10	40	70	110
20	40	65	110
30	45	70	120
40	50	80	150
50	55	95	185
60	65	105	200

FIGURE 5-1. Triglyceride (TG) values in Americans. These values were measured in 10 community studies for fasting TGs in volunteers during the second to seventh decades of life. TG values in women increase until the seventh decade, but in men this rise occurs much earlier, reaching a maximum between the ages of 40 and 50 years. The mean TG levels in middle-aged and older individuals usually do not exceed 150 mg/dL. Distribution curves are not normally distributed, and the 90th percentile for men after age 40 years is approximately 250 mg/dL; for women over 50 years, it is approximately 200 mg/dL [1]. This may be due to gains in adipose tissue mass and frequent metabolic abnormalities in subsets that cause TGs to increase more dramatically with age.

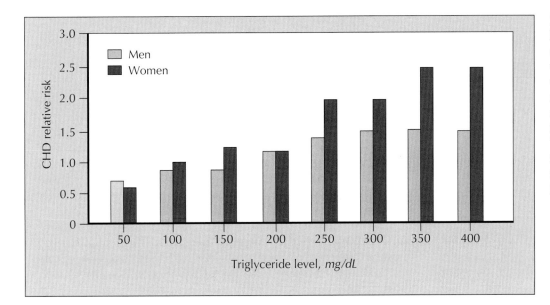

FIGURE 5-2. The incidence of coronary heart disease (CHD)-induced events, such as myocardial infarction and cardiac death, was found to be higher in both men and women with triglyceride levels above the mean for the population. The increase is most obvious as the baseline levels rise from approximately 150 to 350 mg/dL. This relationship of plasma triglycerides to risk of CHD is often stronger in women than in men, as was found in the Framingham Heart Study [2].

TRIGLYCERIDES AND RISK OF VASCULAR DISEASE

Plasma TGs correlate with prevalence and incidence of vascular disease in univariate analysis

Other risk factors are correlated with TG concentrations

By discounting for these confounding relationships with other major risk factors, multivariate analyses have often found little evidence for hypertriglyceridemia as an independent risk factor

FIGURE 5-3. Epidemiologic findings indicate that plasma triglycerides (TGs) strongly correlate with the prevalence and incidence of vascular disease in univariate analysis [3–5]. However, many other risk factors are correlated with TG concentrations. When multivariate analyses are performed, and these confounding relationships are discounted, little evidence remains for hypertriglyceridemia, per se, as an independent risk factor for cardiovascular disease [6,7]. Although TG-rich lipoproteins may not damage the arterial wall directly, the underlying metabolic disorders that cause increased concentrations of plasma TGs may also lead to other lipoprotein abnormalities that are atherogenic.

RISK FACTORS ASSOCIATED WITH PLASMA TRIGLYCERIDES

Low HDL cholesterol

Low apo A-I

Increased LDL cholesterol

Increased apo B

Small dense LDL

Glucose intolerance

Insulin resistance/hyperinsulinemia

Diabetes mellitus

Obesity (abdominal obesity?)

High blood pressure

FIGURE 5-4. Risk factors associated with increased plasma triglycerides (TGs) include low high-density lipoprotein (HDL) cholesterol [8], low apolipoprotein A-I (apo A-I) [6], increased low-density lipoprotein (LDL) cholesterol, and small dense LDL particles [9]. In addition, glucose intolerance with insulin resistance and hyperinsulinemia or definite diabetes mellitus is frequently found [10,11]. Obesity is a common contributing factor to hypertriglyceridemia. The occurrence of intra-abdominal obesity, in particular, appears to be linked to glucose intolerance, high blood pressure, and the lipoprotein abnormalities noted above [12].

RISK OF CHD WITH INCREASING TRIGLYCERIDES

	RELATIVE RISK*	
	MEN	WOMEN
Univariate analysis	1.33	2.02
Adjusted for HDL cholesterol	1.24	1.57

*Risk ratio for CHD in middle-aged persons for each 100 mg/dL rise in serum triglycerides. Data based on meta-analysis of 14 prospective studies [13].

FIGURE 5-5. In a recent meta-analysis of several observational studies, the simple measurement of total plasma triglycerides (TGs) in men has been found to predict an increase in vascular events by 33% for each 100 mg/dL increase in the plasma concentration [13]. A similar rise in plasma TGs for women was associated with an increase in risk of coronary heart disease (CHD) by 100%. Men with

plasma TG levels of 300 mg/dL would be expected to have 66% more CHD than their counterparts with a plasma TG level of 100 mg/dL. For women, a similar increase in plasma TG would be expected to increase risk of CHD by fourfold.

There is a moderate, but highly significant, inverse relationship between plasma TG and high-density lipoprotein (HDL) cholesterol concentrations. When the risk associated with a rise in TGs from 100 to 300 mg/dL is adjusted for the lower HDL cholesterol, the residual effect is a 47% and 113% increased risk of CHD in men and women, respectively. Furthermore, individuals with moderately elevated TGs (range, 200 to 500 mg/dL) often have higher low-density lipoprotein cholesterol levels; the adjustment for this relationship further reduces the risk that can be assigned specifically to elevations in TGs.

The usual daily fluctuations in human plasma levels are much greater for TGs than for cholesterol. This variation would significantly weaken any correlation of TGs with CHD risk. Few studies have accounted for the true biologic variation in TGs and, in fact, virtually all large studies have used single measures for statistical analyses. This may mean that the reported positive relationship between CHD risk and plasma TGs may be significantly stronger than current estimates [14].

DEFINING HYPERTRIGLYCERIDEMIAS

DEFINING HYPERTRIGLYCERIDEMIA

TG CATEGORY	PLASMA TG LEVEL, *mg/dL*
Normal	200
Borderline high	200–400
High	400–1000
Very high	>1000

FIGURE 5-6. Triglyceride (TG) levels below 100 mg/dL are desirable for young individuals (less than 20 years of age) and below 150 mg/dL for middle-aged or older adults. Significant metabolic abnormalities are observed frequently in individuals with TGs exceeding 200 mg/dL. Individuals with borderline high TGs of 200 to 400 mg/dL should be evaluated for other risk factors. Low high-

density lipoprotein (HDL) cholesterol, low-density lipoprotein (LDL) cholesterol above desirable levels, glucose intolerance, and hypertension will often be found in this group. Individuals with high TGs (*ie*, 400 to 1000 mg/dL) often have major gene defects causing the hypertriglyceridemia. Although very low HDL cholesterol is usually found, the LDL cholesterol may also be below the mean for age and gender. In this group and those with very high TGs, secondary disorders such as diabetes mellitus, nephrosis, hypothyroidism, and liver disease should be considered.

Patients with TGs above 1000 mg/dL usually have major gene defects in TG metabolism and other metabolic disorders. Some increased risk of vascular disease is related to the nearly universal finding of very low HDL cholesterol. However, LDL cholesterol may also be very low, and this appears to ameliorate the risk of vascular disease. In all such patients, there is the hazard of developing the "hyperchylomicronemic syndrome," which can lead to pancreatitis, peripheral neuropathy, central nervous system dysfunction, or myocardial compromise. Values expressed are those obtained after a 12-hour fast.

PRIMARY VERSUS SECONDARY HYPERTRIGLYCERIDEMIA	
PRIMARY HYPERTRIGLYCERIDEMIA	SECONDARY HYPERTRIGLYCERIDEMIA
Major gene defects	Metabolic abnormalities
Polygenic syndromes	Drugs

FIGURE 5-7. Primary versus secondary hypertriglyceridemia. Several primary metabolic disorders of lipoprotein metabolism have been well described and have produced moderate to severe hypertriglyceridemia. These are often due to major gene defects, many of which have been defined at a molecular level. Some have a weak or no apparent relationship to vascular disease, including lipoprotein lipase deficiency, apo C-II deficiency, and familial hypertriglyceridemia. Others confer significant increase in risk of cardiovascular disease; these include familial combined hyperlipidemia and dysbetalipoproteinemia. More recently, moderate hypertriglyceridemia has been associated with a series of disorders in chylomicron, very low-density lipoprotein (VLDL), and low-density lipoprotein (LDL) metabolism. Delayed clearance of "chylomicron remnants" and the definition of small dense LDL particles as well as LDL with reduced cholesteryl ester and relative increase in the protein component (hyper apo B) have been defined as syndromes. These often have patterns of familial clustering and are suggested to be genetically determined. Low high-density lipoprotein (HDL) cholesterol, high blood pressure, and hyperinsulinemia appear to be frequent concomitants of these abnormal lipoprotein patterns.

To understand the physiologic basis of these genetic disorders, it is important to consider the structure and metabolism of chylomicrons and VLDL as well as their relationships to the metabolism of LDL and HDL.

A series of metabolic disorders can produce changes in triglyceride metabolism causing elevated plasma VLDL and chylomicrons. These are referred to as the secondary hypertriglyceridemias. Certain drugs may also cause secondary hypertriglyceridemia.

ETIOLOGY OF THE HYPERTRIGLYCERIDEMIAS

GENETIC HYPERTRIGLYCERIDEMIA

No apparent vascular effects
- Lipoprotein lipase deficiency
- Apo C-II deficiency
- Familial hypertriglyceridemia*

Risk event
- Familial combined hyperlipidemia*
- Dysbetalipoproteinemia

*Common occurrences.

FIGURE 5-8. Hypertriglyceridemia due to major gene defects may produce marked elevations of triglycerides (TG) (>1000 mg/dL), yet cause no apparent increase in vascular disease risk. This is true for lipoprotein lipase deficiency and apo C-II deficiency [15–17]. These two disorders impair the very earliest phases of TG clearance and apparently do not lead to the generation of significant remnant lipoproteins. These extremely rare disorders manifest in children. Few adults have been followed into the sixth and seventh decades; therefore, a moderate effect on atherogenesis would not have been detected. The common disorder, familial hypertriglyceridemia, is due to major gene defects primarily associated with the overproduction of TG by the liver without a marked enhancement of apo B-100 secretion [17]. Therefore, there is not the increased number of the very low-density lipoprotein (VLDL) particles available for conversion to remnant lipoproteins and to low-density lipoprotein (LDL).

Familial combined hyperlipidemia is associated with increased numbers of VLDL particles and a concomitant generation of increased remnant lipoproteins and LDL [18,19].

Dysbetalipoproteinemia is also associated with remnant lipoprotein accumulation because the latter two are strongly associated with arteriosclerosis.

It should be noted that both familial hypertriglyceridemia and familial combined hyperlipidemia are descriptive terms for clinical syndromes that are only superficially understood. It seems certain that there will be several molecular defects uncovered that may allow development of subcategories of these disorders with more specific assignment of vascular disease risk than is currently possible.

METABOLIC DISORDERS ASSOCIATED WITH PLASMA TRIGLYCERIDE ELEVATIONS

COMMON

Excess adipose tissue (intra-abdominal fat)
Inadequate insulin action
  Insulin resistance
  NIDDM
  IDDM
Nephrosis
Renal failure
Hypothyroidism
Gout

RARE

Glycogen storage disease
Lipid storage disorders
Autoimmune disorders

FIGURE 5-9. Metabolic disorders associated with plasma triglyceride (TG) elevations. Plasma TGs may be markedly increased by other disorders that change lipid metabolism [20]. Obesity, particularly excess intra-abdominal fat, is associated with increased very low-density lipoprotein (VLDL) levels [21]. Insulin resistance, even with normal fasting plasma glucose, is associated with higher TG levels [22]. Control of blood sugar alone may not normalize TG levels in non–insulin-dependent diabetes mellitus (NIDDM), in which obesity is often a factor. When adequately treated, insulin-dependent diabetes mellitus (IDDM) usually results in desirable TG levels. Nephrosis increases VLDL production [23] and reduces plasma clearance. Hypothyroidism impairs clearance. Hyperuricemia is often associated with higher VLDL production rates [24].

Genetic disorders of glycogen metabolism or tissue phospholipid and glycolipid degradation that lead to abnormal hepatic storage of these substances are strongly associated with increased VLDL for unknown reasons [25]. Rarely, autoantibodies to lipolytic enzymes, apolipoproteins, or endothelial surface components may appear in systemic lupus erythematosus or other autoimmune disorders and interfere with catabolism of VLDL in chylomicrons, resulting in increased plasma TGs.

CHEMICAL SUBSTANCES THAT MAY ELEVATE TRIGLYCERIDES

Alcohol
Estrogen (oral)
Retinoic acid derivatives
Thiazide diuretics
β-adrenergic blockers

FIGURE 5-10. Chemical substances that may elevate triglycerides (TGs). An individual with primary hypertriglyceridemia may experience marked increases in plasma very low-density lipoprotein (VLDL) and chylomicrons if alcohol is consumed in significant quantities [26]. Similarly, estrogen use for contraception or postmenopausal hormonal replacement may also raise TGs [27,28]. This effect is only evident if given as an oral preparation, presumably because of higher concentrations delivered to the liver via the portal venous circulation. The rise in TGs may be particularly dramatic in persons with genetic hypertriglyceridemia.

The use of vitamin A derivatives (when given orally) and isotretinoin may greatly enhance an underlying hypertriglyceridemic state [29]. Thiazide diuretics usually cause minimal change at low doses but may become a factor in higher dosage, particularly in insulin-resistant states [30]. The noncardioselective β-blockers may raise TGs by 25% to 45%, although this effect is much less evident in the cardioselective compounds [31].

TRIGLYCERIDE ELEVATIONS AND ASSOCIATED LIPOPROTEIN ABNORMALITIES

Increased number of LDL particles
Small dense LDL
Hyper apo B
Increased chylomicron remnants
Reduced HDL cholesterol
Reduced apo A-I
Reduced Lp [A-1 only] vs Lp [A-I/A-II] particles

FIGURE 5-11. Triglyceride (TG) elevations and associated lipoprotein abnormalities. The presence of hypertriglyceridemia due to either major genetic disorders or to polygenic effects appears to confer a risk of vascular disease when accompanied by one or more of the lipoprotein abnormalities listed. An increased number of low-density lipoprotein (LDL) particles are found in familial combined hyperlipidemia due to their overproduction as products of very low-density lipoprotein (VLDL) hydrolysis [32,33]. In the presence of hypertriglyceridemia, the number of LDL particles may be greater than indicated by LDL cholesterol levels because the particles tend to become depleted of cholesterol. Consequently, there is a relative increase in the protein component (apo B). The LDL particles are smaller and more dense because of the lipid depletion. This condition has been referred to as "small dense LDL" (pattern B) [34]. When the apo B concentration exceeds approximately the 90th percentile (130 mg/dL), the disorder is referred to as "hyper apo B" [35]. The prolonged circulation of chylomicron remnants that have been partially depleted of their TG component is also associated with increased quantities of VLDL remnants. Reduced high-density lipoprotein (HDL) cholesterol and the apo A-I component has been associated with increased risk in hypertriglyceridemia [36]. The second most common apolipoprotein in HDL, apo A-II, does not appear to provide protection from atherosclerosis and may even impair the function of HDL in its protective role. New techniques for the quantification of HDL particles containing both apo A-I and apo A-II (Lp [A-I/A-II] particles) as well as those not containing apo A-II (Lp [A-I only] particles) seem to indicate that the relative depletion of the Lp (A-I only) may specifically increase atherogenesis.

SYNTHESIS AND METABOLISM OF CHYLOMICRONS AND VERY LOW-DENSITY LIPOPROTEIN

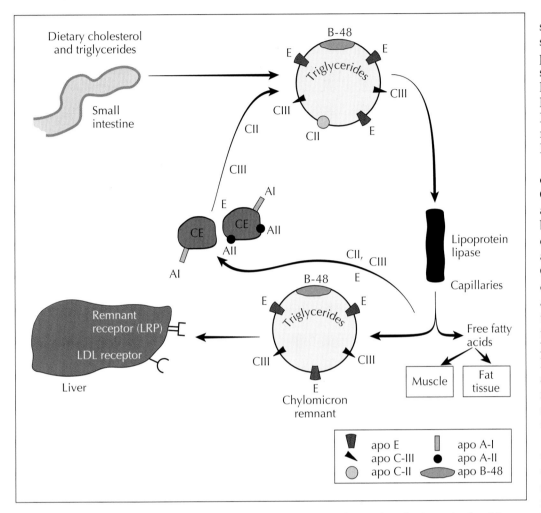

same size that is believed to 1) stabilize the surface, preventing aggregation of lipid particles; and 2) inhibit uptake by cell surfaces, allowing preferential binding to lipoprotein lipase for hydrolysis at the capillary endothelial cell as mediated by apo C-II. The apo C-II and apo C-III proteins are released during lipase action to return to HDL [37].

A third protein, apo E, is also added to chylomicrons through transfer from HDL. Compared with apo C-II and C-III, a lesser amount of this is released from chylomicrons by lipoprotein lipase. Consequent to this enzyme action, remnant particles are generated that are relatively depleted in TGs, apo C-II, and apo C-III, but relatively enriched in cholesteryl esters and apo E. A single copy of apo B-48 and many copies of apo E reside on this remnant particle. On circulation through the liver, there are at least two receptors that have high affinity for apo E; these include the low-density lipoprotein (LDL) receptor and a larger protein referred to as the LDL-receptor related protein (LRP) [38]. Apo B-48 does not have a binding site for either of these receptors.

Uptake in the liver can be regulated by the numbers of apo E and apo C-III molecules. The greater the number of copies of apo E, the higher the affinity of the particle for liver cell surfaces, presumably due to multisite attachment. Increased quantities of apo C-III displace apo E to HDL and reduce the rate of uptake of remnants by the liver.

Hepatic TG lipase is another enzyme on cell surfaces in Disse's spaces. This enzyme may further digest chylomicron remnant TGs and phospholipids. It also removes apo E from the surface of these particles [39]. Its role in the clearance of chylomicron remnant lipoprotein is not fully understood.

FIGURE 5-12. Chylomicron metabolism. Chylomicrons are formed in the intestinal epithelium after absorption of dietary cholesterol, as well as monoglycerides, fatty acids, and other hydrolytic products of dietary fats. The synthesis of apo B-48 and the transfer of newly synthesized triglycerides (TGs) are two essential steps in the generation of chylomicrons. The gene for this protein generates mRNA, which is edited in the intestine to translate only 48% of the gene sequence. The liver lacks this editing system and uses the full transcript (100%) to secrete the entire protein, called apo B-100.

Several additional apolipoproteins are transferred from high-density lipoprotein (HDL) to chylomicrons after arrival in the plasma. These include apo C-II, a small (9 kD) protein essential for activity of lipoprotein lipase. Apo C-III is a negatively charged protein of the

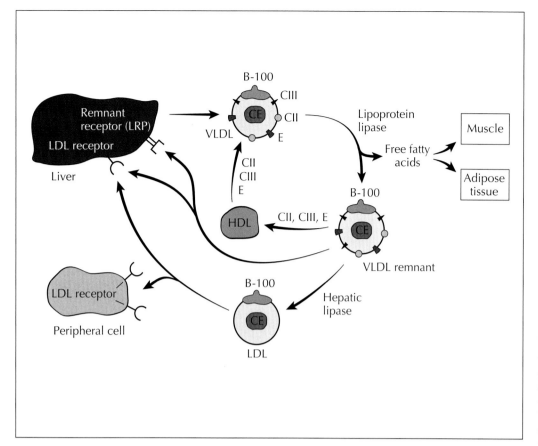

crons involving lipoprotein lipase and the generation of a remnant lipoproteins [37]. Major differences in the fate of VLDL remnant as compared with chylomicron remnant are possible. VLDL remnants have available an additional binding site for the low-density lipoprotein (LDL) receptor via apo B-100. However, they are taken up by liver cells less rapidly than are chylomicron remnants. This may be because they contain fewer apo E molecules per particle—a function of their smaller size and surface area.

The VLDL remnant may alternatively be converted to LDL via the action of hepatic TG lipase, which does not require the presence of apo C-II [40]. The LDL conversion is possible because apo B-100 can adopt a configuration that stabilizes a particle of the size and composition of LDL (apo B-48 does not appear capable of this function). Conversion of VLDL remnants involves removing most of the remaining TG and leaving cholesteryl esters as the major core lipid. In addition, residual apo E, apo C-II, and apo C-III are removed. Most LDL in the plasma of humans appears to be derived from this pathway. Its clearance from the plasma is highly dependent on the LDL receptor because apo B-100 does not bind to the LDL-receptor related protein (LRP). Every cell in the normal human body is capable of expressing LDL receptors. However, most available LDL receptors occur on hepatocytes and, therefore, the liver removes 75% to 80% of LDL.

FIGURE 5-13. Very low-density lipoprotein (VLDL) metabolism. Triglyceride (TG) synthesis in the liver provides for efficient energy transfer into the plasma as VLDL. The VLDL particle is assembled by adding lipid to a large (550,000 D) protein, apo B-100. This protein is a full transcript of the apo B gene. Several copies of apo C-II, apo C-III, and apo E are also added in the liver cell, although additional copies of these latter proteins are transferred from high-density lipoprotein (HDL) to the nascent VLDL after their arrival in the plasma. VLDLs follow a process similar to that discussed in Fig. 5-12 for chylomi-

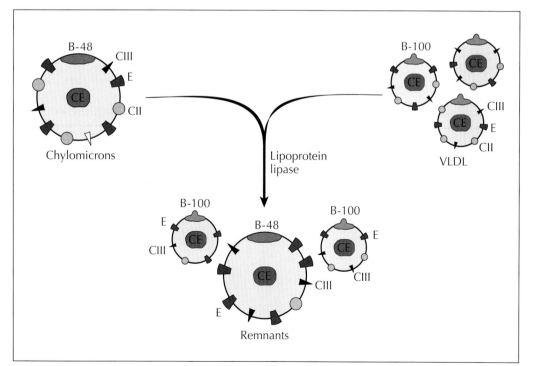

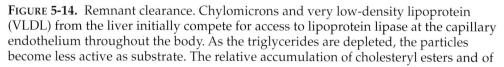

FIGURE 5-14. Remnant clearance. Chylomicrons and very low-density lipoprotein (VLDL) from the liver initially compete for access to lipoprotein lipase at the capillary endothelium throughout the body. As the triglycerides are depleted, the particles become less active as substrate. The relative accumulation of cholesteryl esters and of

apo E results in a population of potentially atherogenic particles that have several available pathways for further catabolism.

The major pathway may be the uptake into the liver through binding of apo E to the low-density lipoprotein (LDL) receptor and to the LDL-receptor related protein. After a fat-containing meal, both chylomicron and VLDL remnants accumulate in plasma, reflecting the competition between these particles for the receptors.

The rate of hepatic uptake is partly determined by the number of apo E molecules per particle. Chylomicron remnants with 10 or more apo E molecules are taken up avidly with a normal residence time of only a few minutes. VLDL remnants with only two to five molecules of apo E per particle are less rapidly cleared (30 to 60 minutes).

The competition of remnants of both types have many implications. High-fat diets may raise the concentration of VLDL remnant. A high intrinsic synthesis of VLDL particles may delay chylomicron remnant clearance [41]. A large circulating mass of remnants of either type may alter both LDL and high-density lipoprotein metabolism.

SPECIFIC DEFECTS IN METABOLISM

FIGURE 5-15. A prolonged life span for chylomicron remnants can be demonstrated in hypertriglyceridemic states. A variety of potential defects in remnant clearance can be postulated.

The best documented mechanisms for remnant accumulation are the genetic defects in apo E, which cause defective binding to both low-density lipoprotein (LDL)-receptor related protein (LRP) and the LDL receptor. These are discussed more fully in the treatment of dysbetalipoproteinemia. Overproduction of very low-density lipoprotein (VLDL) particles is an essential part of this syndrome as defective apo E alone is not sufficient to cause significant hypertriglyceridemia.

The deficiency of fully active LRP would be expected to produce remnant accumulation; however, no definitive case of defective LRP function has been reported. Gene "knock-out" experiments indicated this to be a lethal mutant. The LRP receptor binds a series of proteins and may be essential for the clearance of several important molecules from plasma.

LDL receptor deficiency causes familial hypercholesterolemia that is manifested primarily by elevations in LDL cholesterol; however, such patients often have mild to moderate hypertriglyceridemia as well. This is thought to result from a reduced capacity for VLDL remnant clearance. Increasing LDL receptors with hydroxymethyl glutaryl coenzyme A (HMG-CoA) reductase inhibitors has been shown to increase the rate of chylomicron remnant clearance [42].

Hepatic lipase deficiency in its full phenotypic expression is quite rare. The buildup of small VLDL-sized particles enriched in apo E has been described in the plasma of individual patients with this disorder.

A severe deficiency of HDL cholesterol occurs in Tangier disease due to rapid clearance of HDL particles. In other patients with apo A-I genetic defects, similar low HDL cholesterol syndromes occur. Remnant-like particles have been described in the blood plasma of these rare patients [39].

Overproduction of VLDL particles would also be expected to cause a relative increase in remnants [41]. VLDL remnants should compete with chylomicron remnant clearance because of the common use of apo E as a ligand. In patients with familial combined hyperlipidemia, a strong correlation between VLDL, apo B-100 production, and reduced chylomicron remnant clearance has been demonstrated.

Apo C-III displaces apo E from remnants; when apo C-III is overexpressed in transgenic mice, remnant clearance is markedly retarded [43]. In humans with hypertriglyceridemia, high plasma apo C-III levels are often found. Although no experimental evidence has been reported that demonstrates overproduction of apo C-III in humans to be a cause of reduced clearance of VLDL, chylomicrons, or the remnants of these lipoproteins, this remains a distinct possibility.

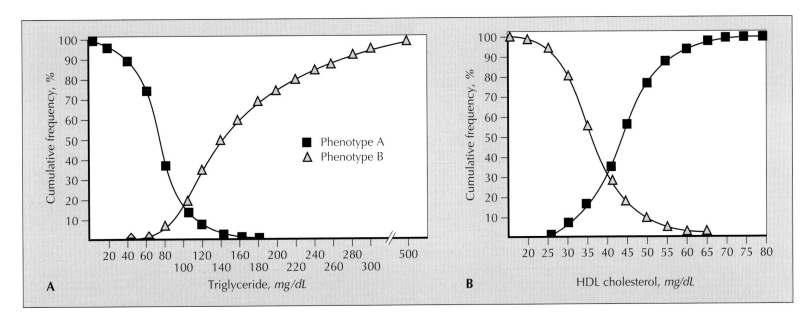

FIGURE 5-16. Small dense low-density lipoprotein (LDL) has been defined by measuring the size of LDL particles. Persons with larger LDL (25.5 nm) have been referred to as phenotype A, and those with small dense LDL (25.5 nm) are called phenotype B [34]. **A,** The majority of people with triglycerides above 200 mg/dL were found to have small dense LDL. **B,** Low high-density lipoprotein (HDL) cholesterol was also strongly associated with the presence of small dense LDL. (*Adapted from* Austin *et al.* [34].)

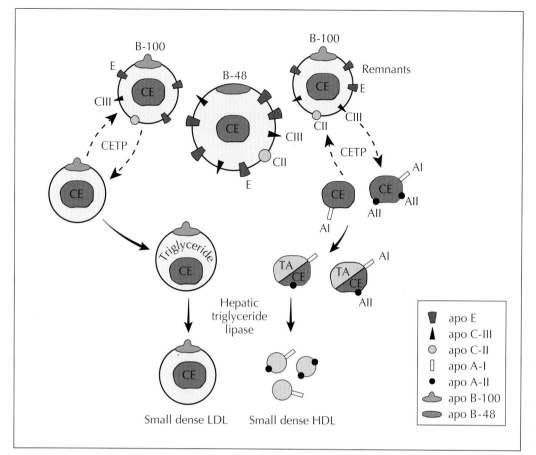

of lipoproteins in plasma [44]. Both LDL and HDL have cholesteryl ester–rich cores that participate in the CETP-mediated exchange for TGs with the remnants. The result is net transfer of cholesteryl esters to the remnants and TG enrichment of LDL and HDL. In individuals with total plasma TGs less than 150 mg/dL, the TG content of LDL and HDL is approximately 5% of the respective mass. In hypertriglyceridemia, TGs may account for 20% or more of the mass in LDL and HDL.

A second, very active lipase (hepatic lipase) is available on the surface of liver cells. This enzyme digests TGs associated with LDL and HDL, reducing the size of these particles [45].

The sequential actions of CETP and hepatic lipase result in the conversion of cholesterol-rich LDL and HDL to smaller, more dense particles.

Although the mechanisms by which small dense HDL is cleared rapidly from the plasma are poorly understood, they are believed to occur mainly via the kidney. The accumulation of TG-rich lipoproteins and their remnants may be the primary event explaining the associated small dense LDL and the reduced mass of HDL (particularly larger HDL-2) found in hypertriglyceridemic patients. These LDL and HDL changes correlate with the prevalence of coronary heart disease.

Figure 5-17. Source of small dense low-density lipoprotein (LDL) and high-density lipoprotein (HDL). Very low-density lipoprotein (VLDL) and chylomicron remnants provide a pool of triglycerides (TGs) for exchange with other lipoproteins. Cholesteryl ester transfer protein (CETP) actively exchanges TG and cholesteryl ester between several classes

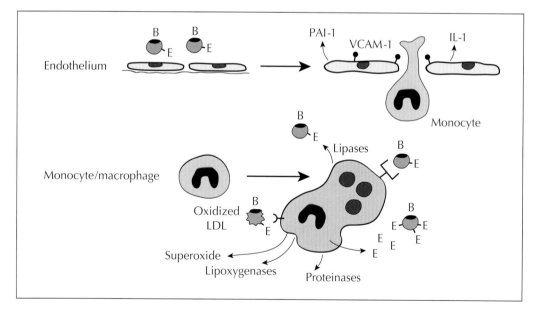

Interleukin-1 (IL-1) secretion is also stimulated. An increase in remnant lipoproteins appears to be the major abnormality of this model.

Once in the intima, the monocytes are activated into macrophages, expressing receptors that bind apo E, thus providing for remnant uptake [48]. In addition, these cells synthesize and secrete apo E [49], which may become associated with nearby lipoproteins and promote their uptake by the available cell surface receptors.

Activated macrophages also secrete lipoprotein lipase, lipoxygenases, and proteinases that may damage both lipid and protein surface components of very low-density lipoprotein and remnant lipoproteins, enhancing the probability of cellular uptake by macrophages via the "scavenger receptors" [50,51] with subsequent formation of foam cells. LDL—low-density lipoprotein; PAI-1—plasminogen activator inhibitor-1.

Figure 5-18. Triglyceride-rich remnant lipoproteins and vascular cells. Studies of rabbit endothelium indicate that diet-induced hyperlipidemia can cause rapid expression of adhesion molecules for leukocytes, particularly vascular cell adhesion molecule-1 (VCAM-1), which binds to the surface antigen VLA-4 of monocytes [46,47].

COAGULATION AND FIBRINOLYSIS IN HYPERTRIGLYCERIDEMIA

Increased factor VIIa
Increased PAI-1
Increased t-PA
Increased platelet activation

FIGURE 5-19. Coagulation and fibrinolysis in hypertriglyceridemia. There are several reports linking plasma triglycerides to various clotting parameters in persons who do not have proven coronary heart disease (CHD). Factor VIIa is correlated with fasting plasma triglyceride (TG) in community studies [52] and is found to be increased by high-fat diets within weeks [53].

In a study of 18 healthy male volunteers, plasminogen activator inhibitor-1 (PAI-1) was found to correlate directly with fasting TG concentrations (r^2=0.3) [54] and inversely with high-density lipoprotein cholesterol (r^2=0.6). Similarly, correlations are found between TGs and PAI-1 in patients with proven CHD [54]. Plasma tissue-type plasminogen activator (t-PA) activity is strongly correlated with PAI-1 [55] and has been observed in hypertriglyceridemia [56].

Increased platelet activation in hypertriglyceridemia has also been strongly implicated by the finding of higher levels of β-thromboglobulin in persons with increased plasma TGs [57].

INHERITED SYNDROMES WITH HYPERTRIGLYCERIDEMIA

DYSBETALIPOPROTEINEMIA

Phenotype	Increased concentrations of VLDL and chylomicron remnants
	VLDL cholesterol/triglyceride >0.3 enriched in apo E rich β mobility on electrophoresis
Frequency	1 per 5000
Inheritance	Polygenic
Probable cause	Apo E defective (E2/E2)
	Increased production of VLDL
Clinical consequence	Increased coronary heart disease
	Tubero-eruptive xanthomata
	Palmar xanthomata

FIGURE 5-20. Dysbetalipoproteinemia is an uncommon disorder of remnant clearance caused by the superimposition of at least two common genetic traits. The first is a defective apo E molecule that has very low binding affinity for remnant receptors. There are three common alleles for apo E, two of which (E3 and E4) bind normally [58,59]. A third common allele, E2, results in a defective protein with weak binding affinity. Approximately 15% of the population has at least one defective allele, and approximately 1% is homozygous for this allele. Dysbetalipoproteinemia is usually a recessive trait (ie, requires two defective alleles). Other less common defective E proteins may have no affinity for the receptor and the clinical disorder may be expressed as a heterozygous defect [59]. Marked elevations in remnants do not usually occur unless there is a concomi-tant overproduction of very low-density lipoprotein (VLDL) that is separately inherited. The coexistence of two traits, each of which exists in 1% to 2% of the population, gives the observed expression of one in 5000 to one in 10,000 persons.

The clinical diagnosis is suggested by elevations of cholesterol and triglycerides to approximately equivalent levels (250 to 800 mg/dL each). There are tubero-eruptive xanthomata on elbows (see Fig. 5-21), knees, or buttocks in 15% to 30% of patients, and some have planar xanthomata along the palmar creases [60].

The isolation of VLDL can confirm the diagnosis because the remnant particles are relatively rich in cholesterol and apo E, with lesser amounts of apo C-II and apo C-III. Consequently, the cholesterol-to-triglyceride mass ratio for isolated VLDL is greater than 0.3 as compared with a ratio of 0.2 obtained for normal VLDL. In addition, the isolated VLDLs have electrophoretic mobility comparable to β-globulins and low-density lipoprotein rather than normal pre-β mobility.

Atherosclerosis is prevalent in both peripheral arteries and in the coronary arteries of affected persons by midlife.

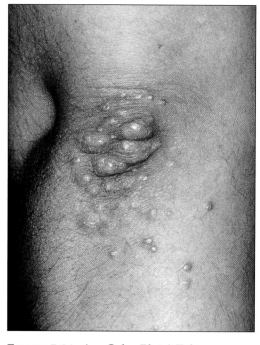

FAMILIAL COMBINED HYPERLIPIDEMIA

Phenotype	Increased VLDL and/or LDL of normal composition; the dominant lipoprotein elevation may present as VLDL *or* LDL
Frequency	1%–2% of population
Inheritance	Autosomal dominant with expression in the third to fourth decade; first-degree relatives may show elevated VLDL and/or LDL
Probable cause	Overproduction of VLDL particles and consequent increased LDL production
Clinical consequences	Increased coronary heart disease

FIGURE 5-21. (*see* Color Plate) Tubero-eruptive xanthomata on the elbow of a patient with dysbetalipoproteinemia. (Courtesy of J. Davignon, MD, Montreal, Canada.)

FIGURE 5-22. Familial combined hyperlipidemia is one of the most common forms of hypertriglyceridemia [61]. It is usually defined as the existence of elevated triglycerides (TGs) or elevated low-density lipoprotein (LDL) cholesterol (exceeding the 95th percentile for age and gender) with one or more first-degree relatives similarly affected. Very low-density lipoprotein (VLDL) is normal in composition and has pre-β mobility on electrophoresis. Children usually have high values of TGs for their age but may not fully express the disorder until the fourth decade of life [62]. LDL may be only moderately elevated at times, particularly when the TG level exceeds 400 mg/dL.

Overproduction of apo B-100 has been well demonstrated in several kindreds who meet the definition for this disorder [63,64]. The association with coronary heart disease in the fifth through seventh decades is well established.

FAMILIAL HYPERTRIGLYCERIDEMIA

Phenotype	Increased VLDL with normal or low LDL; fasting chylomicrons occasionally present
Frequency	1/100
Inheritance	Autosomal dominant
Probable cause	Overproduction of triglycerides without incurred conversion of VLDL to LDL
Clinical consequences	No definite relation to CHD

FIGURE 5-23. Familial hypertriglyceridemia is characterized by increased plasma very low-density lipoprotein (VLDL) triglycerides (TGs) and, in some cases, with TGs above 500 mg/dL, chylomicrons may be present in fasting plasma [61]. The total cholesterol may lie within normal limits because low-density lipoprotein (LDL) cholesterol and high-density lipoprotein (HDL) cholesterol are often at or below the lower limits of normal. Hepatic synthesis of TG is increased, although the higher rate of VLDL particle production seen in familial combined hyperlipidemia is not observed [64,65]. The nascent VLDLs are presumed to be larger and relatively more TG-rich than nascent particles.

HDL cholesterol is reduced and small dense LDL and HDL are usually present. The risk of coronary heart disease (CHD) may be only modestly increased, perhaps due to the low LDL cholesterol.

FIGURE 5-24. (*see* Color Plate) Eruptive xanthomata on the buttocks of a patient with familial hypertriglyceridemia and hyperchylomicronemic syndrome [66]. (Courtesy of J. Davignon, MD, Montreal, Canada.)

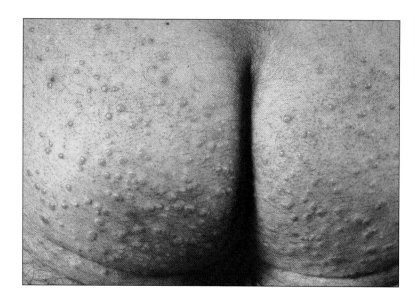

PLURIMETABOLIC SYNDROME ("SYNDROME X")

Glucose intolerance (insulin resistance)
Hypertriglyceridemia
Low HDL cholesterol
High blood pressure
Obesity

FIGURE 5-25. The frequently observed clustering of glucose intolerance and hyperinsulinemia with lipoprotein disorders, hypertension, and obesity has not been explained at a biochemical level [10–12]. Coronary heart disease is believed to result with high frequency in such individuals because each of the traits has been shown separately to be a risk factor [66–68]. HDL—high-density lipoprotein.

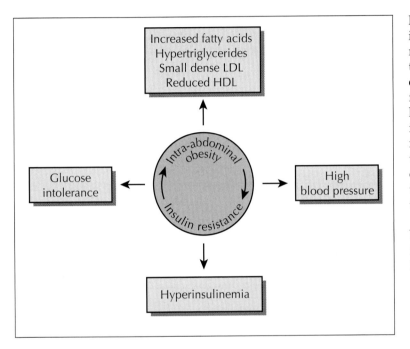

FIGURE 5-26. It has been suggested that insulin resistance is the initiating physiologic derangement with increased fatty acid released from adipose tissue, increased very low-density lipoprotein synthesis, and increased insulin levels. Intra-abdominal obesity may develop in this setting of increased flow of metabolic fuel. High blood pressure may be induced by renal affects of the hyperinsulinemia [67]. Others have suggested that intra-abdominal obesity is the primary event with insulin resistance following in genetically susceptible persons [21]. The increased prevalence of this syndrome in settings of overabundant calories and low levels of exercise strongly supports increased adipose tissue as a major triggering event. The efficacy of weight loss in reversing most of the abnormal physiology also supports obesity as the crucial issue.

Other less noted abnormalities such as hyperuricemia, microalbuminuria, and polycythemia have been found to occur more frequently in this syndrome. HDL—high-density lipoprotein; LDL—low-density lipoprotein.

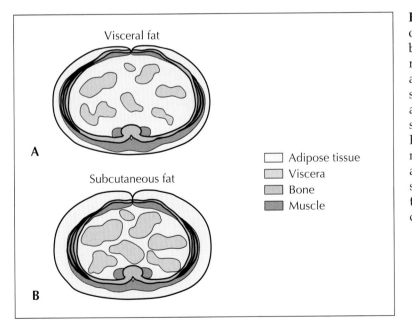

FIGURE 5-27. The concept of intra-abdominal obesity has developed because of observational studies demonstrating a correlation between measures of "central obesity" (waist-hip or waist-thigh ratios) and risk of coronary heart disease [69]. The use of CT of the abdomen allows an improved assessment of central fat illustrating significant independence of visceral as opposed to subcutaneous adipose tissue accumulation [70]. Shown are representative CT scans of two individuals with comparable body mass indices. **A**, Excess visceral fat. **B**, The majority of the fat is present subcutaneously. The blood flow from visceral fat into the portal system and evidence for a relatively enhanced lipolysis with catechol stimuli compared with subcutaneous adipocytes strongly suggests that this type of obesity may have direct metabolic effects, changing glucose and fat metabolism [21].

EFFICACY IN REDUCING VASCULAR DISEASE

TRIGLYCERIDE-REDUCING TRIALS
Stockholm Ischemic Heart Disease Study
Helsinki Heart Study

FIGURE 5-28. Clinical trials with triglyceride (TG)-reducing agents. To date, there have been no clinical trials that have selectively reduced plasma TG levels in an attempt to reduce coronary heart disease events. The diet and drug therapy used in each trial has also altered low-density lipoprotein (LDL) in a meaningful way. Only two trials have 1) used drugs that produce TG reductions as their major mechanism of action; 2) followed sufficient numbers of people with adequate endpoint assessment; and 3) actually measured TGs before and during the study period [71,72]. Only the Helsinki Heart Study [72] measured high-density lipoprotein (HDL) and assessed LDL.

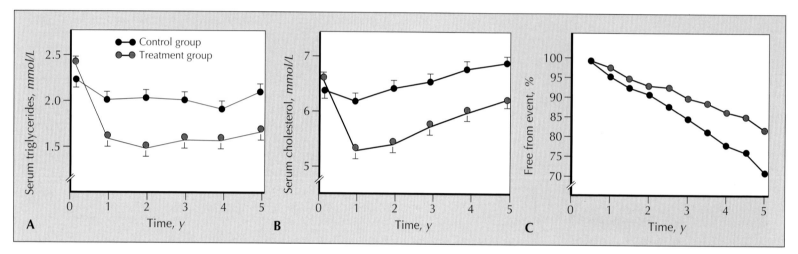

FIGURE 5-29. The Stockholm Ischemic Heart Disease Study was designed to assess plasma lipid reduction as a means of preventing recurrent coronary heart disease (CHD) in those patients who had experienced a myocardial infarction. Five hundred fifty-five men and women under 79 years of age were assigned randomly to either niacin plus clofibrate or to placebo.

A, The total triglyceride (TG) level fell from 2.4 mmol/L (211 mg/dL) to 1.6 mmol/L (140 mg/dL) in the active treatment group. The control group experienced a decline from 2.2 mmol/L (191 mg/dL) to 2.0 mmol/L (176 mg/dL).

B, The total cholesterol level was reduced from 6.6 mmol/L (254 mg/dL) to 5.2 mmol/L (200 mg/dL) initially; by the end of the study, however, the mean plasma cholesterol had risen to 6.1 mmol/L (235 mg/dL). The control group had a steady rise in cholesterol over the 5 years. **C,** The number of persons suffering a recurrent infarction or cardiovascular death was significantly reduced. At the end of the study, only 71% of the control group had not suffered an event whereas 83% of the treated group were event-free. The total mortality was also significantly reduced because of the marked decline in cardiovascular mortality (36%).

The reduction in CHD events was directly related to TG reduction but had no correlation with the decline in cholesterol. However, low-density lipoprotein and high-density lipoprotein (HDL) cholesterol and HDL cholesterol were not measured. Both the drugs used elevated HDL cholesterol significantly, and this probably minimized the change in total plasma cholesterol. (*Adapted from* Carlson and Rosenhamer [71].)

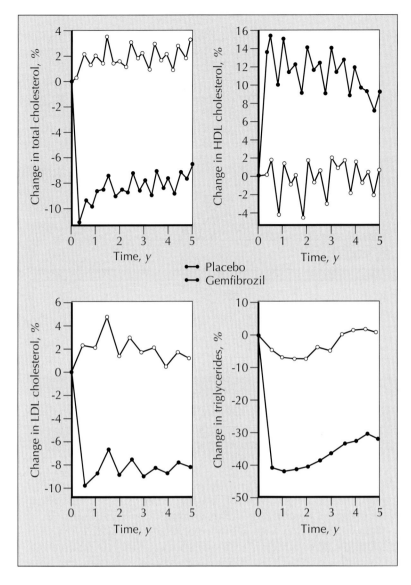

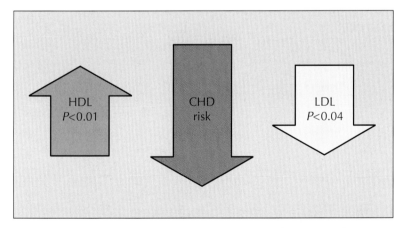

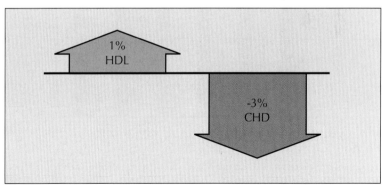

FIGURE 5-30. The Helsinki Heart Study was designed to test the efficacy of gemfibrozil in preventing the first myocardial infarction or cardiovascular mortality in a group of men (*n*=4081) between 40 and 55 years of age who initially had no evidence of coronary heart disease but had a total cholesterol minus high-density lipoprotein (HDL) cholesterol exceeding 200 mg/dL. The men were randomly assigned to take gemfibrozil (600 mg twice daily) or placebo for 5 years [73].

When compared with placebo-treated patients, triglyceride levels were reduced by approximately 35%, and total cholesterol and low-density lipoprotein (LDL) cholesterol levels fell approximately 9%. HDL cholesterol in the gemfibrozil group increased by an average 11% over the 5 years of the study. (*Adapted from* Frick *et al.* [72].)

FIGURE 5-31. In the Helsinki Heart Study, significant correlations with reduced coronary heart disease (CHD) events were associated with an increase in high-density lipoprotein (HDL) cholesterol (*P*<0.01) and a decrease in low-density lipoprotein (LDL) cholesterol (*P*<0.04) LDL cholesterol during 5 years of treatment with gemfibrozil. A large reduction in triglycerides (35%) did not have a significant independent relationship to the observed reduction in cardiac endpoints [73].

FIGURE 5-32. The incidence of myocardial infarction plus mortality from coronary heart disease (CHD) fell 3% for each 1% rise in high-density lipoprotein (HDL) cholesterol achieved in the treated group participating in the Helsinki Heart Study [73].

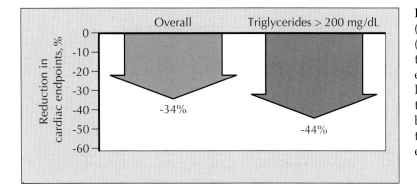

FIGURE 5-33. The overall reduction in major cardiac endpoints (myocardial infarction plus mortality from coronary heart disease (CHD) was 34% in the Helsinki Heart Study. The patients with triglycerides over 200 mg/dL experienced a greater reduction in events (44%). However, these individuals had lower high-density lipoprotein (HDL) cholesterol levels. The increase in HDL cholesterol achieved in those individuals with low HDL cholesterol at baseline correlated strongly with CHD risk reduction, whereas there was a much weaker correlation of CHD events with triglyceride reduction [73].

HELSINKI HEART STUDY

TREATMENT GROUP	BASELINE HDL, *mg/dL*	CHANGE IN HDL, %	CHD EVENTS, *n*	INCIDENCE/1000, *n*
Placebo (*n* = 69)	30.6	+9.0	9	130.4
Gemfibrozil (*n* = 89)	31.0	+33.7*	4	44.9

*Significantly greater than placebo; *P*<0.05.

FIGURE 5-34. In the Helsinki Heart Study, the small groups of patients with hypertriglyceridemia (triglyceride levels above 200 mg/dL), low high-density lipoprotein (HDL) cholesterol levels (below 35 mg/dL), and high low-density lipoprotein (LDL) cholesterol levels (above 160 mg/dL) experienced a 66% reduction in myocardial infarction and mortality from coronary heart disease (CHD) [74].

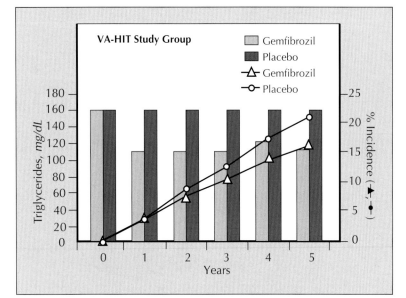

FIGURE 5-35. Results from the Veterans Affairs High-density Lipoprotein Intervention Trial (VA-HIT). In a group of 2531 men with coronary heart disease with low high-density lipoprotein (HDL), intervention with gemfibrozil resulted in a 4% increase in HDL and a 30% reduction in triglycerides (TGs). The relative risk reduction was 22% (*P* = 0.006) as derived from a Cox model. The mean low-density lipoprotein (LDL) and TGs for all participants were in the normal range at entry into the study, 111 and 160 mg/dL, respectively. (*Adapted from* Rubins *et al.* for the VA-HIT Study Group [75].)

RELATIONSHIP BETWEEN TRIGLYCERIDES AND CHD

There is a strong interdependence of elevated TGs and low HDL cholesterol.

High risk of CHD may not occur in the absence of other risk factors, particularly when LDL cholesterol is low (*ie,* < 130 mg/dL).

Certain metabolic disorders raise triglycerides, remnant cholesterol, and/or LDL cholesterol and lower HDL cholesterol.

These disorders are associated with high risk of CHD.

Treatment to reduce TGs offers significant CHD risk reduction when very low-density lipoprotein remnant cholesterol and/or LDL cholesterol are reduced and HDL cholesterol is increased.

FIGURE 5-36. Summary of the relationship between triglycerides (TGs) and coronary heart disease (CHD). HDL—high-density lipoprotein; LDL—low-density lipoprotein.

GENE REGULATION OF APO C-III

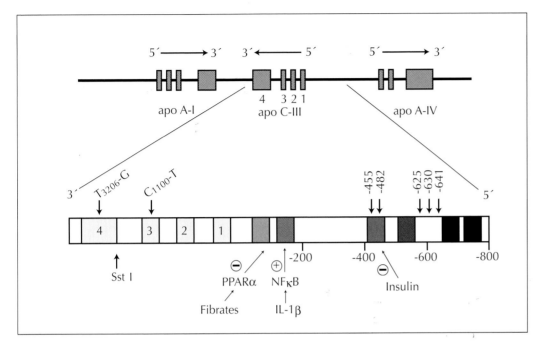

FIGURE 5-37. Regulatory elements in the apo C-III gene. The apo C-III gene is located on human chromosome 11, flanked on one side by the gene for apo A-I and by the gene for apo A-IV on the other [76]. In addition to the SstI polymorphic site in the nontranslated region of exon 4 that has been linked to familial combined hyperlipidemia [77,78], point mutations T3206-G in exon 4 and C110-T in exon 3 have also been

reported to be associated with familial combined hyperlipidemia [79]. In addition, several regulatory sites have been identified in the promoter region of the apo C-III gene that may explain the association of elevated apo C-III concentrations in hypertriglyceridemia and in diabetes mellitus. Chen *et al.* [80] identified an insulin response element in the promoter region of the apo C-III gene in rodents. Another region of the apo C-III promoter has been found to bind the inducible transcription factor NFκB [81]. In HepG2 cells, transcription of an apo C-III promoter reporter construct was shown to be upregulated when NFκB is activated by inflammatory cytokines such as interleukin-1β (IL-1β) [81]. Activation of apo C-III transcription has also been reported to be dependent on the levels of a hepatic nuclear factor (HNF-4) [82,83]. The efficacy of fibric acid derivatives in reducing plasma triglycerides has also been linked to the inhibition of apo C-III gene expression via interaction of PPARα with HNF-4 and a C3P element present in the apo C-III promoter [84].

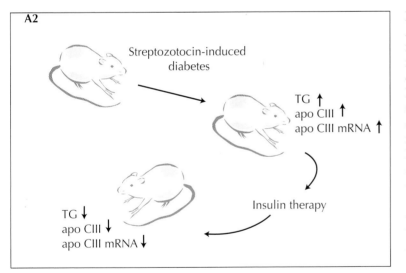

FIGURE 5-38. Insulin response element and apo C-III mRNA [80]. A group of C57BL6 mice were treated with streptozotocin by intraperitoneal injection (200 mg/kg). This resulted in a 2.6-fold increase in plasma glucose, a 1.5-fold increase in plasma triglycerides (TGs), and 1.4-fold increase in apo C-III mRNA in the liver. Within 24 hours of the injection of insulin in a group of streptozotocin-treated mice, plasma glucose was reduced to 10% of the level in the diabetic untreated animal, plasma TG was reduced to 40%, and apo C-III mRNA was reduced to 40%. The levels for all three measurements in the streptozotocin-treated animals that received insulin were significantly lower than those observed in the normal control animals.

The ability of insulin to suppress gene expression was confirmed by inserting the promoter region of the apo C-III gene upstream of the luciferase coding region and subsequently transfecting the plasmid in HepG2 cells. The expression of the luciferase was repressed in a dose-dependent manner by insulin in this in vitro system.

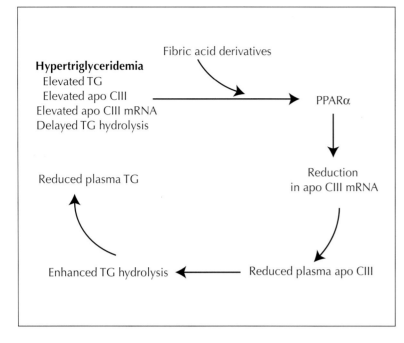

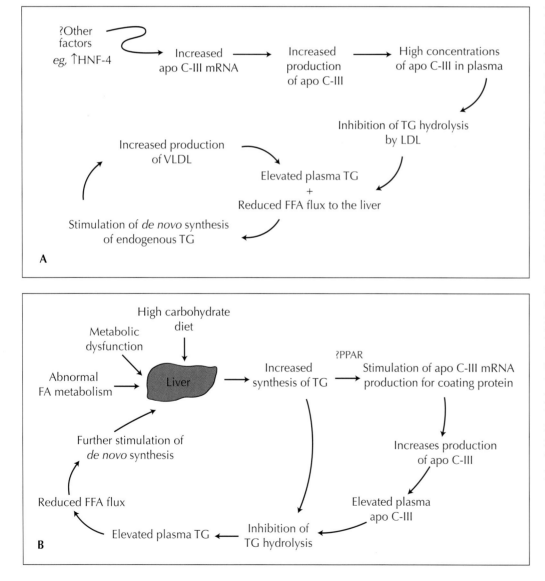

Figure 5-39. Fibric acid derivatives: PPARα, apo C-III gene expression, and hypertriglyceridemia. There is a direct correlation between plasma triglycerides (TGs) and plasma apo C-III [85,86]. Analysis of the very low-density lipoprotein (VLDL) composition in a group of individuals ranging in plasma TG from 50 to 526 mg/dL indicated that the ratio of TG to apoB in VLDL increased from 5 to 20 with increasing plasma TG [87]. While there was a 20-fold difference in VLDL apo C-II, in this group, the number of apo C-II molecules per VLDL particles did not increase. In contrast, there was a 50-fold increase in VLDL apo C-III concentrations with increasing levels of plasma TG [12]. This translates to approximately 20 to 25 molecules of apo C-III for every VLDL particle at the lower range of TG. In individuals with elevated TG, there would be 50 molecules of apo C-III per VLDL particles [87].

The presence of apo C-III on VLDL has been demonstrated to inhibit the activity of lipoprotein lipase [88,89]. In familial apo C-III deficiency, the fractional catabolic rate of VLDL-TG was threefold faster than for normal controls [90]. While we can directly demonstrate increased production of apo C-III in hypertriglyceridemia, studies in transgenic and knockout animal models would support a direct relationship between apo C-III production and hypertriglyceridemia. Overexpression of human apo C-III in the transgenic mouse model is also associated with hypertriglyceridemia [91,92]. In the absence of apo C-III in the knockout mouse, the transient TG elevations following the consumption of a fat-containing meal could not be demonstrated [93].

An 80% reduction in apo C-III mRNA could be demonstrated in the liver of rats treated with bezafibrate for 6 days resulting in a threefold decrease in plasma apo C-III [85]. In primary cultures of human hepatocytes, fenofibric acid lowered apo C-III mRNA in a time- and dose-dependent manner [94]. The net result is a 50% reduction in the amount of apo C-III secreted. There was no change in the level of apo E in this system.

Figure 5-40. Association between apo C-III gene expression and hypertriglyceridemia. **A,** One possible hypothesis for the association between elevated apo C-III concentrations and hypertriglyceridemia is that overexpression of apo C-III mRNA leads to an increased production of apo C-III. With the resulting increase in apo C-III concentrations, triglyceride (TG) hydrolysis by lipoprotein lipase is impaired as reflected by increased plasma TG and reduced free fatty acid (FFA) flux back to liver. The liver responds to the reduced FFA flux by stimulating de novo synthesis of endogenous TG in the form of hepatic VLDL. Increased secretion of very low-density lipoprotein (VLDL). would in turn further exacerbate the hypertriglyceridemic state.

B, Alternately, a number of metabolic states could result in increased production of endogenous TG by the liver. For instance, abnormal fatty acid (FA) metabolism or a high carbohydrate diet could lead to increased synthesis of TG, which in turn could stimulate the production of apo C-III to provide the required complement of protein coat. With the increased concentrations of plasma apo C-III, we would expect further inhibition of lipolytic action. The impaired activity of lipoprotein lipase would contribute to further elevations in plasma TG. LDL—low-density lipoprotein.

ROLE OF APO E IN TRIGLYCERIDE METABOLISM

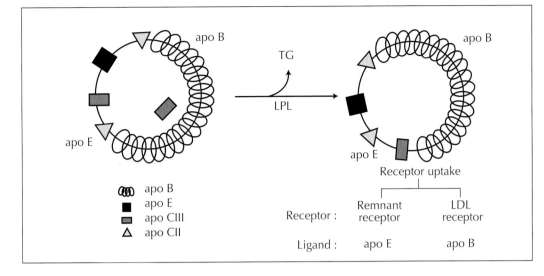

FIGURE 5-41. Apo E and the metabolism of triglyceride (TG)-rich lipoproteins. In addition to the presence of apo B as the structural apolipoprotein, TG-rich lipoproteins also contain a number of exchangeable apolipoproteins: apo C-II, apo C-III, and apo E. While the presence of apo C-II and apo C-III are necessary to modulate the efficient delivery of TG to peripheral tissues, excess amount of apo Cs has been demonstrated to interfere with the receptor-mediated uptake of these particles [95–97]. Depending on the composition of the partially hydrolyzed particles, they may interact with either the low-density

lipoprotein (LDL) receptor or the remnant receptor. The ligands of choice for these receptors are apo B and apo E, respectively. The size of the TG-rich lipoproteins may also play a role in determining the interactions of these particles with the different receptors [98] and may reflect difference in affinities of apo C-III and apo E [99].

Three common alleles (ϵ2, ϵ3, and ϵ4) are responsible for the coding of the three isoforms of apo E found in plasma. Presence of the ϵ2 allele is associated with dysbetal-ipoproteinemia or remnant disease as characterized by the presence of cholesterol-rich remnant lipoproteins and prolonged post-prandial lipemia [100] as compared to the wild type ϵ3 allele. Delayed clearance of postprandial lipoproteins was also been reported in subjects with the ϵ4 allele [101]. In a meta-analysis based on 45 population samples derived from 17 different countries, the presence of the ϵ4 allele is demonstrated to be associated with higher plasma cholesterol levels and triglycerides [102].·

APO E ALLELES AND CAD RISK

FACTOR	PREVALENCE, %	RELATIVE ODDS	POPULATION ATTRIBUTABLE RISK, %
LDL	Men, 30	1.4	11
	Women, 30	1.2	5
HDL < 35	Men, 23	2.4	24
	Women, 5	12.9	37
ϵ4 allele	Men, 24	1.5	11
	Women, 23	2.0	19

FIGURE 5-42. Apo E alleles and coronary artery disease (CAD) risk. Several studies with clinical endpoints have also demonstrated an increased risk for CAD in individuals expressing the ϵ4 allele. In a study of myocardial infarction (MI) survivors and age- and sex-matched healthy controls, the presence of the ϵ4 allele was associated with early age of MI [103,104]. Data from 720 young men between 15 and 34 years old in the Premature Development of Atherosclerosis in Youth (PDAY) indicated that the severity of atherosclerosis was higher in individuals expressing ϵ4 as compared to those expressing ϵ3 and ϵ2 [105]. A survey of men under the age of 40 years who underwent angioplasty revealed a 16-fold greater prevalence of ϵ4 than observed in the general population [106]. More recently, based on the analysis of apo E isoforms in over 1900 participants, the Framingham Offspring Study reported that the prevalence of CHD was associated with the ϵ4 allele in both men and women with relative odds of greater than 1.5 [107]. HDL—high-density lipoprotein; LDL—low-density lipoprotein.

Novel Markers for Coronary Artery Disease and Triglycerides

POTENTIAL MARKERS OF CAD ASSOCIATED WITH ABNORMAL METABOLISM OF TG-RICH LIPOPROTEINS

MEASUREMENTS	TRIALS	FINDINGS
VLDL remnants or IDL	NHLBI Type II Coronary Intervention Study Montreal Heart Study	High concentrations of cholesterol in VLDL remnants or IDL are associated with increased risk for coronary events.
Chylomicron remnants		Following the consumption of a standardized meal containing fat and cholesterol, patients with documented CAD have delayed removal of chylomicron remnants despite normal fasting lipid levels.
Small dense LDL	St. Thomas Atherosclerosis Risk Study	High concentrations of small dense subpopulation of LDL with high protein to cholesterol ratio are associated with increased risk for coronary events.
apo C-III levels in HDL	Cholesterol Lowering and Atherosclerosis Study	Of all patients receiving combination therapy, individuals with the high fraction of plasma apo C-III in the HDL fractions had the most significant disease regression.
HDL	Helsinki Heart Study BECAIT	Interventions that are specifically designed to raise HDL without significant reductions in LDL have been demonstrated to result in significant reductions in the number of clinical events.

FIGURE 5-43. Potential markers of coronary artery disease (CAD) associated with abnormal metabolism of triglyceride (TG)-rich lipoproteins. All these biochemical parameters that have been demonstrated to be predictive of heart disease actually reflect abnormalities in TG metabolism.

As TG-rich lipoproteins are secreted into the circulation, they acquire additional protein components from plasma high-density lipoprotein (HDL), in particular apo C-II, apo C-III, and apo E. While apo C-II is a required activator for the enzyme lipoprotein lipase that is responsible for the hydrolysis of TGs, excess apo C-III will inhibit TG hydrolysis. Partially hydrolyzed TG-rich lipoproteins, either chylomicron remnants or very low-density lipoprotein (VLDL) remnants, can interact with specific receptors and be removed in toto. In the presence of an excess number of TG-rich particles, the competition for the limited number of receptors would result in delayed removal of remnants, both of intestinal and hepatic origin. This would account for the elevated concentration of cholesterol in VLDL remnants and intermediate-density lipoprotein (IDL) observed in the National Heart, Lung, and Blood Institute (NHLBI) Type II Coronary Intervention Study [108] and the Montreal Heart Study [109]. Abnormal postprandial response in CAD would also be explained by the delayed catabolism of TG-rich lipoproteins [110,111].

In the presence of hypertriglyceridemia, excess number of low-density lipoprotein (LDL) favors the exchange of TG from TG-rich lipoproteins for esterified cholesterol from LDL. The enzyme cholesteryl ester transfer protein (CETP) facilitates this remodeling of plasma lipoproteins. The resulting TG-enriched LDL is hydrolyzed by hepatic lipase with the formation of small, dense LDL. High concentrations of a subpopulation of LDL with high protein-to-cholesterol ratio have been demonstrated to be associated with increased risk for coronary events in the St. Thomas Atherosclerosis Risk Study [112].

Apo C-III equilibrates readily among plasma lipoproteins. The preferential association of plasma apo C-III with HDL would reduce the concentrations of apo C-III in the TG-rich VLDL and thus minimize its inhibitory effect on the activity of lipoprotein lipase. This may explain the beneficial effect of the presence of a high apo C-III concentration in high-density lipoprotein (HDL) in the Cholesterol Lowering and Atherosclerosis Study [113] and of the low apo C-III-to-apo B ratio in VLDL observed in the Monitored Atherosclerosis Regression Study [114].

Interventions with fibric acid derivatives that increase HDL cholesterol may also reduce apo C-III levels and improve the catabolism of TG-rich lipoproteins have also been shown to reduce CAD risk [115,116]. BECAIT—Bezafibrate Coronary Atherosclerosis Intervention Trial.

FASTING TRIGLYCERIDES AS AN INDEPENDENT RISK FACTOR FOR CAD

	MEN		WOMEN	
	UNIVARIATE	MULTIVARIATE	UNIVARIATE	MULTIVARIATE
Sample size	46,619	22,499	10,864	6345
Relative risk*	1.31	1.15	1.76	1.37

*Indicates relative risk associated with an increase in triglycerides of 1 mmol/L (88.5 mg/dL).

FIGURE 5-44. Fasting triglycerides (TGs) as an independent risk factor for coronary artery disease (CAD). In a recent meta-analysis of 17 studies in male participants with fasting TG levels, Austin [117] reported a 31% increase in relative risk for cardiovascular disease associated with an increase in plasma TG of 1 mmol/L or 88.5 mg/dL. In a smaller number of studies in women, the increase in relative risk was even higher at 76%. This was comparable to the data reported by Criqui *et al.* [118] that indicated a 54% and 88% increase in relative risk for an increase of 100 mg/dL (1.129 mmol/L) in TG. When adjustments were made for other confounding factors, data from the Lipid Research Clinic Follow-up Study failed to demonstrate a statistically significant contribution for TG. With a larger sample size, despite the reduction in relative risk, statistical significance was demonstrated in the meta-analysis suggesting an independent contribution of elevated TG in the risk for CAD.

This relationship should be taken with some caution, however. The reported association between relative risk and increases in TG levels assumes that the relationship between relative risk and TG levels is linear. This has not been demonstrated. Data from the Framingham Heart Study [119] would suggest that this might not be the case. In men, the relative risk appears to plateau around 300 mg/dL and 400 mg/dL for women.

Elevated TG may also be associated with increased risk for cardiovascular disease mortality. Miller [120] presented 18-year follow-up data on 740 patients, including 518 individuals with documented CAD at baseline. In a multiple logistic regression analysis, patients with a fasting baseline TG of greater than 100 mg/dL (1.12 mmol/L) had significantly reduced chance of survival from coronary events (*P*< 0.001). (*Adapted from* Austin [117].)

METABOLISM OF TRIGLYCERIDE-RICH LIPOPROTEINS, IMMUNE RESPONSE, AND ATHEROSCLEROSIS

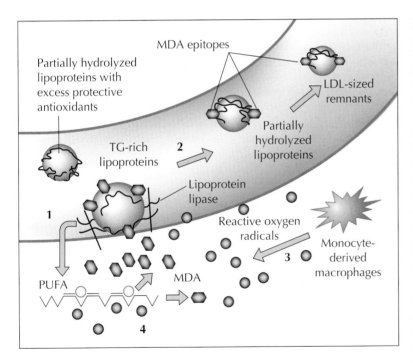

FIGURE 5-45. Transfer of reaction oxygen radicals from diseased endothelium to plasma lipoproteins during triglyceride (TG) hydrolysis. TG-rich lipoproteins interact with lipoprotein lipase (step 1) anchored to along the walls of blood vessels. In the process, they form tight junctions with the endothelium. Fatty acids and monoglycerides are released into the unstirred water layer and pass through the endothelium as an energy supply to the tissues [121]. The TG-rich particles are converted to smaller remnants (step 2) that are released to reenter the circulation [122]. The TG-rich lipoproteins become smaller and more dense as they repeat these interactions, finally becoming low-density lipoprotein (LDL).

In patients with developing atherosclerosis, the subendothelial space is invaded by proliferating monocyte-derived macrophages that are secreting cytokines and reactive oxygen species (ROS) (step 3) [123]. The ROS cleave the double bonds [124] within unsaturated fatty acids (particularly polyunsaturated fatty acids [PUFA]). This generates a series of reactive aldehydes such as malonyl-dialdehyde (MDA) (step 4). MDA forms adducts by reacting with the epsilon amino group of lysine moieties of nearby proteins including the apolipoproteins [125]. Oxidation and modification of the proteins and lipids in the lipoproteins may occur in the plasma space if the release of ROS is sufficient in this location.

These oxidatively damaged lipoproteins should be atherogenic if formed in the intimal space or if released in the circulation. The new epitopes induce antibodies that may provide a protective function through inducing clearance of these damaged lipoproteins into macrophages in spleen, liver, and bone marrow. In the case of the healthy endothelium, there is no excess generation of ROS and the TG-rich lipoproteins would not pick up oxidatively modified epitopes. If there is adequate antioxidant protection in the environment of the particle, the ROS might be quenched, resulting in the formation of a particle with unaltered apolipoproteins and lipids.

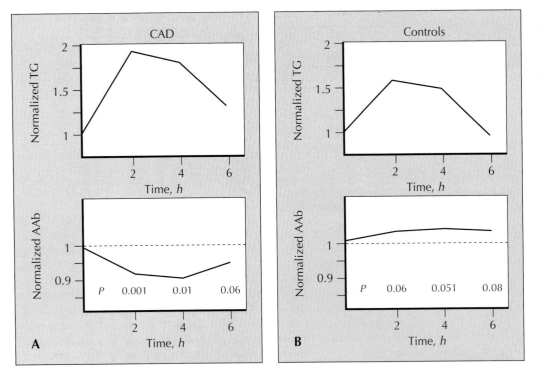

Concomitant with the postprandial rise in plasma triglycerides (TG), individuals with diseased endothelium demonstrated an acute and transient reduction in autoantibody (AAb) levels. A subset of the patients (n=18) who underwent a rigorous 6-month weight reduction program with caloric restriction and supervised aerobic exercise were restudied with the same protocol. Comparable reduction in autoantibody levels were observed after significant reductions in plasma TG and cholesterol. The mean reductions in autoantibody levels were 9% ($P < 0.001$) and 10% ($P < 0.01$) and 6% ($P < 0.06$) at 2, 4, and 6 hours postprandially. Individuals with normal endothelium demonstrated slight increases in autoantibody levels of 4% ($P< 0.051$), 5% (not significant [NS]) and 6% (NS) at 2, 4, and 6 hours postprandially.

It is our hypothesis that the reduction in autoantibody levels observed in the patients with documented coronary artery disease demonstrated the excess generation of oxidatively modified epitopes by the diseased endothelium. The transfer of these epitopes to plasma lipoproteins result in the binding of circulating autoantibodies, thus reducing the level of free autoantibodies detectable by our enzyme-linked assay.

FIGURE 5-46. In vivo generation of oxidatively modified epitopes during postprandial lipemia. We determined circulating levels of autoantibodies against malonly-dialdehyde (MDA)-modified low-density lipoprotein (LDL) following the consumption of a standardized meal containing polyunsaturated fatty acids from soybean. Two groups of subjects were included: 28 men and women with diseased endothelium as demonstrated by history of bypass surgery or angioplasty (**A**) and 17 young individuals with normal endothelium (**B**) [126].

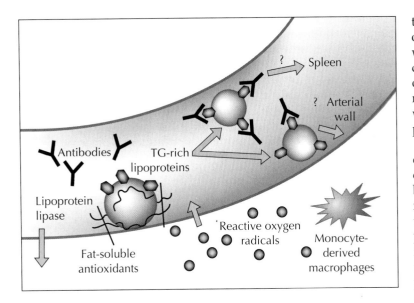

FIGURE 5-47. The role of antibodies to oxidatively modified lipoproteins. In human plasma, antibodies are universally found

that react with various epitopes on proteins that are generated by oxidation. For example, direct reactions of reactive oxygen species with cysteine can lead to formation of cysteic acid. New epitopes can also be produced by indirect reactions, including the initial oxidation of lipids, releasing very reactive compounds such as nonenyl and malonyl dialdehydes. These form covalent bonds with the epsilon amino groups of lysine side chains. Both processes lead to the induction of antibodies to the new adducts.

The role of these antibodies has been the source of significant debate. One school of thought is that these form immune complexes that may accelerate the uptake of damaged lipoproteins by intimal macrophages leading to accelerated foam cell development in the arteriosclerotic lesion. Others have presented evidence that promotion of these antibody concentrations by immunizing young animals with oxidized lipoproteins provides protection from the development of arteriosclerosis. They have suggested that formation of immune complexes in the plasma space could be protective by resulting in the clearance of these altered lipoproteins by macrophages in the spleen, liver, and bone marrow, reducing the chance of uptake by vascular wall. These theories are being investigated in many laboratories.

REFERENCES

1. Lipid Research Clinics Program Epidemiology Committee: Plasma lipid distributions in selected North American populations: the Lipid Research Clinics Program Prevalence Study. *Circulation* 1979, 60:427–438.
2. Castelli W, Garrison RJ, Wilson PWF, *et al.*: Incidence of coronary heart disease and lipoprotein cholesterol levels. The Framingham Study. *JAMA* 1986, 256:2835–2838.
3. The International Committee for the Evaluation of Hypertriglyceridemia as a Vascular Risk Factor (Chairs: Assmann G, Gotto AM Jr, Paoletti R): The hypertriglyceridemias risk and management. *Am J Cardiol* 1991, 68:1A–42A.
4. Bainton D, Miller NE, Bolton CH, *et al.*: Plasma triglyceride and high density lipoprotein cholesterol as predictors of ischemic heart disease in British men. *Br Heart J* 1992, 68:60–66.

5. Assmann G, Schulte H: Role of triglycerides in coronary artery disease: lessons from the Prospective Cardiovascular Munster Study. *Am J Cardiol* 1992, 70:10H–13H.

6. Eisenberg S: Lipoprotein abnormalities in hypertriglyceridemia: significance in atherosclerosis. *Am Heart J* 1987, 113:55–61.

7. Austin MA: Plasma triglyceride and coronary heart disease. *Arterioscler Thromb* 1991, 11:2–14.

8. Davis CE, Gordon D, LaRosa J, *et al.*: Correlations of plasma high-density lipoprotein cholesterol levels with other plasma lipid and lipoprotein concentrations. The Lipid Research Clinics Program Prevalence Study. *Circulation* 1980, 62(suppl IV):IV-24–IV-30.

9. Austin MA, Brunzell JD, Fitch WL, *et al.*: Inheritance of low density lipoprotein subclass patterns in familial combined hyperlipidemia. *Arteriosclerosis* 1990, 10:520–530.

10. Reaven GM: Insulin resistance, hyperinsulinemia, and hyper-triglyceridemia in the etiology and clinical course of hypertension. *Am J Med* 1991, 90:7S–12S.

11. Fontbonne A, Eschwege E: Insulin-resistance, hypertriglyceridemia and cardiovascular risk: the Paris Prospective Study. *Diabetes Metab* 1991, 17:93–95.

12. Kaplan NM: The deadly quartet: upper-body obesity, glucose intolerance, hypertriglyceridemia, and hypertension. *Arch Intern Med* 1989, 149:1514–1520.

13. Austin MA: Triglycerides, small dense LDL and coronary disease. *Atherosclerosis* 1994, 109:259.

14. NIH Consensus Development Panel on Triglyceride, High-Density Lipoprotein, and Coronary Heart Disease: Triglyceride, high-density lipoprotein, and coronary heart disease. *JAMA* 1993, 269:505–510.

15. Ameis D, Kobayashi J, Davis RC, *et al.*: Familial chylomicronemia (type I hyperlipoproteinemia) due to a single missense mutation in the lipoprotein lipase gene. *J Clin Invest* 1991, 87:1165–1170.

16. Ma Y, Henderson HE, Murthy VA, *et al.*: A mutation in the human lipoprotein lipase gene as the most common cause of familial chylomicronemia in French Canadians. *N Engl J Med* 1991, 324:1761–1766.

17. Brewer HB Jr, Rader DJ, Hoeg JM, *et al.*: Recent advances in lipoprotein metabolism and the genetic dyslipoproteinemias. *Adv Exp Med Biol* 1991, 285:237–244.

18. Sniderman A, Brown BG, Stewart BF, *et al.*: From familial combined hyperlipidemia to hyperapoB: unravelling the overproduction of hepatic apolipoprotein B. *Curr Opin Lipid* 1992, 3:137–142.

19. Mahley RW, Weisgraber KH, Innerarity TL, *et al.*: Genetic defects in lipoprotein metabolism: elevation of atherogenic lipoproteins caused by impaired catabolism. *JAMA* 1991, 265:78–83.

20. Durrington PN: Secondary hyperlipidemia. *Br Med Bull* 1990, 46:1005–1024.

21. Fujioka S, Matsuzawa Y, Tokunaga K, *et al.*: Contribution of intra-abdominal fat accumulation to the impairment of glucose and lipid metabolism in human obesity. *Metabolism* 1987, 36:54–59.

22. Brown WV: Lipoprotein disorders in diabetes mellitus. *Med Clin North Am* 1994, 78:143–161.

23. Appel G: Lipid abnormalities in renal disease [clinical conference]. *Kidney Int* 1991, 39:169–183.

24. Palella TD, Fox IH: Hyperuricemia and gout. In *The Metabolic Basis of Inherited Disorders*, edn 6. Edited by Scriver CR, Beaudet AL, Sly WS, *et al.* New York: McGraw Hill Inc; 1989:965–1006.

25. Hers HG, van Hoof F, de Barsy T: Glycogen storage diseases. In *Metabolic Basis of Inherited Disorders*, edn 6. Edited by Scriver CR, Beaudet AL, Sly WS, *et al.* New York: McGraw Hill; 1989:425–452.

26. Pathogenesis of alcohol-induced hypertriglyceridemia. *Nutr Rev* 1987, 45:215–216.

27. Glueck CJ, Scheel D, Fishback J, *et al.*: Estrogen-induced pancreatitis in patients with previously covert familial type V hyper-lipoproteinemia. *Metabolism* 1972, 21:657–666.

28. Davidoff F, Tishler S, Rosoff C: Marked hyperlipidemia and pancreatitis associated with oral contraceptive therapy. *N Engl J Med* 1973, 289:552–555.

29. Marsden J: Hyperlipidemia due to isotretinoin and etretinate: possible mechanisms and consequences. *Br J Dermatol* 1986, 114:401–407.

30. Ames RP: The effects of antihypertensive drugs on serum lipids and lipoproteins. I. Diuretics. *Drugs* 1986, 32:260–278.

31. Hunninghake DB: The effects of cardioselective vasodilating β-blockers on lipids. *Am Heart J* 1991, 121:1029–1032.

32. Ginsberg HN: Lipoprotein physiology and its relationship to atherogenesis. *Endocrinol Metab Clin North Am* 1990, 19:211–228.

33. Havel RJ: Role of triglyceride-rich lipoproteins in progression of atherosclerosis [comment]. *Circulation* 1990, 81:694–696.

34. Austin MA, Breslow JL, Hennekens CH, *et al.*: Low-density lipoprotein subclass patterns and risk of myocardial infarction. *JAMA* 1988, 260:1917–1921.

35. Sniderman A, Shapiro S, Marpole D, *et al.*: Association of coronary atherosclerosis with hyperapobetalipoproteinemia: increased protein but normal cholesterol levels in human plasma low density (β lipoprotein). *Proc Natl Acad Sci U S A* 1980, 77:605–608.

36. Hamsten A: Hypertriglyceridemia, triglyceride-rich lipoproteins and coronary heart disease. *Clin Endocrinol Metab* 1990, 4:895–922.

37. Brewer HB Jr, Gregg RE, Hoeg JM, *et al.*: Apolipoproteins and lipoproteins in human plasma: an overview. *Clin Chem* 1988, 34:B4–B8.

38. Beisiegel U, Weber W, Ihrke G, *et al.*: The LDL receptor related protein, LRP, is an apolipoprotein E binding protein. *Nature* 1989, 341:162–164.

39. Rubinstein A, Gibson JC, Paterniti JR: The effect of heparin induced lipolysis on the distribution of apolipoprotein E among lipoprotein subclasses. *J Clin Invest* 1985, 75:710–721.

40. Goldberg IJ, Le N-A, Paterniti JR, *et al.*: Effect of acute inhibition of hepatic triglyceride lipase on very low density lipoprotein metabolism in the cynomolgus monkey. *J Clin Invest* 1982, 70:1184–1192.

41. Cortner JA, Le N-A, Coates PM, *et al.*: Determinants of fasting plasma triglyceride levels: metabolism of hepatic and intestinal lipoproteins. *Eur J Clin Invest* 1991, 22:158–165.

42. Le N-A, Innis W, Umeakunne K, *et al.*: Accelerated clearance of postprandial lipoproteins with HMG CoA reductase inhibitor. AFCR National Meeting May 5-8, 1995. *J Invest Med* 1995, 43:301A.

43. de Silva H, Lauer SJ, Wang J, *et al.*: Overexpression of human apolipoprotein C-III in transgenic mice results in an accumulation of apolipoprotein B48 remnants that is corrected by excess apolipoprotein E. *J Biol Chem* 1994, 269:2324–2335.

44. Lagrost L, Gandjini H, Athias A, *et al.*: Influence of plasma cholesteryl ester transfer activity on the LDL and HDL distribution profiles in normolipidemic subjects. *Arterioscler Thromb* 1992, 13:815–825.

45. Kuusi T, Saarinen P, Nikkila EA: Evidence for the role of hepatic lipase in the metabolism of plasma HDL$_2$ in man. *Atherosclerosis* 1980, 36:589–593.

46. Hongmei L, Myron I, Cybulsky MA, *et al.*: An atherogenic diet rapidly induces VCAM-1, a cytokine-regulatable mononuclear leukocyte adhesion molecule, in rabbit aortic endothelium. *Arterioscler Thromb* 1993, 13:197–204.

47. de Gruijter M, Hoogerbrugge N, van Rijn MA, *et al.*: Patients with combined hypercholesterolemia-hypertriglyceridemia shown an increased monocyte-endothelial cell adhesion in vitro: triglyceride level as a major determinant. *Metabolism* 1991, 40:1119–1121.

48. Chung BH, Segrest JP: Cytotoxicity of remnants of triglyceride-rich lipoproteins: an atherogenic insult? *Adv Exp Med Biol* 1991, 285:341–351.

49. Wang-Iverson P, Gibson JC, Brown WV: Plasma apolipoprotein E secretion by human monocyte-derived macrophages. *Biochim Biophys Acta* 1985, 834:256–262.

50. Rosenfeld ME, Khoo JC, Miller E, *et al.*: Macrophage-derived foam cells freshly isolated from rabbit atherosclerotic lesions degrade modified lipoproteins, promote oxidation of low-density lipoproteins, and contain oxidation-specific lipid-protein adducts. *J Clin Invest* 1991, 87:90–99.

51. David JB, Bowyer DE: Macrophages modify β-VLDL by proteolysis and enhance subsequent lipid accumulation in arterial smooth muscle cells. *Atherosclerosis* 1989, 77:203–208.

52. Mitropoulos KA, Miller GJ, Reeves BE, *et al.*: Factor VII coagulant activity is strongly associated with the plasma concentration of large lipoprotein particles in middle-aged men. *Atherosclerosis* 1989, 76:203–208.

53. Miller GJ, Martin JC, Mitropoulos KA, *et al.*: Factor VII and dietary fat intake. *Adv Exp Med Biol* 1990, 281:145–149.

54. Hosoai H, Nakamura H: Triglyceride as a risk factor for athero-thrombotic disease through increased plasminogen activator inhibitor. In *Current Advances in Triglycerides and Atherosclerosis.* Edited by Yamamoto A, Nakamura H, Tsuguhiko N. Osaka: Churchill Livingstone; 1994:115–118.

55. Mehta J, Mehta P, Lawson D, *et al.*: Plasma tissue activator inhibitor levels in coronary artery disease: correlation with age and serum triglyceride concentrations. *J Am Coll Cardiol* 1987, 9:263–267.

56. Mussoni L, Mannucci L, Sirtori M, *et al.*: Hypertriglyceridemia and regulation of fibrinolytic activity. *Arterioscler Thromb* 1992, 12:19–25.

57. Hiraga T, Murase T, Tsukada T: Blood coagulation and fibrinolysis in patients with hypertriglyceridemia. In *Current Advances in Triglycerides and Atherosclerosis.* Edited by Yamamoto A, Nakamura H, Tsuguhiko N. Osaka: Churchill Livingstone; 1994:109–114.

58. Zannis VI, Breslow JL: Characterization of a unique human apolipoprotein E variant associated with type III hyperlipopro-teinemia. *J Biol Chem* 1980, 255:1759.

59. Rall SC Jr, Weisgraber KH, Innerarity TL, *et al.*: Structural basis for receptor binding heterogeneity of apolipoprotein E from type III hyperlipoproteinemic subjects. *Proc Natl Acad Sci U S A* 1982, 79:4696.

60. Fredrickson DS, Morganroth J, Levy RI: Type III hyperlipopro-teinemia: an analysis of two contemporary definitions. *Ann Intern Med* 1975, 82:150.

61. Goldstein JL, Schrott HG, Hazzard WR, *et al.*: Hyperlipidemia in coronary artery disease. II. Genetic analysis of lipid levels in 176 families and delineation of a new inherited disorder, combined hyperlipidemia. *J Clin Invest* 1973, 2:1544–1568.

62. Cortner JA, Coates PM, Bennett MJ, *et al.*: Familial combined hyperlipidaemia: use of stable isotopes to demonstrate overpro-duction of very low-density lipoprotein apolipoprotein B by the liver. *J Inherit Metab Dis* 1991, 14:915–922.

63. Janus CK, Nicoll AM, Turner PR, *et al.*: Kinetic basis of the primary hyperlipidemias: studies of apolipoprotein B turnover in geneti-cally defined subjects. *Eur J Clin Invest* 1980, 10:161–172.

64. Kissebah AH, Alfarsi S, Evans DJ: Low density lipoprotein metabo-lism in familial combined hyperlipidemia: mechanisms of the multiple lipoprotein phenotypic expression. *Arteriosclerosis* 1984, 4:614–624.

65. Kesaniemi YA, Vega GL, Grundy SM: Kinetics of apolipoprotein B in normal and hyperlipidemic man: review of current data. In *Lipoprotein Kinetics and Modeling.* Edited by Berman M, Grundy SM, Howard BV. New York: Academic Press; 1982:181–205.

66. Chait A, Robertson HT, Brunzell JD: Chylomicronemia syndrome in diabetes mellitus. *Diabetes Care* 1981, 4:343–348.

67. DeFronzo RA, Ferrannini E: Insulin resistance: a multifaceted syndrome responsible for NIDDM, obesity, hypertension, dyslipi-demia, and atherosclerotic cardiovascular disease. *Diabetes Care* 1991, 14:173–194.

68. Goldschmid MG, Barrett-Connor E, Edelstein SL, *et al.*: Dyslipidemia and ischemic heart disease mortality among men and women with diabetes. *Circulation* 1994, 89:991–997.

69. Bonora E, Zenere M, Branzi P, *et al.*: Influences of body fat and its regional localization on risk factors for atherosclerosis in young men. *Am J Epidemiol* 1992, 135:1272–1278.

70. Leenan R, van der Kooy K, Seidell JC, *et al.*: Visceral fat accumula-tion measured by magnetic resonance imaging in relation to serum lipids in obese men and women. *Atherosclerosis* 1992, 94:171–181.

71. Carlson LA, Rosenhamer G: Reduction of mortality in the Stockholm Ischaemic Heart Disease Secondary Prevention Study by combined treatment with clofibrate and nicotinic acid. *Acta Med Scand* 1988, 223:405–418.

72. Frick MH, Elo H, Haapa K, *et al.*: Helsinki Heart Study: primary prevention trial with gemfibrozil in middle-aged men with dyslipi-demia. *N Engl J Med* 1987, 317:1237–1245.

73. Manninen V, Elo O, Frick MH, *et al.*: Lipid alterations and decline in the incidence of coronary heart disease in the Helsinki Heart Study. *JAMA* 1988, 260:641–651.

74. Manninen V, Huttunen JK, Heinonen OP, *et al.*: Relation between baseline lipid and lipoprotein values and the incidence of coronary heart disease in the Helsinki Heart Study. *Am J Cardiol* 1989, 63:42H–47H.

75. Rubins HB, Robins SJ, Collins D, *et al.* for the VA-HIT Study Group: *N Engl J Med* 1999, 341:410–418.

76. Karathanasis SK, Norum RA, Zannis VI, JL Breslow VI: Linkage of human apolipoproteins A-I and C-III genes. *Nature* 1983, 304:371–373.

77. Dallinga-Thie GM, Bu X-D, van Linde-Sibenius Trip M, *et al.*: Apolipoprotein A-I/C-III/A-IV gene cluster in familial combined hyperlipidemia: effects on LDL-c and apoB and C-III. *J Lipid Res* 1996, 37:136–147.

78. Dallinga-Thie GM, van Linde-Sibenius Trip M, Rotter JI, *et al.*: Complex genetic contribution of the apoAI-CIII-AIV gene cluster to familial combined hyperlipidemia: identification of different susceptibility haplotypes. *J Clin Invest* 1997, 99:953–961.

79. Xu C-F, Talmud P, Schuster H, *et al.*: Association between genetic variation at the apo AI-CIII-AIV gene cluster and familial combined hyperlipidemia. *Clin Genet* 1994, 46:385–397.

80. Chen M, Breslow JL, Li W, Leff T: Transcriptional regulation of the apoC-III gene by insulin in diabetic mice: correlation with changes in plasma triglyceride levels. *J Lipid Res* 1994, 35:1918–1924.

81. Gruber PJ, Torres-Rosado A, Wolak ML, Leff T: ApoC-III gene tran-scription is regulated by a cytokine-inducible NFκB element. *Nucleic Acid Res* 1994, 22: 2417–2422.

82. Reue K, Leff T, Breslow JL: Human apoC-III gene expression is regulated by positive and negative cis-acting elements and tissue-specific protein factors. *J Biol Chem* 1988, 263:6857–6864.

83. Ladias JAA, Hadzopoulou-Cladaras M, Kardassis D, *et al.*: Transcriptional regulation of human apolipoprotein genes apoB, apoC-III and apoA-II by members of the steroid hormone receptor superfamily HNF-4, ARP-1, EAR-2 and EAR-3. *J Biol Chem* 1992, 267:15849–15860.

84. Hertz R, Bishara-Shieban J, Bar-Tana J: Mode of action of peroxi-some proliferators as hypolipidemic drugs: suppression of apoC-III. *J Biol Chem* 1995, 270: 13470–13475.

85. Schonfeld G, George PK, Miller J, *et al.*: Apolipoprotein C-II and C-III levels in hyperlipoproteinemia. *Metabolism* 1979, 28:1001–1010.

86. Bukberg P, Le N-A, Gibson JC, *et al.*: Direct measurement of apoC-III specific activity in 125I-labeled VLDL by immunoaffinity chro-matography. *J Lipid Res* 1983, 24:1251–1260.

87. Le N-A, Gibson JC, Ginsberg HN: Independent regulation of plasma apo C-II and C-III concentrations in very low density and high density lipoproteins: implications for the regulation of the catabolism of these lipoproteins. *J Lipid Res* 1988, 29:669–677.

88. Havel RJ, Shore VG, Shore B, Bier DM: Role of specific glycopep-tides of human serum lipoproteins in the activation of LPL. *Circ Res* 1970, 27: 375–381.

89. Brown WV, Baginsky ML: Inhibition of lipoprotein lipase by an apoprotein of human VLDL. *Biochem Biophys Res Commun* 1972, 46:375–381.

90. Ginsberg HN, Le N-A, Goldberg IJ, *et al.*: Apolipoprotein B metabolism in subjects with deficiency of apoC-III and A-I: evidence that apoC-III inhibits catabolism of TG-rich lipoproteins by LPL in vivo. *J Clin Invest* 1986, 78:1287–1295.

91. Ito Y, Azrolan N, O'Connell A, *et al.*: Hypertriglyceridemia as a result of human apoC-III expression in transgenic mouse. *Science* 1990, 249:790–793.

92. Ebara T, Ramakrishnan R, Steiner G, Shachter NS: Chylomicronemia due to apoC-III overexpression in apoE-null mice: ApoC-III induced hypertriglyceridemia is not mediated by effects on apoE. *J Clin Invest* 1997, 99:2672–2681.

93. Maeda N, Li H, Lee D, *et al.*: Targeted disruption of the apoC-II gene in mice results in hypotriglyceridemia and protection from postprandial hypertriglyceridemia. *J Biol Chem* 1994, 269:23610–23616.

94. Staels B, Vu-Dac N, Kosykh VA, *et al.*: Fibrates downregulate apoC-III expression independent of induction of peroxisomal acyl CoA oxidase: a potential mechanism for the hypolipidemic action of fibrates. *J Clin Invest* 1995, 95:705–712.

95. Shelburne F, Hanks J, Myers W, Quarfordt S: Effect of apoproteins on hepatic uptake of triglyceride emulsions in the rat. *J Clin Invest* 1980, 65:652–658.

96. Windler E, Havel RJ: Inhibitory effect of C apolipoproteins from rats and humans on the uptake of TG-rich lipoproteins and their remnants by the perfused rat liver. *J Lipid Res* 1985, 26:556–565.

97. Kowal RC, Herz J, Weisgraber KH, *et al.*: Opposing effect of apoE and C on lipoprotein binding to low density lipoprotein receptor-related protein. *J Biol Chem* 1990, 265:10771–10779.

98. Rensen PCN, Herijgers N, Netscher MH, *et al.*: Particle size determines the specificity of apoE-containing TG-rich emulsions for the LDL receptor versus hepatic remnant receptor in vivo. *J Lipid Res* 1997, 38:1070–1084.

99. Breyer ED, Le N-A, Li X, *et al.*: ApoC-III displacement of apoE from VLDL: effect of particle size. *J Lipid Res* 1999, 40:1875–1882.

100. Hazzard WR, Bierman EL: Delayed clearance of chylomicron remnants following vitamin A-containing oral fat loads in borad-b-disease (type III hyperlipoproteinemia). *Metabolism* 1976, 25:777–801.

101. Bergeron N, Havel RJ: Prolonged postprandial responses of lipids and apolipoproteins in TG-rich lipoproteins in individuals expressing an ε4 allele. *J Clin Invest* 1996, 7:65–72.

102. Dallongeville J, Lussier-Cacan S, Davignon J: Modulation of plasma TG levels by apoE phenotype: a meta-analysis. *J Lipid Res* 1992, 33: 447–454.

103. Lenzen HJ, Assman G, Buchwalsky R, Schulte H: Association of apoE polymorphism, LDL, and CAD. *Clin Chem* 1986, 32:778–781.

104. Kuusi T, Nieminen MS, Ehnholm C, *et al.*: ApoE polymorphism and coronary artery disease: increased prevalence of E4 in angiographically verified coronary patients. *Arteriosclerosis* 1989, 9: 237–241.

105. Hixson JE for the PDAY Research Group: ApoE polymorphism affect atherosclerosis in young males. *Arterioscl Thromb* 1991, 11:1237–1244.

106. Van Bockxmeer FM, Mamotte CD: Apolipoprotein e4 homozygosity in young men with coronary artery disease. *Lancet* 1992, 340: 879–880.

107. Wilson PWF, Myers RH, Larson MG, *et al.*: ApoE alleles, dyslipidemia, and coronary heart disease: the Framingham Offspring Study. *JAMA* 1994, 272:1666–1671.

108. Levy RI, Brensike JF, Epstein SE, *et al.*: The influence of changes in lipid values induced by cholestyramine and diet on progression of coronary artery disease: results of the NHLBI Type II Coronary Intervention Study. *Circulation* 1984, 69:325–337.

109. Phillips NR, Waters D Havel RJ: Plasma lipoproteins and progression of coronary artery disease of coronary artery disease evaluated by angiography and clinical events. *Circulation* 1993, 88: 2762–2770.

110. Groot PHE, van Stiphout WAHJ, Krauss XH, *et al.*: Postprandial lipoprotein metabolism in normolipidemic man with and without coronary artery disease. *Arterioscler Thromb* 1991, 11:653–662.

111. Sharrett AR, Chambless LE, Heiss G, *et al.*: Association of postprandial triglyceride and retinyl palmitate responses with asymptomatic carotid atherosclerosis in middle-aged men and women: the ARIC Study. *Arterioscler Thromb Vasc Biol* 1995, 15: 2122–2129.

112. Watts GF, Lewis B, Brunt JNH, *et al.*: Effects on coronary artery disease of lipid-lowering diet, or diet plus cholestyramine in the St. Thomas Atherosclerosis Regression Study (STARS). *Lancet* 1992, 339:563–569.

113. Blankenhorn DH, Alaupovic P, Wickham E, *et al.*: Prediction of angiographic change in native human coronary arteries and aorto-coronary bypass grafts: lipids and nonlipid factors. *Circulation* 1990, 81:470–476.

114. Hodis HN, Mack WJ, Azen SP, *et al.*: Triglyceride- and cholesterol-rich lipoproteins have a differential effect on mild-, moderate, and severe lesion progression as assessed by quantitative coronary angiography in a controlled trial of lovastatin. *Circulation* 1994, 90:42–49.

115. Manninen V, Elo MO, Frick MH, *et al.*: Lipid alterations and decline in the incidence of coronary heart disease in the Helsinki Heart Study. *JAMA* 1988, 260: 641–651.

116. Ericsson C-G : Results of the Bezafibrate Coronary Atherosclerosis Intervention Trial (BECAIT) and an update on trials now in progress. *Eur Heart J* 1998, 19(Suppl H): H37–H41.

117. Austin MA: Epidemiology of hypertriglyceridemia and cardiovascular disease. *Am J Cardiol* 1999, 83:13F–16F.

118. Criqui MH, Heiss G, Cohn R, *et al.*: Plasma triglyceride level and mortality from coronary heart disease. *N Engl J Med* 1993, 328:1220–1225.

119. Castelli WP: The triglyceride issue: a view from Framingham. *Am Heart J* 1986, 112: 432–437.

120. Miller M: Is hypertriglyceridemia an independent risk factor for coronary heart disease? The epidemiological evidence. *Eur Heart J* 1998, 19: H18–H22.

121. Dominiczak MH: Glucose homeostasis and fuel metabolism. In *Medical Biochemistry*. Edited by Baynes J, Dominiczak MH. Mosby: London; 1999; 243–266.

122. Eisenberg S, Sehayak E: Remnant lipoproteins and their metabolism. *Baillieres Endocrinol Metab* 1995, 9:739–753.

123. Fantone JC, Ward PA: Role of oxygen-derived free radicals and metabolites in leukocyte-dependent inflammatory reactions. *Am J Pathol* 1982, 107:397–418.

124. Esterbauer H, Jurgens G, Quehenberger O, Koller E: Autooxidation of human low density lipoprotein: loss of polyunsaturated fatty acids and vitamin E and generation of aldehydes. *J Lipid Res* 1987, 28:495–509.

125. Steinbrecher UP: Oxidation of human low-density lipoprotein results in derivatization of lysine residues of apolipoprotein B by lipid peroxide decomposition products. *J Biol Chem* 1987, 262:3603–3608.

126. Le N-A, Li X, Sung K, Brown WV: Evidence for the in vivo generation of oxidatively modified epitopes in patients with documented CAD. *Metabolism* 2000, 49:1271–1277.

LOW-DENSITY LIPOPROTEINS IN ATHEROGENESIS

Sampath Parthasarathy

It is well established that high levels of plasma cholesterol, particularly those associated with low-density lipoprotein (LDL), increase the risk of developing atherosclerosis. It is also clear that lowering plasma cholesterol levels can arrest or even reverse the progression of the disease [1,2].

Very low-density lipoprotein (VLDL), synthesized and secreted by the liver, is the precursor of plasma LDL. Lipolysis of VLDL by lipoprotein lipase, accompanied by the removal of various apoproteins and lipid classes that include free fatty acids, ultimately generates LDL [3]. The net result is a smaller lipoprotein that retains apolipoprotein (apo) B-100 and most of its cholesterol esters. However, LDL is comprises a variety of discrete subclasses of different densities and sizes in the plasma [4]. These subfractions differ in their size, lipid composition, and buoyant densities. Currently, a small, dense subfraction of LDL has been suggested to be more atherogenic than large subfractions [5]. However, there is only one apoprotein per particle regardless of the subfraction. The conversion of VLDL to LDL occurs exclusively in the plasma compartment. The factors that determine the formation or interconversions of subfractions are not known. Recently, the human apo B-100 gene has been expressed in mice that develop atherosclerosis when consuming a cholesterol-enriched diet [6].

The liver plays a major role in the removal of LDL from the plasma. There are receptor-dependent and receptor-independent pathways for the LDL clearance [7]. The receptor-independent pathway is currently poorly understood. The LDL-receptor–dependent pathway has been studied extensively, and elaborate regulatory pathways have been described [8–10]. Recently, a mouse model lacking in the LDL receptor gene has been created; this animal develops severe atherosclerosis when consuming a diet rich in fat [11].

Mutations in the receptor generally adversely affect the uptake and removal of plasma LDL [8]. Consequently, LDL accumulates in the plasma, accounting for the increase in plasma cholesterol. Liver transplantation and gene delivery through viral transfections are experimental approaches to introduce normal copies of the receptor gene and, thus, to decrease plasma LDL levels.

Altered synthesis and production of VLDL and mutations in the apo B-100 gene also affect plasma LDL levels. Mutations in the apo B-100 gene result in hypo- and hyperbetalipoproteinemia with lower or higher plasma LDL and cholesterol levels.

Low-density lipoprotein particles in the plasma can undergo several alterations. The apo B-100 gene can bind covalently via disulfide linkage to apo(a), generating the Lp(a) particle [12,13]. The apo(a) protein is a glycoprotein that adds considerably to the molecular weight of the apo B-100–apo(a) complex. Elevated plasma Lp(a) levels are found in over 15% of the populations, and such elevations are regarded as a contributing factor to the development of atherogenic and thrombogenic disorders. Apo(a) is structurally similar to plasminogen and as a result may interfere with thrombolytic mechanism(s).

The LDL molecule also can undergo other types of modifications, such as glycation and oxidation [14–16]. Glycation can directly affect the apoprotein by modification of critical lysine residues; oxidation of the lipids of LDL generates lipid peroxides; these or the products derived from their degradation can covalently modify the lysine residues of the apoprotein [17]. Although the presence of lipid peroxides in plasma lipoproteins is known, their site of origination is still speculative.

The fatty streak or the early atherosclerotic lesion is well characterized by cells derived from circulating monocytes [18]. These cells differentiate into tissue macrophages, take up cholesterol from LDL, and convert them to cholesterol esters to give the phenotypic expression of "foam cells." It is believed that specific chemotactic factors are involved in the recruitment of monocytes into the artery wall, and hypercholesterolemia somehow contributes to the presence of such factors. However, neither the factors that determine the specific location of the hypercholesterolemic response nor those that initiate monocytes to differentiate into macrophages in the artery wall are well characterized [15].

The uptake of LDL by macrophages is too slow, at least in vitro, to generate foam cells [19]. Macrophages possess too few LDL receptors, and these are downregulated by the cholesterol internalized with LDL when excess LDL particles are presented. When the positive charge on the lysine residues of the apoprotein of the LDL particle is converted to a negative charge (eg, acetylation or by the addition of aldehydes derived from lipid peroxidation, such as malondialdehyde), the lipoprotein is taken up rapidly by macrophages, resulting in increased lipid accumulation in the cells [20]. This is due to the expression of a new class of receptors, termed *scavenger receptors*, that appear as monocytes differentiate into macrophages [21]. Currently, two types of scavenger receptors, class A and class B, have been identified to interact with various forms of oxidized LDL. The receptor proteins include the classic acetyl LDL receptor, CD36, macrosialin, FCRII-B$_2$, LOX-1, and SR-B1. Many of these have been purified,

sequenced, and cloned. Their presence in the macrophage-rich arterial lesion has also been demonstrated. Recently, mice overexpressing the scavenger receptor proteins and the knockout mice completely lacking them have been generated [22–25]. However, it appears that any one specific scavenger receptor may not be solely involved in the uptake of modified lipoproteins.

The oxidative modification of LDL represents one of the in vivo modifications of LDL that renders the lipoprotein capable of uptake by the macrophage scavenger receptors. When the lipids of LDL are oxidized, several products are generated that are capable of modifying the apoprotein to yield a negatively charged particle [16,26]. In addition, the lipid peroxidation products themselves have a variety of potent proatherogenic properties, including the ability to induce the expression of monocyte chemotactic factors, growth factors, and cytokines [27,28]. Thus, an LDL molecule that has undergone a minimum degree of oxidation so that it still is capable of interaction with the LDL receptor (minimally oxidized LDL or minimally modified LDL) exhibits a number of atherogenic properties, which are attributable to its lipid components.

The presence of oxidized LDL has been demonstrated in vivo, and mechanistic studies have shown that prevention of LDL oxidation can reduce the uptake of LDL in vivo [29]. The extent and/or the precise mechanism(s) by which oxidation of LDL occurs in vivo is currently under intense investigation. It is believed that high plasma LDL may lead to high intimal LDL concentrations, where it may interact with the extracellular matrix components, thus prolonging the residence time and increasing its chances of undergoing oxidative modification.

Several recent studies have shown that antioxidants such as vitamin E can ameliorate the progression of experimental atherosclerosis in animals [29–32]. Epidemiologic and prospective studies also indicate that these antioxidants can decrease the risk of coronary heart disease [33,34]. Antioxidant clinical trials in humans have not been encouraging, and a direct demonstration of a palliative effect of antioxidants in humans is still lacking. However, these trials were not directly conducted to address the role of oxidative stress in the initiation of atherosclerosis; thus they are subject to numerous criticisms [35,36].

Based on the evidence that liver clears oxidized LDL very rapidly, it was suggested that the oxidation might predominantly occur at the subendothelial space [15,16]. However, an intriguing possibility that oxidative clearance of LDL in the plasma compartment might occur in exercisers and in younger women who have high plasma estradiol levels has recently been suggested [36,37]. Such oxidations may raise the level of antioxidant enzymes in the artery wall and might generate antibodies against oxidized LDL, both of which might protect against atherosclerosis [38,39].

STRUCTURE OF LOW-DENSITY LIPOPROTEIN

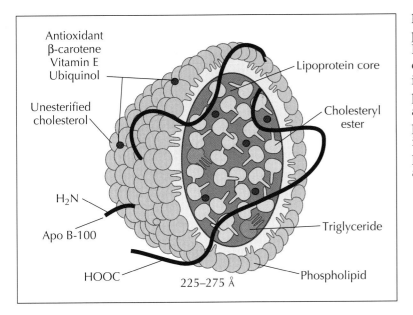

FIGURE 6-1. The structure of a low-density lipoprotein (LDL) particle. LDL is the major cholesterol-carrying plasma lipoprotein. Each particle with a mass exceeding 3,000,000 D has 1500 molecules of cholesteryl esters in its core. There is very little triglyceride in the core of normal LDL particles. Considerable amounts of plasma tocopherols, carotenoids, and other lipophilic antioxidants are also present. Other lipophilic molecules, including drugs and proteins, may also be associated with the lipoprotein. Its surface is composed of free cholesterol and phospholipids (predominantly phosphatidylcholine and sphingomyelin) and a single protein, apolipoprotein (apo) B-100.

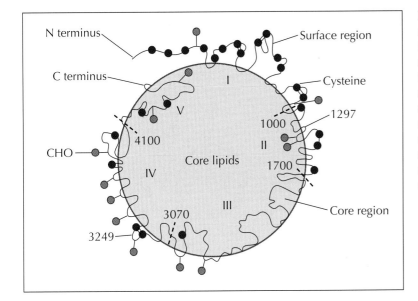

FIGURE 6-2. Representation of apolipoprotein (apo) B-100 on low-density lipoprotein (LDL). Apo B-100 consists of 4536 amino acids (molecular weight, approximately 540,000 D) and weaves in and out of the LDL surface. Apo B is susceptible to proteolysis (especially by thrombin and kallikrein) during isolation. The thrombin cleavage sites are represented in the figure at amino acid 1297 and 3249. The amphipathic nature of apo B makes some regions buried in the core and some exposed to the outside. Isolated apo B is very insoluble in aqueous solutions. There are at least 20 potential *N*-glycosylation sites and several heparin binding sites. The receptor-binding domain of apo B appears to be located near amino acid 3300. Apo B does not exchange among lipoproteins. (*Adapted from* Yang *et al.* [40].)

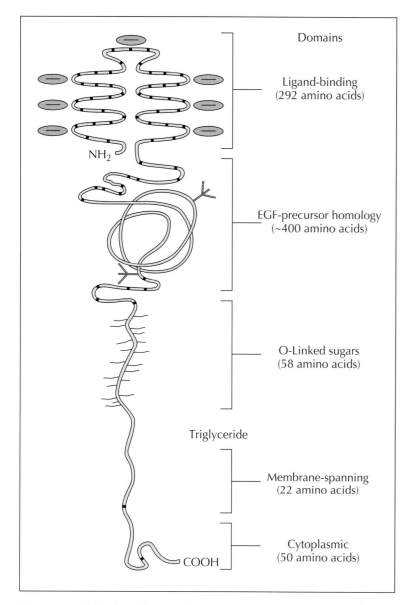

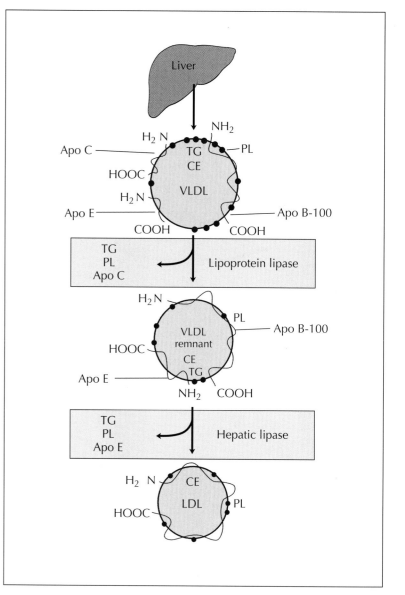

FIGURE 6-3. The low-density lipoprotein (LDL) receptor (apolipoprotein [apo] B/E receptor). The LDL receptor is a single protein with five functional domains. The carboxyl terminal of 50 amino acids provides a cytoplasmic domain that is believed to play an important role in the internalization of the lipoprotein. The membrane-spanning domain has 22 amino acids. The third domain of 58 amino acids is rich in serine and threonine residues (18 residues) and has several O-linked sugars. The largest domain has over 400 amino acids and is 35% homologous to the precursor of epidermal growth factor (EGF). The cysteine-rich N-terminal domain consists of 292 amino acids that include several negatively charged amino acids that generate regions for binding to either a single apo E molecule or an apo B-100 molecule. The requirements for apo B-100 binding are more stringent than for apo E binding. (*Adapted from* Brown and Goldstein [8].)

FIGURE 6-4. Formation of low-density lipoprotein (LDL) in the plasma. Very low-density lipoprotein (VLDL), secreted by the liver, is subject to hydrolysis by lipoprotein lipase so that triglycerides (TGs) are depleted but cholesteryl esters (CEs) are retained in the particle. Apolopoprotein (apo) C and phospholipids (PLs) are also markedly reduced during lipase action. The resulting remnant particle is internalized by the liver via the apo E–mediated uptake and by the LDL receptor and by the separate "remnant receptors." In humans, the remnants may undergo further hydrolysis by hepatic lipase, with further depletion of apo E, phospholipids, and triglycerides. Consequently, there is considerable size reduction, leaving an LDL particle predominantly enriched in cholesterol esters with a single apoprotein, apo B-100.

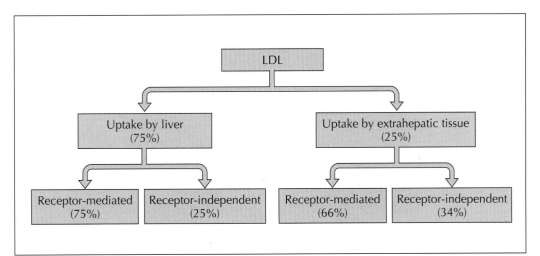

FIGURE 6-5. Removal of low-density lipoprotein (LDL) from the plasma. Circulating LDL is cleared from the plasma by the liver (25%) and by extrahepatic tissues (25%). The clearance is mediated by both receptor-dependent (>70%) and receptor-independent pathways. The pathways that contribute to the clearance of LDL by LDL receptor–independent mechanisms are poorly understood. Modifications that occur in the plasma (glycation or oxidation) may account for LDL receptor–independent clearance mechanisms. Deficiency in the LDL receptors always results in hypercholesterolemia. About 35% to 50% of plasma LDL is cleared daily in normal persons.

FACTORS THAT INFLUENCE THE LEVEL OF HEPATIC LDL RECEPTOR ACTIVITY

ACTIVATORS	SUPPRESSORS
Thyroxine	Mutations in LDL receptor gene
Cholesterol deprivation	Cholesterol feeding
Starvation (dogs and rats)	Starvation (rabbits)
17-α-Ethinyloestradiol	Nonfat diet of casein and wheat starch
Bile acid sequestrants	Saturated fat
Inhibitors of (hepatic) HMG-CoA reductase	
Unsaturated fat	

FIGURE 6-6. Factors that influence the level of hepatic low-density lipoprotein (LDL) receptor activity. HMG-CoA—hydroxymethyl glutaryl-coenzyme A.

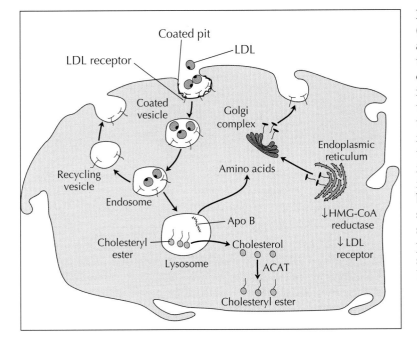

FIGURE 6-7. Receptor-mediated clearance of low-density lipoprotein (LDL). The LDL receptor is synthesized in the endoplasmic reticulum and processed in the Golgi complex. It is exported to the surface in the mature form to the plasma membrane, where it collects in the coated pits. LDL binds to its receptor in the coated pits and is internalized in the coated vesicles. After acidification and uncoating, the resulting endosomes are delivered to the lysosomes for degradation of the lipid and protein components. The receptor dissociates from the LDL and is recycled to the surface. Apo B is hydrolyzed to constituent amino acids and cholesterol esters are degraded to free cholesterol and transported to endoplasmic reticulum. This free cholesterol serves several regulatory functions. It is esterified by acyl coenzyme A:cholesterol acyl transferase (ACAT) for storage as cytoplasmic cholesteryl ester droplets. The free cholesterol suppresses activities of the key enzymes of cholesteryl biosynthetic pathway (hydroxymethyl glutaryl-coenzyme A [HMG-CoA] synthase and reductase) and suppresses the synthesis of new LDL receptor protein. (*Adapted from* Brown and Goldstein [8].)

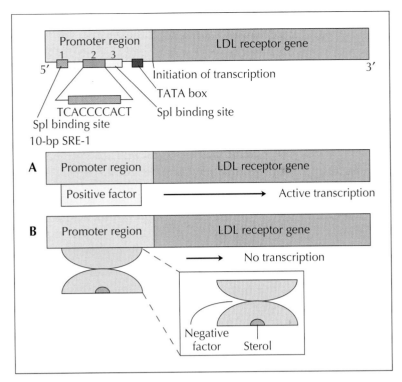

FIGURE 6-8. The low-density lipoprotein (LDL) receptor gene is subject to feedback regulation by cholesterol and its metabolic products. It is suppressed when the cellular cholesterol accumulates. When the cellular cholesterol is low, more receptor is synthesized. According to a current hypothesis [9,10], an active form of cholesterol (an oxidized cholesterol derivative) binds to a regulatory protein(s), which in turn binds to the regulatory elements of the LDL receptor gene. The target for this regulation is a 10–base pair (bp) sequence in the 5' flanking region. This stretch, termed the sterol regulatory element (SRE), binds to SRE-binding proteins (SREBP), which in turn bind to sterols and control the transcription of the gene.

Two SREBPs (SREBP-1 and SREBP-2) control cholesterol homeostasis. Several studies [9,10] showed that a novel proteolytic mechanism may control the activities of SREBPs. The SREBPs are embedded in the nuclear and endoplasmic reticulum membranes. The amino terminal of SREBP-1 contains DNA binding and transcriptional activation domains. **A,** In the absence of sterols, this domain is cleared proteolytically and transcriptional activation of LDL receptor occurs. **B,** When there is an accumulation of cellular cholesterol, proteolytic activity is decreased and the active fragment is no longer generated. (*Adapted from* Wang *et al.* [9] and Briggs *et al.* [41].)

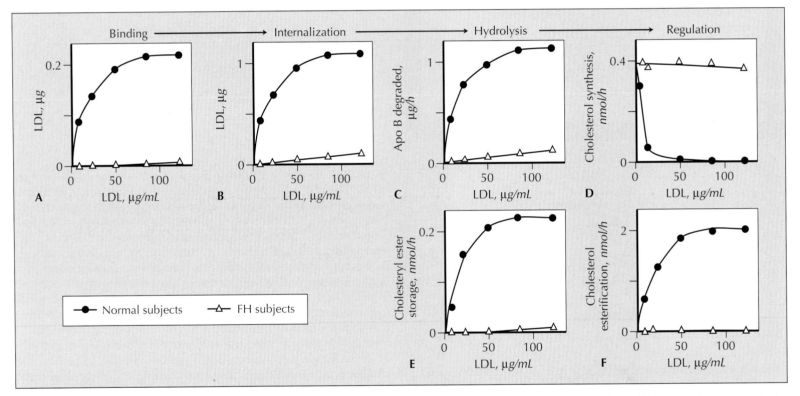

FIGURE 6-9. Low-density lipoprotein (LDL) receptor deficiency: classification of LDL receptor mutations. Mutations in the LDL receptor gene affecting the functional LDL receptor lead to the abnormal phenotype specified by the disease familial hypercholesterolemia (FH). Individuals who inherited two mutant alleles are more severely affected (FH homozygotes, one in 1 million) than those with one mutant allele (FH heterozygotes, one in 500). Both have high plasma cholesterol levels. The FH mutation is an outstanding example of a single-gene mutation that often results in early atherosclerosis. Myocardial infarction, angina pectoris, and even sudden death occur frequently before age 15 years in homozygotes.

In cells from FH-homozygote patients 1) there is failure to bind and internalize LDL, and 2) there is no effect on acyl coenzyme A:cholesterol acyl transferase (ACAT) or hydroxymethyl glutaryl-coenzyme A (HMG-CoA) reductase activities when the cells are incubated with LDL (in normal cells, ACAT is activated and HMG-CoA reductase is suppressed under these conditions).

A to **C,** Cells in patients with FH showing little binding and degradation of LDL. **D,** Synthesis of cholesterol in FH cells is unaffected but is suppressed in normal individuals. **E** and **F,** No increase in cholesteryl ester mass or cholesterol esterification is shown. (*Adapted from* Brown and Goldstein [8] and Goldstein *et al.* [42].)

A. CLASSIFICATION OF LDL RECEPTOR MUTATIONS

Class I	These "null" alleles (R-O) fail to produce detectable receptors; this mutation is very common.
Class II	The synthesized receptors do not undergo proper posttranslational modification and are degraded, never to reach the cell surface.
Class III	Receptors are produced and processed at normal rates but are unable to bind LDL efficiently.
Class IV	Receptors have defective internalization and do not localize at the coated pits.
Class V	Receptors internalize but do not recycle.

FIGURE 6-10. Classification of low-density lipoprotein (LDL) receptor mutation. **A** and **B**, Each class of LDL receptor mutations affects different regions in the gene and thus interferes with different steps in the process by which the receptor is synthesized, processed, and translocated. ER—endoplasmic reticulum.

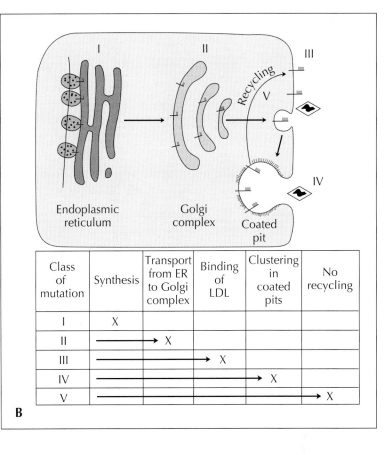

Class of mutation	Synthesis	Transport from ER to Golgi complex	Binding of LDL	Clustering in coated pits	No recycling
I	X				
II	→	X			
III	→		X		
IV	→			X	
V	→				X

B

ATHEROGENIC LIPOPROTEINS

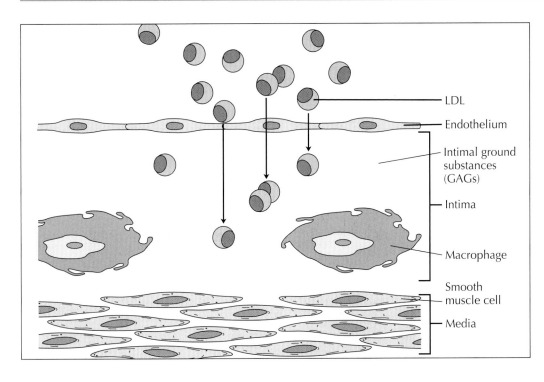

LDL

Endothelium

Intimal ground substances (GAGs)

Intima

Macrophage

Smooth muscle cell

Media

FIGURE 6-11. Infiltration and entrapment of low-density lipoprotein (LDL) in the arterial wall. Circulating LDLs migrate through the endothelial barrier of the arterial wall and penetrate into the intima. A portion of the LDL is entrapped in the subendothelial space as a result of its interaction with extracellular matrix components. These include the proteoglycans and other intimal glycosaminoglycans (GAGs), which have high affinity for apolipoprotein B. This entrapment increases the residence time of LDL in the artery and renders the LDL susceptible to modifications such as oxidation and aggregation. Aggregates of LDL have been identified in association with matrix components. (*Adapted from* Grundy [43].)

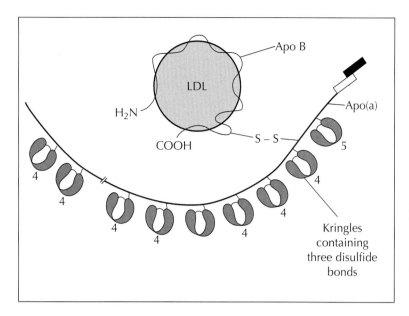

FIGURE 6-12. Lipoprotein(a) [Lp(a)] represents a distinct genetic form of low-density lipoprotein (LDL) wherein apolipoprotein (a) [apo(a)] is linked to apo B-100 via cysteine K4$_{36}$of apo(a) and an unknown cysteine from the carboxyl end of apo B by disulfide linkage. The apo(a) is a glycoprotein that exhibits considerable genetically determined polymorphism among individuals producing a wide range of molecular weights, from 300 to 800 kD. Apo(a) is strikingly similar to plasminogen.

Although three of the five kringles present in plasminogen (K1, K2, and K3) are absent in apo(a), K4 is repeated several times. A number of epidemiologic studies have shown a link between elevated levels of Lp(a) and cardiovascular disease [44]. It may have both atherogenic and antithrombolytic potential. Apo(a) has been found in the macrophage-rich atherosclerotic lesion. The mechanism(s) by which Lp(a) might contribute to cardiovascular diseases is currently theoretical. Recently, mice strains that over-express human apo(a) have been developed [45]. These animals develop accelerated atherosclerosis when fed atherogenic diets. (*Adapted from* Scanu and Fless [13].)

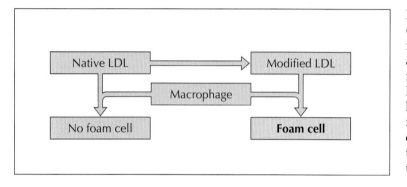

FIGURE 6-13. Why do we need modified low-density lipoprotein (LDL)? Macrophages have few receptors for LDL; therefore in vitro incubation of macrophages with LDL does not lead to cellular lipid accumulation. The few receptors that may be present will be down-regulated in the presence of high cholesterol and extracellular LDL levels. Homozygous familial hyperlipidemic patients and Watanabe heritable hyperlipidemic rabbits that do not have functional LDL receptors develop accelerated atherosclerosis with macrophage foam cell–rich fatty streak lesions. Incubations of macrophages with negatively charged LDL molecules, such as acetyl LDL, lead to enhanced uptake of the lipoprotein and large amounts of lipid accumulation.

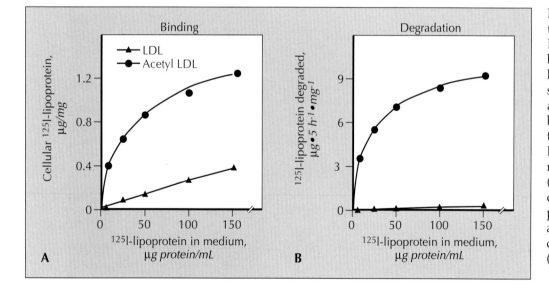

FIGURE 6-14. Modified low-density lipoprotein (LDL) concept: degradation of acetyl LDL and accumulation of cholesteryl ester by macrophages. **A** and **B,** Macrophages have very few receptors for LDL and consequently do not take up and degrade large amounts of LDL. Thus, macrophages incubated with LDL do not accumulate cholesteryl esters. However, when lysine residues of LDL are acetylated using acetic anhydride, a negatively charged lipoprotein is generated (acetyl LDL). The acetyl LDL is taken up and degraded by the scavenger receptor pathway. Macrophages incubated with acetyl LDL accumulate large amounts of cholesterol in the form of cholesteryl ester. (*Adapted from* Goldstein *et al.* [19].)

INCREASE IN INTRACELLULAR CHOLESTEROL CONTENT IN MACROPHAGES INCUBATED WITH ACETYL LDL

ADDITION TO THE MEDIUM	CHOLESTEROL CONTENT OF THE CELL, µg/mg cell protein
None	28
LDL, 25 µg/mL	33
Acetyl LDL, 25 µg/mL	105

FIGURE 6-15. Increase in intracellular cholesterol content in macrophages incubated with acetyl low-density lipoprotein (LDL). Cultured mouse peritoneal macrophages were incubated in Roswell Park Memorial Institute (RMPI) medium for 24 hours in cell culture dishes at 37°C. Cells were washed with Hank's buffer and cellular lipids were extracted by organic solvents for the determination of cholesterol. Numbers given are from a typical experiment.

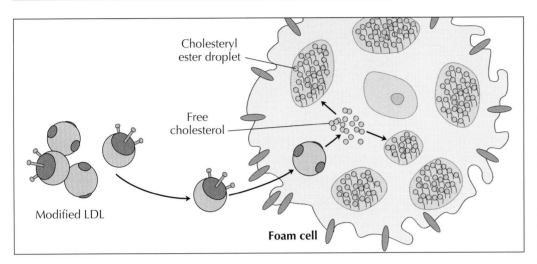

FIGURE 6-16. Foam cell formation. Foam cells derive their name by the foamy appearance caused by lipid accumulation and are the hallmark of early atherosclerotic, fatty streak lesions. The predominant cell type that accumulates lipids is the macrophage, although smooth muscle cell–derived foam cells also occur. Increased chemotactic activity may account for the presence of monocytes or macrophages in the artery. However, the factors that aid in the differentiation of monocytes into differentiated tissue macrophages are yet unknown. Modified lipoproteins are recognized and internalized by the scavenger receptors on the macrophages; there is no feedback regulation of the uptake by this mechanism. The accumulated cellular cholesterol is readily converted to cholesteryl ester and stored as large cytoplasmic lipid droplets. Recently, methods have been developed to isolate and study foam cells from the atherosclerotic artery [46]. (*Adapted from Grundy [43].*)

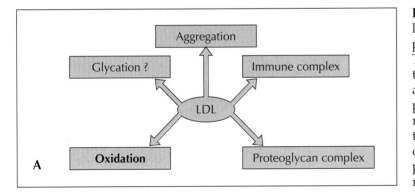

FIGURE 6-17. Factors involved in increased uptake of low-density lipoprotein (LDL) by macrophages. **A,** Several changes in the LDL particle can bring about its increased uptake by macrophages. These include particle aggregation (phospholipase C or elastase-treatments and vortexing), formation of immune complexes with anti–apolipoprotein (apo) B antibodies, complexes with sulfated polysaccharides such as dextran sulfate, and glycation of lysine residues in the presence of high glucose and oxidation. Although these changes are presumably unrelated to each other, glycation can lead to enhanced oxidation; oxidation itself may lead to particle aggregation, and complex formation with extracellular matrix components may affect oxidation. **B,** A variety of receptors may be involved in the uptake of these modified forms of LDL. SR—scavenger receptor.

B. ROLE OF MONOCYTE OR MACROPHAGE RECEPTORS IN THE UPTAKE OF LIPOPROTEINS

RECEPTORS	LIGANDS
Apo B/E receptor (LDL receptor)	Self-aggregated LDL
	Aggregates of LDL with other macromolecules
Acetyl LDL receptor (SR-AI, SR-AII)	Chemically modified forms of LDL, *eg*, acetyl LDL and oxidized LDL
Oxidized LDL receptors	Oxidized LDL
	Acetyl LDL?
Fc receptor	Immune complexes of lipoprotein-antibody complexes
CD$_{36}$	Lipid components of oxidized LDL
SR-BI, SR-BII	HDL, LDL, lipids?
Other scavenger receptors	Glycated LDL and other modified lipoproteins

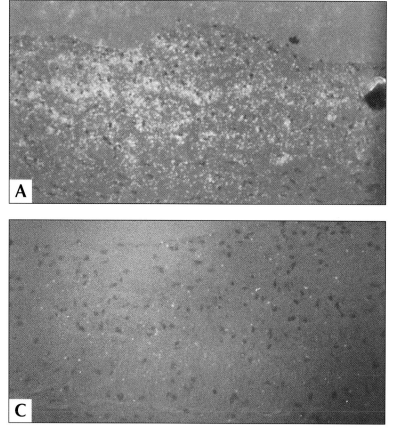

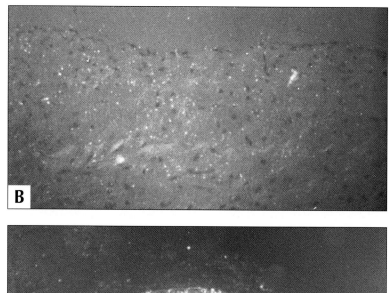

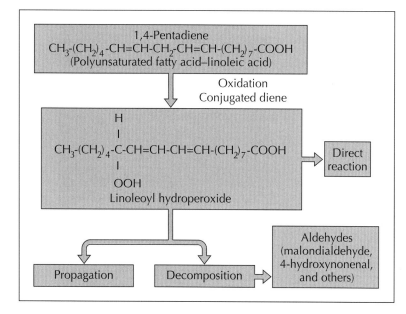

FIGURE 6-18. (*see* Color Plates) The abundant expression of scavenger receptor and the absence of low density-lipoprotein (LDL) receptor in the atherosclerotic lesion. Macrophages possess very few LDL receptors, and these are presumably downregulated in cholesterol-enriched foam cells. Scavenger receptors, on the other hand, are not subject to downregulation and take up massive amounts of cholesterol. **A,** Antisense probe for the scavenger receptor shows good hybridization, indicating the presence of the scavenger receptor. **B,** In this control set-up for *panel A*, the sense probe for the scavenger receptor does not hybridize. **C,** Antisense probe for the LDL receptor shows no hybridization, indicating the absence of the

LDL receptor. **D,** In this positive control for *panel C*, the antisense probe for the LDL receptor shows hybridization for the adrenal tissue from a normal rabbit, indicating that the probe is appropriate.

Scavenger receptors represent a family of receptors (related or unrelated to each other) that may mediate the recognition and uptake of modified lipoproteins. Currently, the acetyl LDL receptors, the $Fc\gamma R_{11}-B_2$, CD_{36}, and an uncharacterized 95-kD protein, may represent such receptors. Furthermore, scavenger receptors may mediate the uptake of damaged albumin, oxidized high-density lipoprotein, glycosylated proteins, and others. (*From* Yla Herttuala *et al.* [24]; with permission.)

LIPID PEROXIDATION AND OXIDIZED LOW-DENSITY LIPOPROTEIN

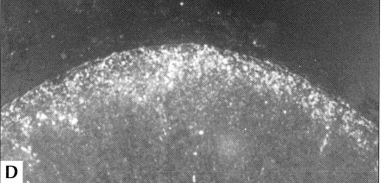

FIGURE 6-19. Peroxidation of polyunsaturated fatty acids. Oxidation of low density-lipoprotein (LDL) is suggested to generate a modified LDL. The oxidation affects the fatty acid molecules of lipids associated with LDL. Unsaturated fatty acids have two or more double bonds separated by a CH_2 bond. When oxidized, the unsaturated fatty acids undergo molecular rearrangement, generating peroxy fatty acids that have a conjugated double bond with no CH_2 bond separating the two double bonds. These readily decompose, particularly in the presence of redox metals such as iron and copper, and generate aldehydes and other products that can react with amino groups of lysine residues. The peroxy and alkoxy radicals generated during the decomposition also promote the propagation of lipid peroxidation.

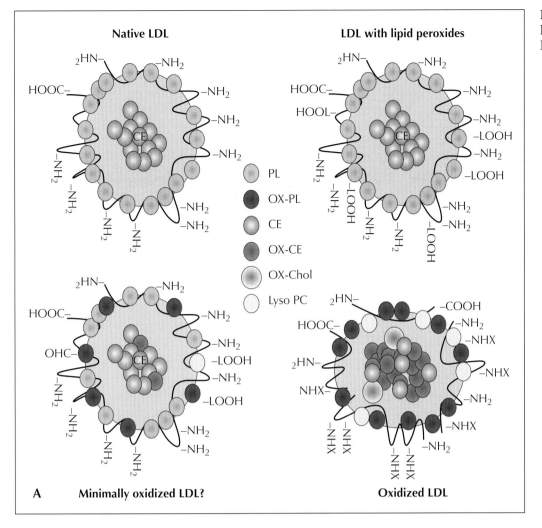

FIGURE 6-20. Types of oxidized low-density lipoprotein (LDL) (**A** and **B**). (*Adapted from* Parthasarathy *et al.* [47].)

Native LDL

LDL with lipid peroxides

PL
OX-PL
CE
OX-CE
OX-Chol
Lyso PC

A Minimally oxidized LDL?

Oxidized LDL

B. TYPES OF OXIDIZED LOW-DENSITY LIPOPROTEIN	
TYPE	CHARACTERISTICS
Native LDL	Degraded via the LDL receptor Does not generate foam cells with macrophages Contains vitamin E, carotenoids, and other antioxidants
Seeded LDL	Contains lipid peroxides generated by cells Degraded via the LDL receptor Contains vitamin E, carotenoids, and other antioxidants May be more readily oxidized compared with native LDL Biologically active?
Mildly oxidized LDL	Contains lipid peroxidases generated by the oxidation of LDL-associated lipids Contains intact apo B-100 and is degraded via the LDL receptor May contain lower amounts of vitamin E, carotenoids, and other antioxidants Is more readily oxidized further Biologically active Immunogenic lipids
Oxidized LDL	Contains lipid peroxides and their degradation products generated by the oxidation of LDL-associated lipids Contains proteolyzed and modified apo B-100 and is degraded via scavenger receptors Not recognized by the LDL receptor Causes lipid accumulation in the macrophages from generating foam cells Contains very low levels of vitamin E, carotenoids, and other antioxidants Biologically active Immunogenic

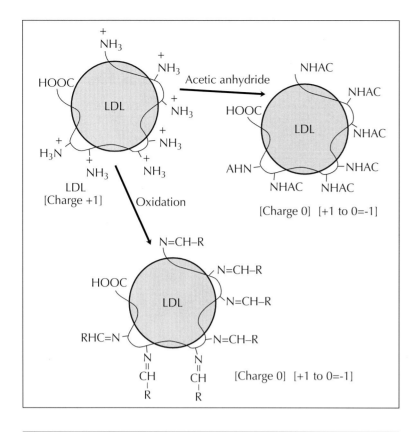

FIGURE 6-21. Acetylation and oxidation generate more negatively charged low-density lipoprotein (LDL). Aldehydes including malondialdehyde (MDA) and 4-hydroxynonenal (4-HNE) are generated during the oxidation of LDL. Both acetylation and aldehyde conjugation of lysine residues of apolipoprotein B neutralize the positive charge on the amino group and generate negatively charged lipoproteins. It is estimated that an extensive (>70%) number of lysines have to be acetylated for scavenger receptor recognition. Considerably less derivatization by MDA is required (15%) for receptor recognition. Oxidation of LDL generally results in approximately 40% to 50% loss of lysine amino groups. Other modifications besides aldehyde addition (Schiff-base formation) may, however, account for some of the loss in lysines.

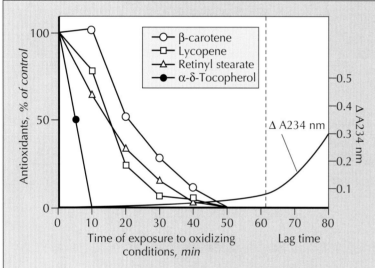

FIGURE 6-22. Consumption of antioxidants and formation of conjugated dienes during the oxidation of low-density lipoprotein (LDL). Antioxidants protect LDL against oxidation. When LDL is exposed to oxidation conditions, the antioxidants present in LDL react with the peroxides and quench the propagation of lipid peroxidation. Until almost all the antioxidants are consumed, the oxidation occurs at a slow rate. In this figure, which represents a hypothetical oxidation of LDL by cupric ions, the lag time denotes the approximate time at which the antioxidants are lost and the rapid propagation of lipid peroxidation ensues. However, there are circumstances under which the antioxidants may promote oxidation and, thus, become pro-oxidants. For example, the oxidation of LDL may be enhanced by antioxidants if mediated by cellular peroxidases [48].

The precise requirement of antioxidants to prevent the oxidation of LDL may vary depending on the nature of the LDL particle. Fatty acid composition, the amount of peroxides associated with LDL, the size of the particle, its lipid composition, and other factors may determine the rate of LDL oxidation. (*Adapted from* Esterbauer *et al.* [49].)

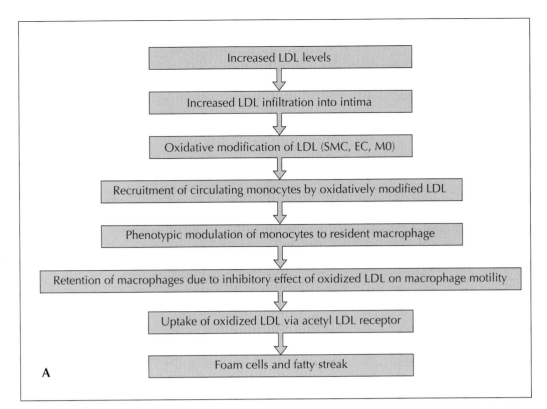

A

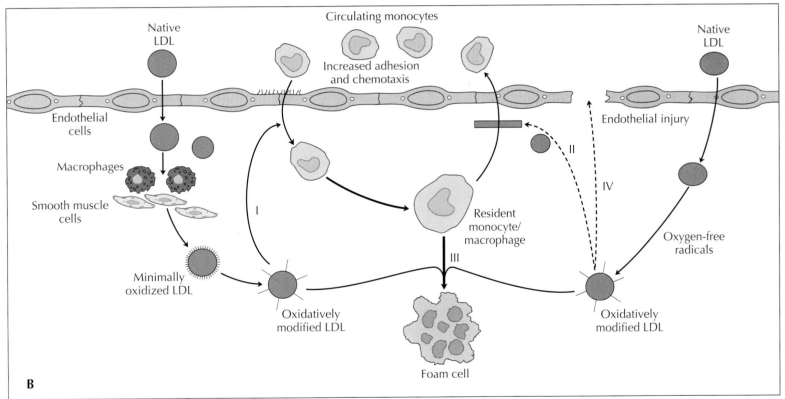

B

FIGURE 6-23. A, Elevated levels of plasma low-density lipoprotein (LDL) alone may be sufficient to initiate the fatty streak lesion. High levels of plasma LDL may increase the availability of LDL in the intima. Free or matrix-bound LDL may undergo oxidation by cells such as endothelial cells (EC), smooth muscle cells (SMCs), or macrophages (M0s). The mildly oxidized LDL may increase the chemotactic recruitment of monocytes by inducing the expression of monocyte chemotactic protein-1 (MCP-1) or by generating lysophospholipids (more extensively, oxidized LDL). Monocytes may differentiate into macrophages, and components of oxidized LDL may promote retention of macrophages in the artery. Macrophages and oxidized LDL may then interact via scavenger pathways leading to foam cell formation. **B,** LDL may enter the artery wall and may be trapped by specific interactions with extracellular matrix components. Cells of the artery may inhibit the oxidation of LDL by mechanisms not yet characterized. Superoxide generation, 15-lipoxygenase activity, and other pathways may contribute to the oxidation. Minimally oxidized LDL (with intact apolipoprotein (apo) B-100) possesses components that have potent biologic properties; these include their ability to induce MCP-1 and granulocyte macrophage colony–stimulating factor. Further increase in oxidation generates oxidized LDL in which apo B-100 is extremely proteolyzed and altered. The maximally oxidized LDL also possesses components that are chemotactic to monocytes and T lymphocytes. Lipids from oxidized LDL also inhibit the chemotaxis of differential macrophages. Macrophages take up oxidized LDL via scavenger receptors and accumulate cholesterol esters, thus accounting for foam cells. There are over 20 postulated mechanisms by which the oxidized LDL may contribute to atherogenesis. Most of the proatherogenic effects of oxidized LDL are mediated by its lipid components. (*Adapted from* Steinberg [50] and Quinn *et al.* [51].)

PHYSICAL AND CHEMICAL PROPERTIES OF OXIDIZED LDL

Increased negative charge and density
Decreased uptake via LDL receptor
Increased uptake via scavenger receptor
Decreased vitamin E and antioxidants
Decreased polyunsaturated fatty acids
Decreased phosphatidylcholine and increased
     lysophosphatidylcholine
Increased cholesterol oxidation products
Increased fatty acid oxidation products
Fragmentation of apolipoprotein B
Loss of amino acids (histidine, lysine, and proline)
Increased apoprotein fluorescence
Altered immunoreactivity and antigenicity

FIGURE 6-24. Physical and chemical properties of oxidized low-density lipoprotein (LDL). (*Adapted from* Parthasarathy and Rankin [52].)

SOME PROATHEROGENIC EFFECTS OF OXIDIZED LDL

SOME PROATHEROGENIC EFFECTS OF LOW-DENSITY LIPOPROTEIN

Oxidized LDL:

Is degraded at a faster rate than native LDL by macrophage leading to lipid accumulation

Is chemotactic to monocytes, smooth muscle cells, and T lymphocytes and induces T-cell activation and monocyte differentiation

Inhibits macrophage motility, potentially trapping macrophages in the artery

Inhibits endothelium-dependent relaxation factor (nitric oxide) synthesis

Inhibits the migration of endothelial cells

Induces the expression of adhesion molecules on the endothelium

Minimally oxidized LDL:

Enhances monocyte adhesion to endothelium

Induces the expression of monocyte chemotactic protein-1 and granulocyte-macrophage colony–stimulating factors

Components of oxidized LDL:

Are cytotoxic to cells

Induce interleukin-1 synthesis and secretion by macrophages

Induce smooth muscle cell proliferation

Enhance procoagulatory activity

Induce apoptosis in cells

Enhance platelet aggregation

FIGURE 6-25. Some proatherogenic effects of oxidized low-density lipoprotein (LDL). Oxidized LDL used in these studies is not homogeneous and does not represent any specific preparation. The lipoproteins used may vary in their content of oxidized lipids and their decomposition products. Oxidized LDL also has other proatherogenic effects on platelet function, on the relaxation of endothelium, and on smooth muscle cells.

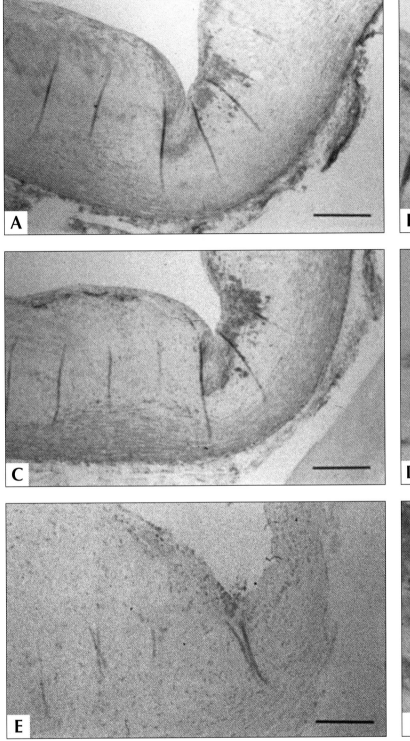

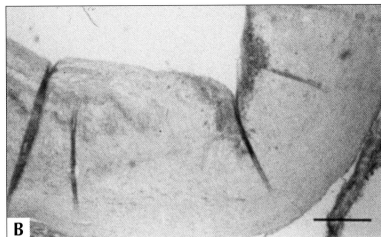

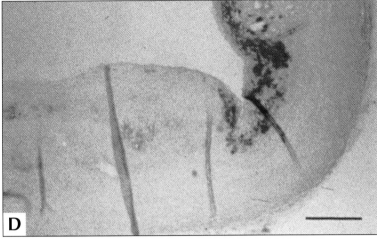

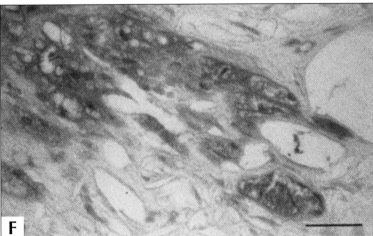

FIGURE 6-26. (*see* Color Plates) The presence of oxidatively modified proteins in the atherosclerotic lesion. Oxidized low-density lipoprotein (LDL) has been isolated from atherosclerotic lesions. As further evidence for the oxidation hypothesis, immunohistochemistry was employed using antibodies that would recognize modified lysine residues. Antibodies were generated against modified LDL (malondialdehyde-LDL, 4-hydroxynonenal LDL, and oxidized LDL) and atherosclerotic lesions were immunostained with them. The areas that reacted positively with specific antibodies (immunostained with antibody against malondialdehyde [**A**], 4-hydroxynonenal LDL [**B**], and oxidized LDL [**C**]) in the lesion were also rich in macrophages (**D**), thus providing evidence that modified lipoproteins are present in the atherosclerotic lesion in the proximity of macrophages. The presence of these "oxidation markers" has been demonstrated in the lesions of rabbits, humans, monkeys, and apolipoprotein B–deficient, high-fat fed transgenic mice. **E,** Control section in which the antibody is preblocked with the antigen before being tested with the tissue. **F,** Magnified section showing intracellular accumulation of the antigen-antibody stain.

Autoantibodies to oxidized LDL occur in the sera of several species. The prevalence and titer of these antibodies may have a positive correlation with increased risk for coronary heart disease. (*From* Palinski *et al.* [53].)

SCAVENGER RECEPTORS

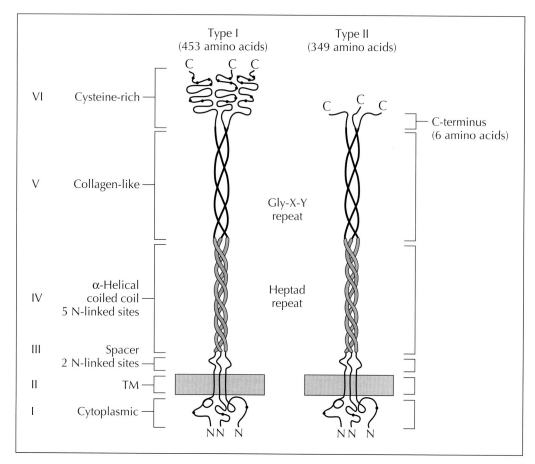

FIGURE 6-27. Scavenger receptor (type I and type II). The scavenger receptor is biochemically and genetically distinct from the low-density lipoprotein (LDL) receptor. It is expressed in macrophages, endothelial cells, and smooth muscle cells. It recognizes acetyl LDL, oxidized LDL, and several polyanionic molecules such as polyinosinic acid, fucoidan, and bacterial lipopolysaccharide. Unlike the LDL receptor, the expression of the scavenger receptor is not regulated by cellular cholesterol, thus permitting massive uptake of cholesterol when modified lipoproteins are presented to the cell. The presence of this receptor has been demonstrated in human and rabbit atherosclerotic lesions.

The type I scavenger receptor has six domains and 453 amino acids. The protein is made of domain I, a 50-amino-acid N-terminal cytoplasmic domain; domain II, a 26-amino-acid transmembrane domain; and extracellular domains III, IV, V, and VI consisting of 32, 163, 72, and 110 amino acids, respectively. Domain IV has a distinguishing feature of heptad repeat units. Domain V has collagen-like repeats of Gly-X-Y sequences and is presumably involved in ligand binding. Domain VI is a cysteine-rich domain that is absent in the type II receptor. The receptor in the reduced form is a 77-kD glycoprotein that in the unreduced form forms a 220-kD ligand-binding trimer. It is suggested that additional scavenger receptors that bind to oxidized LDL are present in macrophages. TM—thrombomodulin. (*Adapted from* Kodama *et al.* [22] and Rohrer *et al.* [54].)

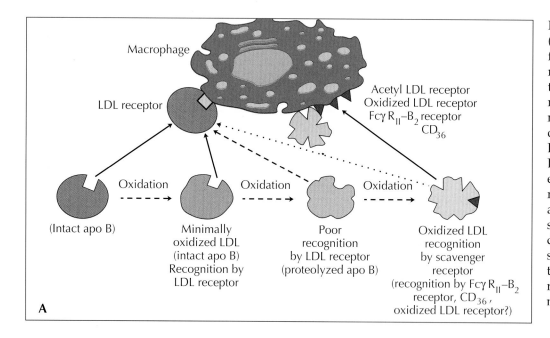

FIGURE 6-28. Low-density lipoprotein (LDL) and scavenger receptor activities as a function of time in culture. **A,** LDL and minimally oxidized LDL are recognized by the LDL receptor. Incubation of macrophages with these lipoproteins does not result in lipid accumulation. Further oxidation results in poor recognition by the LDL receptor. More extensively oxidized LDL is recognized by the macrophage scavenger receptors and other uncharacterized receptors. Extensively oxidized LDL may also be recognized by CD_{36}, $Fc\gamma R_{11}B_2$, and several other surface proteins. During the differentiation of monocytes in culture, scavenger receptors are induced. The relative contribution of different scavenger receptors in the uptake of oxidized LDL has not been established. (*continued*)

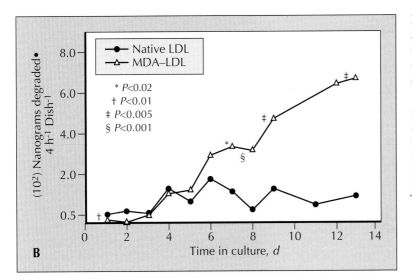

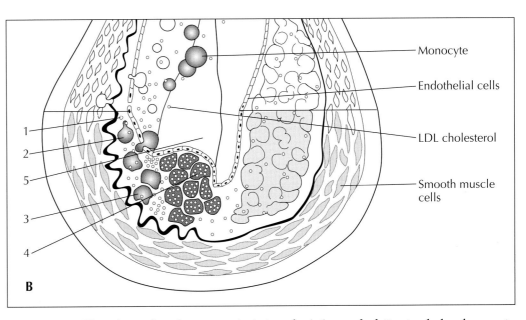

FIGURE 6-28. (*continued*) **B,** Freshly isolated monocytes do not have a high degree of expression of the acetyl LDL receptor, and they take up modified lipoproteins poorly. Upon culturing, they take up increased amounts of the acetyl LDL, and the cellular expression of the receptor increases.

Cultured THP-1 line of monocytes can be induced to express scavenger receptor (acetyl LDL receptor) by exposure to differentiating agents such as phorbol myristate acetate (PMA). Smooth muscle cells and fibroblasts can also be induced to express the acetyl LDL receptor upon suitable stimulation. apo—apolipoprotein; MDA—malondialdehyde. (Part A *adapted from* Fogelman *et al.* [55].)

OXIDATION, ANTIOXIDANTS, AND ATHEROSCLEROSIS

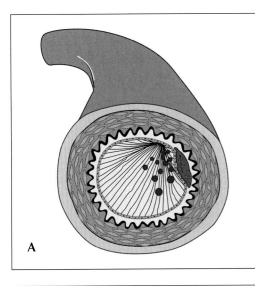

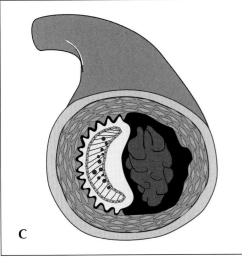

FIGURE 6-29. The atherosclerotic process. **A,** Artery depicting early fatty streak development. **B,** *1,* low-density lipoproteins (LDL) becomes oxidized within the arterial subendothelial space. *2,* Circulating monocytes are recruited to the subendothelial space by chemoattractants, including oxidized LDL. *3,* These monocytes undergo differentiation, becoming macrophages, which are scavenger cells that recognize and accumulate oxidized LDL. *4,* The lipid-laden macrophages then become foam cells, which cluster under the endothelial lining to form a bulge into the artery. *5,* This bulge is called a *fatty streak* and is the first overt sign of atherosclerotic change. **C,** Cross-section of an artery with an atherosclerotic lesion with a narrowed lumen. (*Courtesy of* Merrell Dow Pharmaceuticals Inc., Cincinnati, OH.)

EFFECT OF ANTIOXIDANTS ON EXPERIMENTAL ATHEROSCLEROSIS

ANTIOXIDANT	EXPERIMENTAL SYSTEM	DECREASE IN LESION AREA, %
Probucol	WHHL rabbit	50–60
Probucol	Cholesterol-fed rabbit	75
Butylated hydroxytoluene	Cholesterol-fed rabbit	70
Diphenylenediamine	Cholesterol-fed rabbit	71
Vitamin E	Cholesterol-fed macaque	Change in carotid stenosis: 35
Vitamin E	Humans	Reduction in nonfatal MI

FIGURE 6-30. Effect of antioxidants on experimental atherosclerosis. The Watanabe heritable hyperlipidemic (WHHL) rabbit represents an animal model in which the plasma cholesterol and low-density lipoprotein (LDL) levels are very high because of a deficiency in LDL receptors. Cholesterol feeding, on the other hand, induces a novel lipoprotein β–very low-density lipoprotein that may be directly taken up by macrophages without the prerequisite for an oxidative step. Human clinical intervention trials have now been carried out. MI—myocardial infarction.

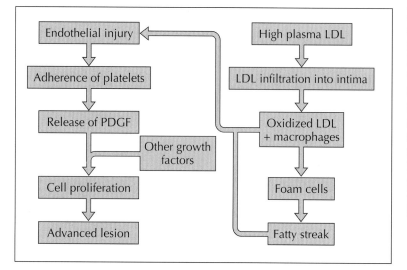

FIGURE 6-31. Postulated link between lipid-infiltration hypothesis and the endothelial injury hypothesis. The fatty streak lesions have an intact endothelium. The monocytes can penetrate the endothelium, differentiate into macrophages, and become foam cells. Thus the lipid-infiltration hypothesis itself may be sufficient to account for the fatty streak lesions. The oxidized low-density lipoproteins (LDLs) present in the intima or the oxidized and damaging components released from the foam cell macrophages may injure the endothelium. Thus, platelets may adhere to the exposed intima, thus advancing the fatty streak lesion to the advanced lesions. Oxidized LDL may also induce the proliferation of smooth muscle cells and prevent endothelial cell migration, thus affecting the "healing" process. PDGF—platelet-derived growth factor. (*Adapted from* Steinberg [50].)

STEPS IN THE ATHEROSCLEROTIC PROCESS THAT MIGHT BE AFFECTED BY OXIDATIVE STRESS

Fatty streak formation	Monocyte binding to the endothelium
	Monocyte and T-cell chemotaxis
	Monocyte transformation into macrophages
	Further oxidation of LDL
	Foam cell formation
Intimal medial thickness	Migration of smooth muscle cells
	Secretion of smooth muscle cell growth–promoting activities
	Smooth muscle cell proliferation
	Extracellular lipid accumulation
	Extracellular matrix production
Plaque rupture	Calcification
	Apoptosis
	Activation of matrix metalloproteinases
	Activation of procoagulant activities and thrombus formation

FIGURE 6-32. Steps in the atherosclerotic process that might be affected by oxidative stress. LDL—low-density lipoprotein.

References

1. Lowering blood cholesterol to prevent heart disease. *JAMA* 1985, 253:2080–2086.

2. Tyroler H: Lowering plasma cholesterol levels decreases risk of coronary heart disease: an overview of clinical trials. In *Hypercholesterolemia and Atherosclerosis*. Edited by Steinberg D, Olefsky JM. New York: Churchill Livingstone, 1987:99–116.

3. Havel RJ: The role of liver in atherogenesis. *Arteriosclerosis* 1985, 2:569–575.

4. Krauss RM: The tangled web of coronary risk factors. *Am J Med* 1990, 2(suppl A):36–41.

5. Krauss RM: Dense low density lipoproteins and coronary artery disease [review]. *Am J Cardiol* 1995, 75(suppl B):53–75.

6. Veniant MM, Pierotti V, Newland D, *et al.*: Susceptibility to atherosclerosis in mice expressing exclusively apolipoprotein B48 or apolipoprotein B100. *J Clin Invest* 1997, 100:180–188.

7. Pittman RC, Carew TE, Attie AD, *et al.*: Receptor-dependent and receptor-independent degradation of low density lipoprotein in normal and in receptor-deficient mutant rabbits. *J Biol Chem* 1982, 257:7994–8000.

8. Brown MS, Goldstein JL: A receptor-mediated pathway for cholesterol homeostasis. *Science* 1986, 232:34–47.

9. Wang X, Briggs MR, Hua X, *et al.*: Nuclear protein that binds sterol regulatory element of low density lipoprotein receptor promoter. II. Purification and characterization. *J Biol Chem* 1993, 268:14497–14504.

10. Yang J, Sato R, Goldstein JL, *et al.*: Sterol-resistant transcription in Cho 61b caused by gene rearrangement that truncates SREBP-2. *Genes Dev* 1994, 8:1910–1919.

11. Ishibashi S, Brown MS, Goldstein JL, *et al.*: Hypercholesterolemia in low density lipoprotein receptor knockout mice and its reversal by adenovirus-mediated gene delivery. *J Clin Invest* 1993, 92:883–893.

12. Scanu AM: Lipoprotein(a): its inheritance and molecular basis of its atherothrombotic role. *Mol Cell Biochem* 1992, 113:127–131.

13. Scanu AM, Fless GM: Lipoprotein(a): heterogeneity and biological relevance. *J Clin Invest* 1990, 85:1709–1715.

14. Gugliucci Creriche A, Stahl AJ: Glycation and oxidation of human low density lipoproteins reduces heparin binding and modifies charge. *Scand J Clin Lab Invest* 1993, 53:125–132.

15. Steinberg D, Parthasarathy S, Carew TE, *et al.*: Beyond cholesterol. Modifications of low-density lipoprotein that increase its atherogenicity. *N Engl J Med* 1989, 320:915–924.

16. Parthasarathy S: *Modified Lipoproteins in the Pathogenesis of Atherosclerosis*. Austin, TX: RG Landes Publishers, CRC Press Inc; 1994.

17. Steinbrecher UP: Oxidation of human low density lipoprotein results in derivatization of lysine residues of apolipoprotein B by lipid peroxide decomposition products. *J Biol Chem* 1987, 262:3603–3608.

18. Gerrity RG: The role of the monocyte in atherogenesis. *Am J Pathol* 1981, 103:181–190.

19. Goldstein JL, Ho YK, Basu SK, *et al.*: Binding site on macrophages that mediates uptake and degradation of cetylated low density lipoproteins, producing massive cholesterol deposition. *Proc Natl Acad Sci U S A* 1979, 76:333–337.

20. Haberland ME, Fogelman AM, Edwards PA: Specificity of receptor-mediated recognition of malondialdehyde-modified low density lipoproteins. *Proc Natl Acad Sci U S A* 1982, 79:1712–1716.

21. Brown MS, Goldstein JL: Atherosclerosis. Scavenging for receptors [news]. *Nature* 1990, 343:508–509.

22. Kodama T, Freeman M, Rohrer L, *et al.*: Type I macrophage scavenger receptor contains alpha-helical and collagen-like coiled coils. *Nature* 1990, 343:531–535.

23. Takahashi K, Naito M, Kodama T, *et al.*: Expression of macrophage scavenger receptors in various human tissues and atherosclerotic lesions. *Clin Biochem* 1992, 25:365–368.

24. Yla Herttuala S, Rosenfeld MR, Parthasarathy S, *et al.*: Gene expression in macrophage-rich human atherosclerotic lesions. 15-lipoxygenase and acetyl low density lipoprotein receptor messenger RNA colocalize with oxidation specific lipid-protein adducts. *J Clin Invest* 1991, 87:1146–1152.

25. Sakaguchi H, Takeya M, Suzuki H, *et al.*: Role of macrophage scavenger receptor in diet-induced atherosclerosis in mice. *Lab Invest* 1998, 78:423–434.

26. Parthasarathy S, Steinberg D, Witztum JL: The role of oxidized low-density lipoproteins in the pathogenesis of atherosclerosis. *Annu Rev Med* 1992, 43:219–225.

27. Cushing SD, Berliner JA, Valente AJ, *et al.*: Minimally modified low density lipoprotein induces monocyte chemotactic protein 1 in human endothelial cells and smooth muscle cells. *Proc Natl Acad Sci U S A* 1990, 87:5134–5138.

28. Ku G, Thomas CE, Akeson AL, *et al.*: Induction of interleukin 1 β expression from human peripheral blood monocyte-derived macrophages by 9-hydroxyoctadecadienoic acid. *J Biol Chem* 1992, 267:14183–14188.

29. Carew TE, Schwenke DC, Steinberg D: Antiatherogenic effect of probucol unrelated to its hypocholesterolemic effect: evidence that antioxidants *in vivo* can selectively inhibit low density lipoprotein degradation in macrophage-rich fatty streaks and slow the progression of atherosclerosis in the Watanabe heritable hyperlipidemic rabbit. *Proc Natl Acad Sci U S A* 1987, 84:7725–7729.

30. Sparrow CP, Doebber TW, Olszewski J, *et al.*: Low density lipoprotein is protected from oxidation and the progression of atherosclerosis is slowed in cholesterol-fed rabbits by the antioxidant N,N'-diphenyl-phenylenediamine. *J Clin Invest* 1992, 89:1885–1891.

31. Verlangieri AJ, Bush MJ: Effects of d-alpha-tocopherol supplementation on experimentally induced primate atherosclerosis. *J Am Coll Nutr* 1992, 11:131–138.

32. Kita T, Nagano Y, Yokode M, *et al.*: Prevention of atherosclerotic progression in Watanabe rabbits by probucol. *Am J Cardiol* 1988, 62(suppl B):13–19.

33. Gaziano JM, Manson JE, Buring JE, *et al.*: Dietary antioxidants and cardiovascular disease. *Ann N Y Acad Sci* 1992, 669:249–258.

34. Gey KF, Puska P: Plasma vitamins E and A inversely correlated to mortality from ischemic heart disease in cross-cultural epidemiology. *Ann N Y Acad Sci* 1989, 570:268–282.

35. Stephens NG, Parsons A, Schofield PM, *et al.*: Randomized controlled trial of vitamin E in patients with coronary disease: Cambridge Heart Antioxidant Study (CHAOS). *Lancet* 1996, 347(suppl A):781–786.

36. Shern-Brewer R, Santanam N, Wetzstein C, *et al.*: Exercise and cardiovascular disease: a new perspective. *Arteriosclerosis Thromb Vasc Biol* 1998, 18:1181–1187.

37. Santanam N, Shern-Brewer R, McClatchey R, *et al.*: Estradiol as an antioxidant: incompatible with its physiological concentrations and function. *J Lipid Research* 1998, 39:2111–2118.

38. Ramasamy S, Parthasarathy S, Harrison DG: Regulation of endothelial nitric oxide synthase gene expression by oxidized linoleic acid. *J Lipid Res* 1998, 39;268–276.

39. Palinski WS, Miller E, Wiztum JL: Immunization of LDL receptor-deficient rabbits with homologous malondialdehyde-modified reduces atherogenesis. *Proc Natl Acad Sci U S A* 1995, 92:821–825.

40. Yang C, Gu Z, Weng S, *et al.*: Structure of apolipoprotein B-100 of human low density proteins. *Arteriosclerosis* 1989, 9:96–108.

41. Briggs MR, Yokoyama C, Wang X, *et al.*: Nuclear protein that binds sterol regulatory element of low density lipoprotein receptor promoter. I. Identification of the protein and delineation of its target nucleotide sequence. *J Biol Chem* 1993, 268:14490–14496.

42. Goldstein JL, Brown MS, Anderson RG, *et al.*: Receptor-mediated endocytosis: concepts emerging from the LDL receptor system [review]. *Annu Rev Cell Biol* 1985, 1:1–39.

43. Grundy SM: *Cholesterol and Atherosclerosis: Diagnosis and Treatment.* Philadelphia: JB Lippincott; 1990.

44. Austin MA, Hokanson JE: Epidemiology of triglycerides, small dense low-density lipoprotein, and lipoprotein(a) as risk factors for coronary heart disease [review]. *Med Clin North Am* 1994, 78:99–115.

45. Callow MJ, Stoltzfus LJ, Lawn RM, *et al.*: Expression of human apolipoprotein B and assembly of lipoprotein(a) in transgenic mice. *Proc Natl Acad Sci U S A* 1994, 91:2130–2134.

46. Rosenfeld ME, Khoo JC, Miller E, *et al.*: Macrophage-derived foam cells freshly isolated from rabbit atherosclerotic lesions degrade modified lipoproteins, promote oxidation of low-density lipoproteins, and contain oxidation-specific lipid-protein adducts. *J Clin Invest* 1991, 87:90–99.

47. Parthasarathy S, Santanam S, Augé N: Antioxidants and Low density Lipoprotein Oxidation. In *Antioxidant Status, Diet, Nutrition, and Health.* Edited by Papas A. Boca Raton, FL: CRC Press; 1999:347–369.

48. Santanam N, Parthasarathy S: Paradoxical actions of antioxidants in the oxidation of low-density lipoprotein by peroxidases. *J Clin Invest* 1995, 95:2594–2600.

49. Esterbauer H, Striegl G, Puhl H, *et al.*: Continuous monitoring of *in vitro* oxidation of human low density lipoprotein. *Free Radic Res Commun* 1989, 6:67–75.

50. Steinberg D: Metabolism of lipoproteins and their role in atherogenesis. *Atheroscler Rev* 1988, 18:1–23.

51. Quinn MT, Parthasarathy S, Steinberg D, *et al.*: Oxidatively modified low density lipoproteins: a potential role in recruitment and retention of monocyte/macrophages during atherogenesis. *Proc Natl Acad Sci U S A* 1987, 84:2995–2998.

52. Parthasarathy S, Rankin SM: Role of oxidized low density lipoprotein in atherogenesis. *Prog Lipid Res* 1992, 31:127–143.

53. Palinski W, Rosenfeld ME, Yla Herttuala S, *et al.*: Low density lipoprotein undergoes oxidative modification in vivo. *Proc Natl Acad Sci U S A* 1989, 86:1372–1376.

54. Rohrer L, Freeman M, Kodama T, *et al.*: Coiled-coil fibrous domains mediate ligand binding by scavenger receptor type II. *Nature* 1990, 343:570–572.

55. Fogelman AM, Haberland ME, Seager J, *et al.*: Factors regulating the activities of the low density lipoprotein receptor and the scavenger receptor on human monocyte-macrophages. *J Lipid Res* 1981, 22:1131–1141.

HIGH-DENSITY LIPOPROTEIN METABOLISM

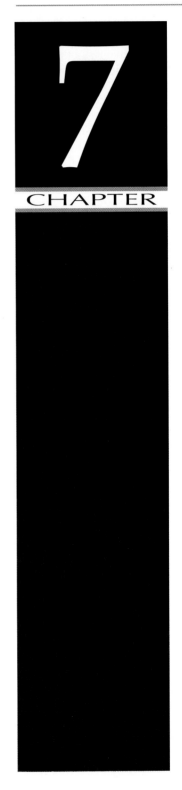

7

CHAPTER

H. Bryan Brewer, Jr.

High-density lipoprotein (HDL) cholesterol concentrations are inversely associated with coronary heart disease (CHD) in humans [1,2]. The initial descriptions of this inverse relationship in the early 1950s [3–5] were "rediscovered" in the 1970s [6–9]. The major mechanism proposed for the protective effect of HDL is reverse cholesterol transport, a process in which excess cholesterol from peripheral cells is transported back to the liver for removal from the body [10]. The higher the plasma levels of HDL, the more efficient is the transport to the liver of excess cholesterol from peripheral cells.

A number of genetic diseases are associated with both increased or decreased levels of plasma HDL [11,12]. Elevated levels of HDL have been proposed to be associated with a decreased risk of premature cardiovascular disease and include apolipoprotein (apo) A-1 gene overexpression and familial hyperalphalipoproteinemia. In contrast, elevated plasma HDL levels due to cholesteryl ester transport protein deficiency (CETP) have recently been recognized to be associated with an increased risk of cardiovascular disease. Several different genetic diseases are characterized by low plasma levels of HDL. Structural defects in the apo A-1 gene complex, familial hypoalphalipoproteinemia, Tangier disease, as well as patients with the lipid triad and the metabolic syndrome have an increased risk of early heart disease. However, patients with lecithin cholesterol acyltransferase deficiency or fish eye disease and selected kindreds with familial hypoalphalipoproteinemia are not at increased risk for premature cardiovascular disease.

Several clinical trials are underway to determine the efficacy of raising plasma HDL cholesterol levels to reduce cardiovascular morbidity and mortality. Although limited evidence is available, many experts in the field of lipoprotein metabolism and atherosclerosis believe that raising HDL concentrations will reduce the risk of cardiovascular disease. The treatment of individuals with hypoalphalipoproteinemia at risk for CHD includes exercise, caloric restriction if not at ideal body weight, and elimination of cigarette smoking. If these lifestyle changes do not adequately increase the HDL levels, selected individuals may require drug therapy. Nicotinic acid, statins, and the fibrates are among the most effective drugs in raising HDL concentrations.

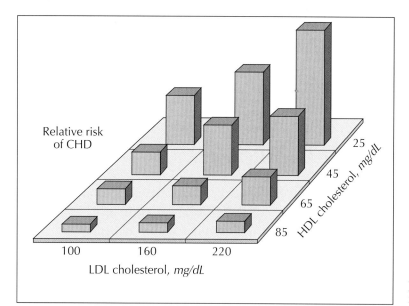

FIGURE 7-1. The Framingham Heart Study: risk of coronary heart disease (CHD) by high-density lipoprotein (HDL) and low-density lipoprotein (LDL) cholesterol. Epidemiologic studies have definitely established that total and LDL cholesterol concentrations are directly correlated with clinical coronary atherosclerosis [13]. The inverse association of HDL cholesterol concentrations with CHD endpoints have also been established in both cross-sectional and prospective epidemiologic studies [14]. In the Framingham Heart Study, the interrelationship between LDL and HDL cholesterol concentrations and the relative risk of developing CHD has been well documented [2]. For individuals with HDL cholesterol concentrations of 45 mg/dL or less, the risk of CHD increases as the LDL cholesterol concentrations increase. However, patients with elevated HDL cholesterol concentrations are protected against the development of vascular disease. This protection is striking at 65 mg/dL, and at 85 mg/dL, even high concentrations of LDL do not predispose to increased CHD risk. Therefore, high plasma HDL cholesterol levels often confer a remarkably lower risk for developing CHD.

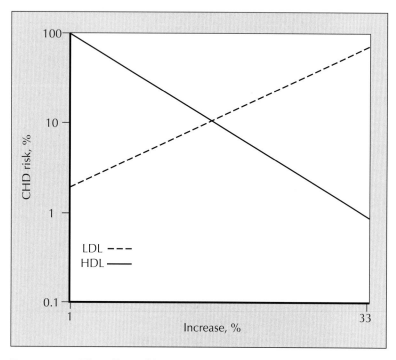

FIGURE 7-2. The effect of low-density lipoprotein (LDL) and high-density lipoprotein (HDL) change on coronary heart disease (CHD) risk. A review of both epidemiologic and clinical trial data indicates that a 1% reduction in the concentration of LDL cholesterol reduces subsequent cardiovascular disease risk by 2%. However, raising HDL cholesterol concentrations appears to be even more effective in reducing CHD risk. Increasing HDL concentrations by 1% is associated with a 3% reduction in clinical CHD endpoints. Data are plotted on a log scale.

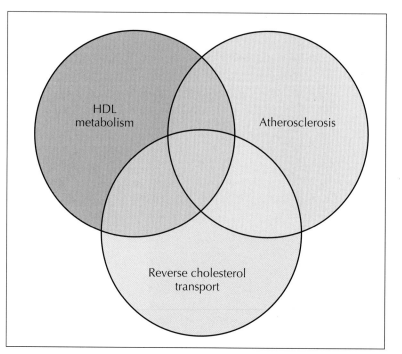

FIGURE 7-3. Venn diagram illustrating the relationships of high-density lipoprotein (HDL) metabolism, reverse cholesterol transport, and atherosclerosis. The concept of reverse cholesterol transport has been closely linked with plasma HDL. Thus, HDL metabolism, reverse cholesterol transport, and human atherogenesis are intimately interrelated. However, it should be pointed out that HDL metabolism, reverse cholesterol transport, and atherogenesis may reflect only a convergence of three distinct processes (Venn diagram). The inverse association of HDL with atherosclerosis is due, at least in part, to mechanisms independent of reverse cholesterol transport. For example, HDL can affect vasomotor tone, which may be important to coronary artery vasospasm [15,16], and HDL may protect low-density lipoprotein from oxidation or aggregation, which has been proposed to be important in the development of atherosclerosis [16–20]. Therefore, the processes involved in the deposition of cholesterol into vascular tissues and the development of coronary heart disease are multifactorial, and defects in reverse cholesterol transport may play a pivotal role in the atherosclerosis process.

HDL STRUCTURE AND METABOLISM

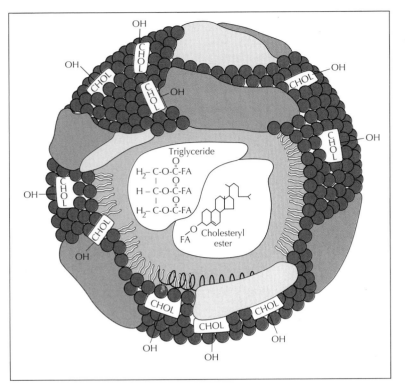

FIGURE 7-4. Schematic model of a plasma high-density lipoprotein particle. The surface of the lipoprotein particle is covered by phospholipids with the polar head groups of the phospholipids interacting with the aqueous environment. The protein components of the lipoprotein, designated apolipoproteins, as well as cholesterol (CHOL) are intercalated between the polar head groups of the phospholipids. The neutral lipids, cholesteryl esters and triglycerides, fill the core of the lipoprotein particle. Several different apolipoproteins are present on the lipoprotein particle. The apolipoproteins are associated with the lipoprotein particle by protein–protein as well as protein–lipid interactions. Apolipoproteins function in lipoprotein metabolism as ligands for receptors, cofactors for enzymes, and structural proteins for lipoprotein particle biosynthesis [21].

APOLIPOPROTEINS IN HIGH-DENSITY LIPOPROTEINS			
MAJOR APOLIPOPROTEINS	MINOR APOLIPOPROTEINS	APPROXIMATE MOLECULAR WEIGHT, kD	MAJOR SITE OF SYNTHESIS
Apo A-I		28	Liver, intestine
Apo A-II		18	Liver
	Apo A-IV	45	Intestine
	Apo E	34	Liver
	Apo C-I	7	Liver
	Apo C-II	10	Liver
	Apo C-III	10	Liver

FIGURE 7-5. High-density lipoproteins (HDLs) are a polydisperse collection of lipoprotein particles that contain two major and five minor apolipoproteins (apos). The sizes of the apos range from 7000 to 45,000 D. Apo A-I and apo A-II, the two major apos in HDL, are present almost exclusively in HDL. Apo E as well as apo C-I, apo C-II, and apo C-III are also present in chylomicrons and very low-density lipoproteins (VLDLs). Apo A-IV may be present in chylomicrons and VLDL. ApoA-IV may be present in chylomicrons. VLDL and a major fraction of apo A-IV is poorly lipidated and isolated in the very high-density lipoprotein (VHDL) fraction (density, 1.21 to 1.25 g/mL).

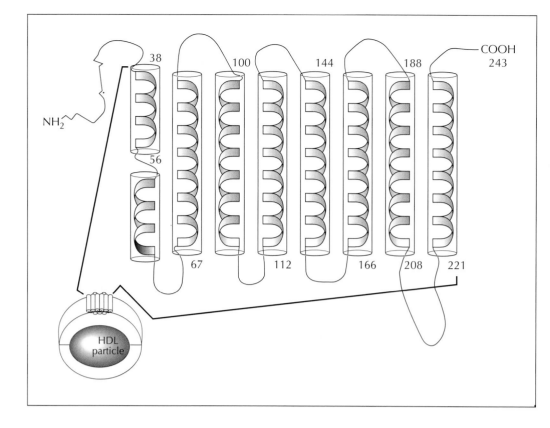

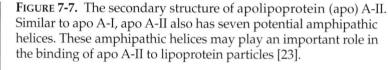

FIGURE 7-6. The secondary structure of apolipoprotein (apo) A-I. Apo A-I is present at the aqueous–lipid interface of high-density lipoprotein (HDL) particles. ApoA-I has been proposed to bind to these particles by virtue of antiparallel arrays of amphipathic helices. These nine coiled structures have hydrophobic amino acids on one side of the helices that permit the binding of the protein to lipid [22]. The hydrophilic aspects of the helices are then presented to the free water in plasma and lymph. The antiparallel arrays have also been proposed to be important for interaction with other apos, enzymes, and cellular receptors [23].

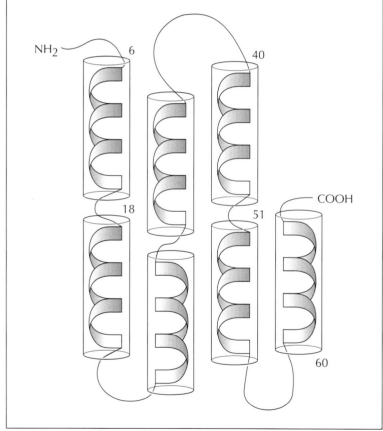

FIGURE 7-7. The secondary structure of apolipoprotein (apo) A-II. Similar to apo A-I, apo A-II also has seven potential amphipathic helices. These amphipathic helices may play an important role in the binding of apo A-II to lipoprotein particles [23].

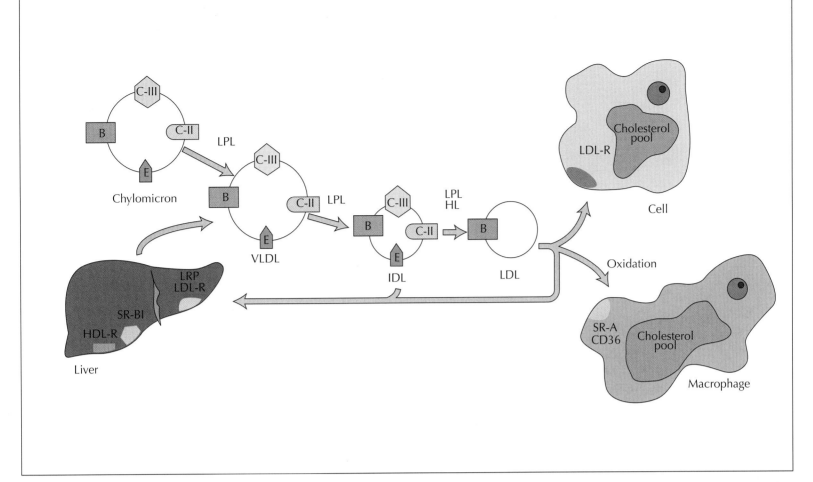

FIGURE 7-8. Interrelationship of the metabolism of chylomicrons, very low-density lipoprotein (VLDL), intermediate density lipoprotein (IDL), and low-density lipoprotein (LDL). The metabolism of all of the major plasma lipoproteins is interrelated and involves the interplay of lipolytic enzymes, apolipoproteins (apos), receptors, and transfer proteins. An overview of the metabolism of the major apo B–containing lipoproteins secreted by the intestine and liver is shown. Triglyceride-rich chylomicrons are secreted from the intestine and function to transport dietary lipids to peripheral tissues and the liver. The triglycerides on chylomicrons undergo hydrolysis by lipoprotein lipase and the particles are converted to remnants with a hydrated density of VLDL and IDL. VLDL is secreted by the liver, and the triglycerides that are present on VLDL also undergo hydrolysis by lipoprotein lipase. With triglyceride hydrolysis, VLDL undergoes stepwise delipidation with the formation of particles with a hydrated density of IDL and finally LDL. Chylomicron and VLDL remnants are cleared from the plasma by interacting with the hepatic LRP (LDL receptor–related protein) and LDL receptors (LDL-R). The interaction of LDL with cellular receptors initiates receptor-mediated endocytosis and degradation of LDL in the liver and peripheral cells in the body.

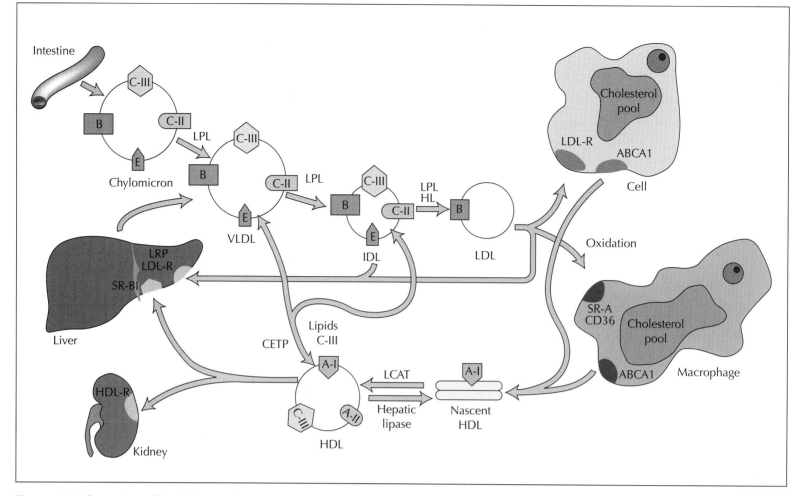

FIGURE 7-9. Overview of high-density lipoprotein (HDL) metabolism and reverse cholesterol transport. Four major pathways are involved in the synthesis of mature HDL. Nascent or pre-HDL, which are composed primarily of apolipoprotein (apo) A-I phospholipid disks, are secreted from the human intestine and liver. Lipids and apolipoprotein constituents of HDL are acquired from the intravascular metabolism and remodeling of both-triglyceride rich chylomicrons and hepatic very low-density lipoprotein (VLDL), which converts nascent HDL to mature HDL. Nascent HDL plays a pivotal role in lipoprotein metabolism and reverse cholesterol transport by facilitating the efflux of excess cholesterol from the membranes of peripheral cells including macrophages by interaction with the ABCA1 transporter [24]. The free cholesterol on nascent HDL is esterified to cholesteryl esters by lecithin cholesterol acyltransferase (LCAT). With the formation of cholesteryl esters, the nascent HDL are converted to spherical lipoproteins with a hydrated density of HDL_3. HDL_3 are converted to the larger HDL_2 by the acquisition of lipids and apolipoproteins (*eg*, apo C-III) released during the stepwise delipidation and remodeling of the triglyceride-rich chylomicrons and VLDL and by the esterification of the cholesterol removed from peripheral tissues. HDL transports cholesterol back to the liver by two pathways. The first pathway involves a direct delivery of cholesterol to the liver by a newly recognized receptor, SR-BI [24–26], that functions to remove cholesteryl esters selectively from lipoproteins without holoparticle uptake and degradation. Additionally, HDL particles are taken up intact and degraded by receptors primarily in the liver and kidney. In the second pathway, HDL cholesteryl esters are exchanged for triglycerides in the apo B–containing lipoproteins (VLDL, intermediate-density lipoprotein [IDL], low-density lipoprotein [LDL]) by the cholesteryl ester transfer protein (CETP) [27]. A significant fraction of cholesteryl esters present in HDL are transferred back to the liver by the LDL pathway. Thus, cholesterol may be transported back to the liver directly by HDL or following exchange to VLDL-IDL-LDL. It also has been proposed that a variable portion of tissue cholesterol is transported to the liver by HDL particles containing apo E, which may interact with both the hepatic LRP(LDL receptor–related protein) and LDL receptors (LDL-R). HDL-R—high-density lipoprotein receptors; HL—hepatic lipase; LPL—lipoprotein lipase.

ABCA1 TRANSPORTER

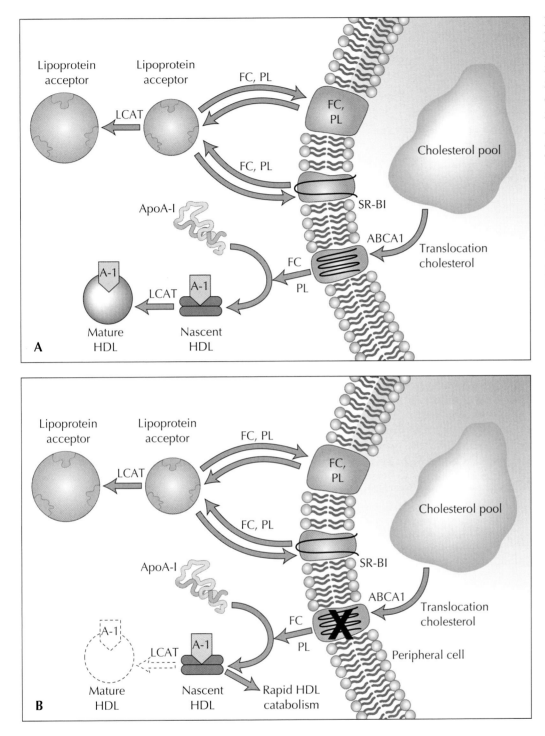

FIGURE 7-10. The ABCA1 transporter. Poorly lipidated apolipoprotein (apo) A1 interacts with the ABCA1 transporter to facilitate the removal of excess cholesterol from peripheral cells. The nascent high-density lipoprotein (HDL) formed following the interaction of apo A1 with the ABCA1 transporter on the cell membrane is converted to mature HDL by the LCAT (A). The genetic defect in Tangier disease (B) is a structural mutation in the ABCA1 transporter. The defect in the ABCA1 transporter results in decreased efflux of cholesterol from the cell and reduced lipidation of apo A1. The poorly lipidated HDL is rapidly degraded by the kidney, leading to the low plasma HDL levels characteristic of Tangier disease [28].

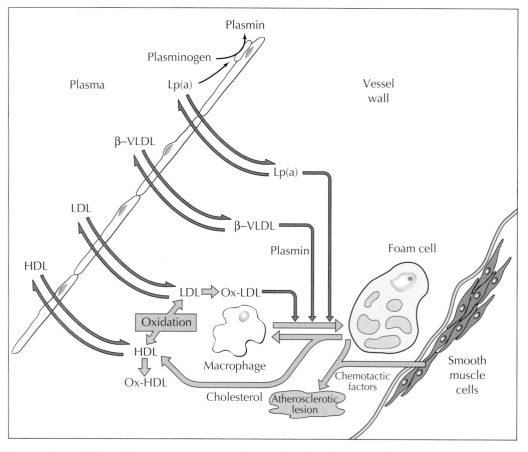

cardiovascular disease. Increased plasma concentrations of these lipoproteins are associated with increased diffusion into the vessel wall. The major atherogenic lipoprotein, LDL, requires oxidative modification to be taken up by the macrophage with the formation of foam cells. Elevated levels of β-VLDL and Lp(a) in the vessel wall are also associated with foam cell formation. Lp(a) may also contribute to the development of atherosclerosis by competition with plasminogen for the plasminogen receptor [29]. Thus, the atherogenic potential of Lp(a) may result from both uptake by the macro-phage with foam cell formation and its thrombotic potential as a competitor of plasminogen. Foam cell formation, macrophage activation, lipid oxidation, and endothelial cell injury all lead to the release of chemotactic factors that contribute to the development of the atherosclerotic lesion. The major antiatherogenic lipoprotein, high-density lipoprotein (HDL), protects against the development of foam cells and atherosclerosis by several potential mechanisms. One major proposed mechanism is reverse cholesterol transport, whereby HDL facilitates the removal of cholesterol from the foam cells and transports this cholesterol out of the vessel wall and back to the liver where it can be removed from the body. In addition, HDL may protect LDL from being oxidized (Ox) in the vessel wall.

FIGURE 7-11. Role of the plasma lipoproteins in the development of the atherosclerotic lesion. The development of the atherosclerotic lesion involves the interaction of lipoproteins with macrophages with the formation of foam cells, which are characteristic of early atherosclerosis. Elevated levels of three major classes of plasma lipoproteins—low-density lipoprotein (LDL), β–very low-density lipoprotein (B-VLDL) (remnant lipoproteins), and lipoprotein (a) (Lp[a])—have been associated with an increased risk of early

FAMILIAL HYPERALPHALIPOPROTEINEMIA

FAMILIAL HYPERALPHALIPOPROTEINEMIAS

Familial hyperalphalipoproteinemia with a **decreased** risk of premature cardiovascular disease
  Familial Apo A-I gene overexpression
  Familial hyperalphalipoproteinemia
Familial hyperalphalipoproteinemia with an **increased** risk of premature cardiovascular disease
  Cholesteryl ester transfer protein deficiency

FIGURE 7-12. Familial hyperalphalipoproteinemia, which is characterized by elevated plasma levels of high-density lipoprotein, has been proposed to be associated with a decreased and an increased risk of premature cardiovascular disease. Three genetic forms of familial hyperalphalipoproteinemia have been recognized.

FEATURES OF A KINDRED WITH FAMILIAL APO A-I GENE OVEREXPRESSION

Clinical features	No xanthomas or xanthelasma
Lipids	Plasma cholesterol increased
	Plasma triglycerides normal to increased
Lipoproteins	Chylomicrons normal
	VLDL increased
	LDL normal
Lipoprotein metabolism	HDL markedly increased
Cardiovascular disease	Selective increased synthesis of apo A-I
	Proposed decreased risk of premature cardiovascular disease

FIGURE 7-13. A single kindred has been reported with familial hyperalphalipoproteinemia, which was shown by apolipoprotein (apo) A-I and apo A-II kinetics studies to be caused by a selective increase in synthesis of apo A-I with normal apo A-II synthesis. The proband had no clinical manifestations as a result of elevated high-density lipoprotein (HDL) cholesterol levels. The apo A-I structural gene was normal and the increase in HDL was caused by increased plasma levels of apo A-I. Apo A-I and apo A-II in HDL were catabolized at a normal rate. The proband represents a unique example of selective overexpression of the apo A-I gene leading to elevated levels of HDL cholesterol. Analysis of the kindred was consistent with protection against the development of premature cardiovascular disease [30]. LDL—low-density lipoprotein; VLDL—very low-density lipoprotein.

CLINICAL LIPOPROTEIN AND APOLIPOPROTEIN PROFILE OF THE PROBAND WITH FAMILIAL APO A-I GENE OVEREXPRESSION

	APO A-I OVEREXPRESSION, mg/dL	CONTROLS, mg/dL
Plasma cholesterol	271	162±28
Plasma triglycerides	255	72±30
VLDL cholesterol	24	9±8
LDL cholesterol	117	139±40
HDL cholesterol	130	53±10
Apo A-I	241	136±15
Apo A-II	34	34±6
Apo B	103	120±20

FIGURE 7-14. Clinical lipoprotein and apolipoprotein profile of a 62-year-old female proband with overexpression of the apolipoprotein (apo) A-I gene, which results in markedly increased plasma levels of apo A-I and high-density lipoprotein (HDL) cholesterol. Plasma apo A-II levels are normal, and the increase in HDL cholesterol is due to an increase in apo A-I containing HDL. LDL—low-density lipoprotein; VLDL—very low-density lipoprotein.

FEATURES OF FAMILIAL HYPERALPHALIPOPROTEINEMIA

Clinical features	No xanthomas or xanthelasma
Lipids	Plasma cholesterol increased
	Plasma triglycerides normal
Lipoproteins	Chylomicrons normal
	VLDL normal
	LDL normal
	HDL markedly increased
Gene defect	Unknown
Cardiovascular disease	Proposed decreased risk of premature cardiovascular disease

FIGURE 7-15. Familial hyperalphalipoproteinemia is associated with an increase in high-density lipoprotein (HDL) cholesterol with relatively normal plasma low-density lipoprotein (LDL) cholesterol concentrations. The mode of inheritance has not been definitely determined; however, elevated HDL cholesterol is present in several members of the kindreds consistent with a familial inheritance of the elevated HDL cholesterol. There are no distinguishing clinical features and individuals with familial hyperalphalipoproteinemia have been reported to be protected against the development of premature cardiovascular disease. Some initially reported kindreds with familial hyperalphalipoproteinemia have been shown to have cholesteryl ester transfer protein (CETP) deficiency. VLDL—very low-density lipoprotein.

CLINICAL LIPOPROTEIN AND APOLIPOPROTEIN PROFILE OF A PROBAND WITH FAMILIAL HYPERALPHALIPOPROTEINEMIA

	HYPERALPHALIPOPROTEINEMIA, mg/dL	CONTROLS, mg/dL
Plasma cholesterol	282	162±28
Plasma triglycerides	79	72±30
VLDL cholesterol	12	9±8
LDL cholesterol	65	139±40
HDL cholesterol	200	53±10
Apo A-I	195	136±15
Apo A-II	35	34±6
Apo B	110	120±20

FIGURE 7-16. The apolipoprotein and lipoprotein profile of a 52-year-old female proband with familial hyperalphalipoproteinemia is characterized by increased plasma concentrations of apolipoprotein (apo) A-I and high-density lipoprotein (HDL) cholesterol. Kindreds with familial hyperalphalipoproteinemia have a reduced risk of premature cardiovascular disease. LDL—low-density lipoprotein; VLDL—very low-density lipoprotein.

FEATURES OF PROBANDS WITH CETP DEFICIENCY

Clinical features	No xanthomas or xanthelasma
Lipids	Plasma cholesterol increased
	Plasma triglycerides normal
Lipoproteins	Chylomicrons normal
	VLDL increased
	LDL decreased
	HDL markedly increased
Gene defect	Structural defect in the CETP gene
Cardiovascular disease	Risk of premature cardiovascular disease is still controversial

FIGURE 7-17. Cholesteryl ester transfer protein (CETP) deficiency is associated with a marked increase in high-density lipoprotein (HDL). To date the majority of patients with CETP deficiency have been reported from kindreds in Japan. There are no characteristic clinical features of CETP deficiency and the diagnosis may be suspected by a markedly elevated HDL cholesterol level. Mutations in the CETP gene result in CETP deficiency. Results of recent studies have been consistant with an increased risk of premature cardiovascular disease in individuals with CETP deficiency [31–34]. LDL—low-density lipoprotein; VLDL—very low-density lipoprotein.

CLINICAL LIPOPROTEIN AND APOLIPOPROTEIN PROFILE OF A PROBAND FROM A KINDRED WITH CETP DEFICIENCY

	CETP DEFICIENCY, mg/dL	CONTROLS, mg/dL
Plasma cholesterol	251	162±28
Plasma triglycerides	98	72±30
VLDL cholesterol	15	9±8
LDL cholesterol	59	139±40
HDL cholesterol	177	53±10
Apo A-I	268	136±15
Apo A-II	39	34±6
Apo B	81	120±20

FIGURE 7-18. Clinical lipoprotein and apolipoprotein profile of a 38-year-old male proband with cholesteryl ester transfer protein (CETP) deficiency. The marked elevations of plasma high-density lipoprotein (HDL) and apolipoprotein (apo) A-I are the most characteristic features of CETP deficiency. LDL—low-density lipoprotein; VLDL—very low-density lipoprotein.

FAMILIAL HYPOALPHALIPOPROTEINEMIA

CLASSIFICATION OF THE GENETIC DEFECTS IN FAMILIAL HYPOALPHALIPOPROTEINEMIA

Hypoalphalipoproteinemia with an *increased* risk of premature cardiovascular disease:
Apo A-I gene defects
Familial hypoalphalipoproteinemia
Hypertriglyceridemia-hypoalphalipoproteinemia syndrome
Tangier disease
Hypoalphalipoproteinemia with *no increased* risk of premature cardiovascular disease:
Lecithin:cholesterol acyltransferase deficiency
Familial hypoalphalipoproteinemia

FIGURE 7-19. Several different familial dyslipoproteinemias have been recognized that are characterized by low high-density lipoprotein (HDL) cholesterol levels. Not all individuals with familial hypoalphalipoproteinemia are at risk for the development of early heart disease, and the genetic defects are categorized based on the presence or absence of an increased risk of premature cardiovascular disease. The challenge for the physician is to identify 1) those individuals with low HDL cholesterol levels who are at an increased risk for the development of premature cardiovascular disease and require treatment from those probands of kindreds, with 2) familial hypoalphalipoproteinemia patients who are not at risk.

FIGURE 7-20. The apolipoprotein (apo) A-I:apo C-III:apo A-IV gene cluster. The tandem array of the genes for apos A-I, C-III, and A-IV on chromosome 11 account for the molecular defects observed in the different kindreds with defects in the A-I gene only, or genetic defects that also include C-III or C-III and A-IV.

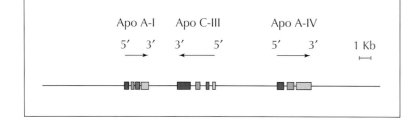

FEATURES OF KINDREDS WITH APO A-I GENE DEFECTS

Clinical feature	Planar xanthomas
Lipids	Plasma cholesterol normal
	Plasma triglycerides normal to decreased
Lipoproteins	Chylomicrons normal
	VLDL normal to decreased
	LDL normal to decreased
	HDL markedly decreased
Gene defect	Gene defect in the apo A-I gene; apo A-I + apo C-III genes; or apo A-I + apo C-III + apo A-IV genes
Cardiovascular disease	Increased risk of premature cardiovascular disease

FIGURE 7-21. A clinical feature that is unique in patients with mutations that results in loss of apolipoprotein (apo) A-I synthesis is planar xanthomas (*see* Fig. 7-23). The plasma lipids may be relatively normal and the characteristic lipoprotein change is a markedly decreased high-density lipoprotein (HDL) cholesterol level. The genetic defects reported have included structural mutations in the apo A-I gene [35–37], rearrangements in the apo A-I and apo C-III gene that lead to loss of both apo A-I and apo C-III [38], as well as deletions of the genome containing all three of the genes coding for apo A-I, apo C-III, and apo A-IV [39]. The kindred with apo A-I and apo C-III deficiency have reduced levels of very low-density lipoprotein (VLDL) and triglyceride-rich lipoproteins. Most kindreds that have a genetic defect leading to a deficiency of plasma apo A-I have an increased risk of premature cardiovascular disease. LDL—low-density lipoprotein.

CLINICAL LIPOPROTEIN AND APOLIPOPROTEIN PROFILE OF A PROBAND WITH A STRUCTURAL DEFECT IN THE APO A-I GENE

	APO A-I GENE DEFECT, *mg/dL*	CONTROLS, *mg/dL*
Plasma cholesterol	187	162±28
Plasma triglycerides	129	72±30
VLDL cholesterol	26	9±8
LDL cholesterol	152	39±40
HDL cholesterol	9	53±10
Apo A-I	0	136±15
Apo A-II	20	34±6
Apo B	123	120±20

FIGURE 7-22. Lipoprotein and apolipoprotein (apo) profile present in a 28-year-old male with a structural defect in the apo A-I gene resulting in a deficiency of plasma apo A-I and markedly reduced high-density lipoprotein (HDL) cholesterol levels. Premature cardiovascular disease was present in this proband, illustrating the increased risk of coronary heart disease in patients with a deficiency of apo A-I and HDL. LDL—low-density lipoprotein; VLDL—very low-density lipoprotein.

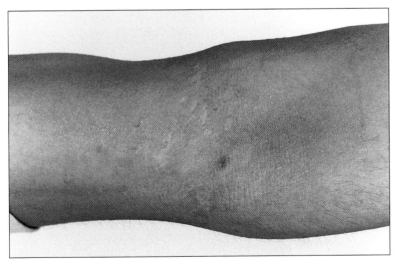

FIGURE 7-23. (*see* Color Plate) Flat planar xanthomas are characteristic of patients with markedly reduced plasma high-density lipoprotein (HDL) cholesterol due to structural defects in the apolipoprotein (apo) A-I gene. These xanthomas are usually present on the arms and trunk and have an orange hue.

FEATURES OF KINDREDS WITH FAMILIAL HYPOALPHALIPOPROTEINEMIA AND INCREASED RISK OF PREMATURE CARDIOVASCULAR DISEASE

Clinical features	No xanthomas or xanthelasma
Lipids	Plasma cholesterol normal
	Plasma triglycerides normal
Lipoproteins	Chylomicrons normal
	VLDL normal
	LDL normal
	HDL decreased
Gene defect	Unknown
Cardiovascular disease	Increased risk of premature cardiovascular disease

FIGURE 7-24. Kindreds with familial hypoalphalipoproteinemia with normal triglycerides may have an increased risk of premature cardiovascular disease. There are no characteristic clinical features and the plasma lipids and lipoproteins are often normal except for the reduced plasma levels of high-density lipoprotein (HDL) cholesterol. The genetic defects leading to familial hypoalphalipoproteinemia have not been identified. Patients with coronary heart disease with "normal lipids" may be members of kindreds with familial hypoalphalipoproteinemia. LDL—low-density lipoprotein; VLDL—very low-density lipoprotein.

LIPOPROTEIN AND APOLIPOPROTEIN PROFILE OF A PROBAND WITH FAMILIAL HYPOALPHALIPOPROTEINEMIA

	HYPOALPHALIPOPROTEINEMIA, mg/dL	CONTROLS, mg/dL
Plasma cholesterol	78	162±28
Plasma triglycerides	64	72±30
VLDL cholesterol	5	9±8
LDL cholesterol	51	139±40
HDL cholesterol	22	53±10
Apo A-I	50	136±15
Apo A-II	22	34±6
Apo B	57	120±20

FIGURE 7-25. Lipoprotein and apolipoprotein (apo) profile of a 38-year-old male proband with familial hypoalphalipoproteinemia with decreased plasma high-density lipoprotein (HDL) cholesterol levels, apo A-I, and apo A-II. This kindred was characterized by patients with low HDL cholesterol levels and premature cardiovascular disease. LDL—low-density lipoprotein; VLDL—very low-density lipoprotein.

FEATURES OF A PROBAND WITH THE FAMILIAL HYPERTRIGLYCERIDEMIA-HYPOALPHALIPOPROTEINEMIA SYNDROME

Clinical features	No xanthomas or xanthelasma
Lipids	Plasma cholesterol normal to increased
	Plasma triglycerides increased
Lipoproteins	Chylomicrons normal
	VLDL increased
	LDL normal to decreased
	HDL decreased
Lipoprotein metabolism	Increased catabolism of HDL
Gene defect	Unknown
Cardiovascular disease	Increased risk of premature cardiovascular disease

FIGURE 7-26. A common dyslipoproteinemia observed in patients with established coronary heart disease is elevated triglycerides, dense low-density lipoprotein (LDL), and decreased high-density lipoprotein (HDL) cholesterol. There are no characteristic clinical features, and patients have a significantly increased risk of premature heart disease. The lipid and lipoprotein profile may vary depending on the diet and lifestyle; however, the hypertriglyceridemia and hypoalphalipoproteinemia are persistent. The increased risk for the development of premature coronary heart disease may be due to the combination of the elevated atherogenic remnants of triglyceride-rich particles, dense LDL, and low HDL. VLDL—very low-density lipoprotein.

LIPOPROTEIN AND APOLIPOPROTEIN PROFILE OF A PROBAND WITH ESTABLISHED CORONARY HEART DISEASE

	HYPERTRIGLYCERIDEMIA–HYPOALPHALIPOPROTEINEMIA SYNDROME, mg/dL	CONTROLS, mg/dL
Plasma cholesterol	250	162±28
Plasma triglycerides	383	72±30
VLDL cholesterol	86	9±8
LDL cholesterol	139	139±40
HDL cholesterol	25	53±10
Apo A-I	85	136±15
Apo A-II	22	34±6
Apo B	210	120±20

FIGURE 7-27. Clinical lipoprotein and apolipoprotein (apo) profile of a 42-year-old proband with established coronary heart disease and a lipoprotein profile characteristic of the familial hypertriglyceridemia-hypoalphalipoproteinemia syndrome with low plasma high-density lipoprotein (HDL) cholesterol and high triglyceride levels. LDL—low-density lipoprotein; VLDL—very low-density lipoprotein.

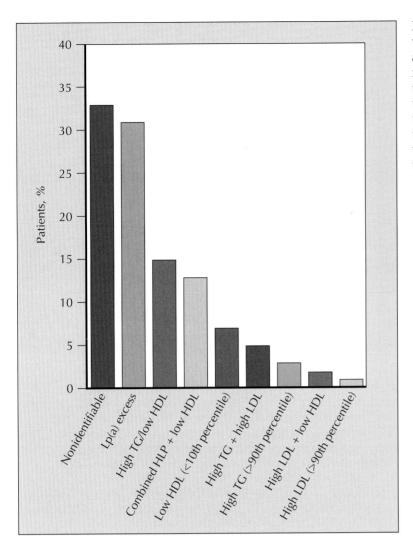

FIGURE 7-28. Frequency of genetic dyslipoproteinemias in patients with established coronary artery disease. An evaluation of patients admitted with the diagnosis of premature myocardial infarction revealed that 67% of patients had an underlying genetic dyslipoproteinemia [40]. A depressed high-density lipoprotein (HDL) cholesterol concentration was present in 42% of these patients. The hypertriglyceridemia-hypoalphalipoproteinemia syndrome (high triglyceride [TG], low HDL) was present in 15% of the probands with established coronary artery disease. HLP—hyperlipoproteinemia; Lp(a)–lipoprotein (a).

FEATURES OF KINDREDS WITH TANGIER DISEASE

Clinical features	Cloudy corneas
	Orange tonsils
	Intermittent neuropathy
Lipids	Plasma cholesterol normal to decreased
	Plasma triglycerides increased
Lipoproteins	Chylomicrons normal
	VLDL increased
	LDL normal to decreased
	HDL markedly decreased
Lipoprotein metabolism	Increased catabolism of HDL
Gene defect	Unknown
Cardiovascular disease	Mild increased risk of premature cardiovascular disease

FIGURE 7-29. Tangier disease is characterized by cloudy corneas, intermittent peripheral neuropathy, and orange tonsils. Hypertriglyceridemia, low in low-density lipoprotein (LDL) cholesterol, and a severe reduction in high-density lipoprotein (HDL) cholesterol are the typical changes in plasma lipids and lipoproteins observed in patients with Tangier disease. The decreased HDL levels are due to increased catabolism of apo A-I and apo A-II [41]. The genetic defect in Tangier disease is a mutation in the ABCA1 transporter [28]. There is a mildy increased risk of cardiovascular disease in patients with Tangier disease [42,43]. VLDL—very low-density lipoprotein.

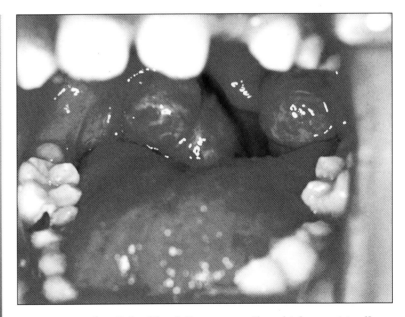

FIGURE 7-30. (*see* Color Plate) Orange tonsils, which are virtually pathognomonic of Tangier disease, are the result of massive lipid accumulation in the lymphoid tissues. Histologic analysis of the tonsilar tissue reveals cholesterol-loaded macrophages.

LIPOPROTEIN AND APOLIPOPROTEIN PROFILE OF A PROBAND WITH TANGIER DISEASE

	TANGIER DISEASE, mg/dL	CONTROLS, mg/dL
Plasma cholesterol	43	162±28
Plasma triglycerides	408	72±30
VLDL cholesterol	81	9±8
LDL cholesterol	5	139±40
HDL cholesterol	7	53±10
Apo A-I	15	136±15
Apo A-II	4	34±6
Apo B	89	120±20

FIGURE 7-31. The lipoprotein and apolipoprotein (apo) profile of a 32-year-old proband from a kindred with Tangier disease. Plasma apo A-I, apo A-II, high-density lipoprotein (HDL) cholesterol, as well as low-density lipoprotein (LDL) cholesterol are decreased and triglycerides are increased. VLDL—very low-density lipoprotein.

FEATURES OF KINDREDS WITH CLASSIC LCAT DEFICIENCY

Clinical features	Cloudy corneas
	Renal disease
	Hemolytic anemia
Lipids	Plasma cholesterol normal
	Plasma triglycerides increased
Lipoproteins	Chylomicrons normal
	VLDL increased
	LDL normal to decreased
	HDL markedly decreased
Lipoprotein metabolism	Increased catabolism of HDL
Gene defect	Structural defect in LCAT gene
Cardiovascular disease	No increased risk of premature cardiovascular disease

FIGURE 7-32. Patients with familial classic lecithin:cholesterol acyltransferase (LCAT) deficiency have cloudy corneas, hemolytic anemia, and mild to severe renal disease. The lipid and lipoprotein profiles are characterized by hypertriglyceridemia and markedly decreased levels of high-density lipoprotein (HDL) cholesterol. The molecular defect is a structural mutation in the LCAT gene. Structural mutations in the LCAT gene with a small amount of residual LCAT activity have a different clinical phenotype with no renal disease or hemolytic anemia, but patients with severe cloudy corneas are designated as having CLC fish eye disease. There is no apparent increased risk of premature cardiovascular disease in patients with classic familial LCAT deficiency or fish eye disease. LDL—low density lipoprtein; VLDL—very low-density lipoprotein.

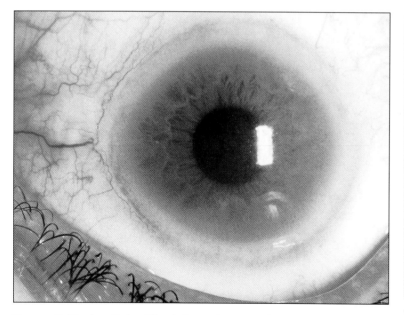

FIGURE 7-33. (*see* Color Plate) Opacification of the cornea is a striking clinical feature of patients with familial lecithin:cholesterol acyltransferase deficiency. The corneal opacification reflects the loss of reverse cholesterol transport from tissues of these patients.

LIPOPROTEIN AND APOLIPOPROTEIN PROFILE OF A PROBAND WITH CLASSIC LCAT DEFICIENCY

	LCAT DEFICIENCY, mg/dL	CONTROLS, mg/dL
Plasma cholesterol	169	162±28
Plasma triglycerides	675	72±30
VLDL cholesterol	72	9±8
LDL cholesterol	90	139±40
HDL cholesterol	7	53±10
Apo A-I	30	136±15
Apo A-II	5	34±6
Apo B	4	120±20

FIGURE 7-34. Plasma lipoproteins and apolipoproteins (apos) of a 29-year-old proband with familial lecithin:cholesterol acyltransferase (LCAT) deficiency demonstrating decreased plasma high-density lipoprotein (HDL) cholesterol, plasma apo A-I, and apo A-II as well as increased plasma triglycerides. Despite the low plasma HDL cholesterol levels, patients with classic LCAT deficiency have no increased risk of premature cardiovascular disease. LDL—low-density lipoprotein; VLDL—very low-density lipoprotein.

DIETARY FAT COMPOSITION AND CARDIOVASCULAR DISEASE RISK

DIET AND THE PATHOGENESIS OF ATHEROSCLEROSIS

FACTOR	EFFECT
Saturated fat, cholesterol	↑LDL cholesterol
Salt, heavy ethanol consumption	Hypertension
Central obesity	Dyslipidemia, hypertension, insulin resistance and hyperinsulinemia, glucose intolerance and NIDDM

FIGURE 8-3. Diet and the pathogenesis of atherosclerosis. The various dietary factors that influence atherogenesis appear to function by different mechanisms. For example, saturated fat and dietary cholesterol increase plasma low-density lipoprotein (LDL) cholesterol levels, which in turn cause lipid accumulation in the artery wall and modulate other biologic mechanisms involved in atherogenesis. Salt and heavy ethanol consumption increase cardiovascular risk by increasing blood pressure, whereas light (one or two drinks per day) ethanol consumption may reduce risk. Central obesity, which results from caloric intake that chronically exceeds energy expenditure in genetically susceptible individuals, is associated with several intermediate markers of atherosclerotic disease. These include dyslipidemia, hypertension, insulin resistance and hyperinsulinemia, and impaired glucose tolerance, including non–insulin-dependent diabetes mellitus (NIDDM). These all improve when body weight is lost and is stabilized at lower levels.

DIETARY COMPOSITION OF PEOPLE IN THE WESTERN HEMISPHERE

MEAN FOOD ENERGY AND FAT/SATURATED FAT INTAKE FROM USDA SURVEYS FOR SELECTED SEX/AGE GROUPS

	MEN AGED 19–50					WOMEN AGED 19–50				
	MEAN ENERGY INTAKE, KCAL	ENERGY FAT, %	SATURATED FAT, %	MEAN TOTAL FAT/G	MEAN SATURATED FAT G	MEAN ENERGY INTAKE	ENERGY FAT, %	ENERGY SATURATED FAT, %	MEAN TOTAL FAT G	MEAN SATURATED FAT G
HFCS spring 1965	2875	43.7		143.6		1785	41.9		85.5	
NFCS 1977 to 1978	2423	41.4		113.3		1590	40.9		73.8	
CSFII 1985	2548	41.5	13.3	105.7		1655	36.7	13.5	68.8	
CSFII 1986						1582	36.4	13.3	65.4	
NFCS 1987 to 1988	2272	37.3	13.4	95.4	34.4	1543	36.2	13.0	63.3	22.9
CSFII 1989 to 1991	2349	35.4	12.5	93.7	33.1	1616	34.4	12.0	63.2	22.1
CSFII 1994	2659	33.7	11.3	100.8	34.1	1699	32.5	10.9	62.7	21.0
CSFII 1985	2667	33.1	11.3	100.6	34.6	1758	32.8	11.1	65.5	22.1

FIGURE 8-4. Secular trends in dietary fat consumption and age-adjusted mean serum cholesterol in the United States using data from the US Department of Agriculture (USDA). The mean fat intake (expressed as a percentage of calories) and the mean serum cholesterol level in the United States have fallen progressively in both men and women from the 1960s through 1995. The sources of the data are designated in the table. At the same time, there has been a progressive decline in coronary heart disease (CHD) morbidity and mortality (data not shown). If this downward trend in both saturated fat intake and serum cholesterol values continues, mean cholesterol levels in both genders should reach a goal of approximately 200 mg/dL by the year 2010 CSFII—Continuing Survey of Food Intake II; HFCS—Nationwide Consumption Survey; NFCS—Household Food Consumption Survey.

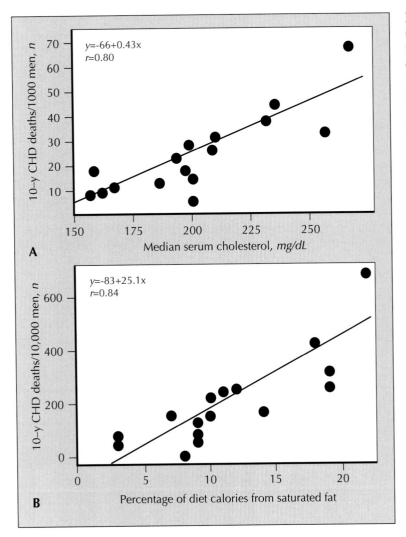

A

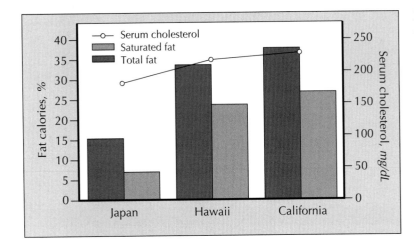

B

FIGURE 8-5. Comparison of the rates of coronary heart disease (CHD) mortality and serum cholesterol levels in residents of countries consuming different average amounts of dietary fat and cholesterol. In 16 population groups from seven countries [1,2], there was a linear relationship between 10-year CHD mortality rates and median serum cholesterol levels (**A**).

A similar relationship was demonstrated between CHD mortality rates and percentage of calories from fat (**B**). For example, in those countries where the consumption of fat constituted about 40% of calories and saturated fat accounted for about 20% of calories such as in Finland, the United States, and the Netherlands, there were higher average serum cholesterol levels and increased mortality from CHD as compared with countries such as Japan and Greece, where saturated fat consumption was less than 10% of calories and serum cholesterol levels were lower. (**A** *adapted from* Keys *et al.* [2]; **B** *adapted from* Keys *et al.* [3].)

FIGURE 8-6. Correlation between increasing dietary fat and serum cholesterol, in populations migrating to countries with different dietary habits. In the Ni-Hon-San Study, dietary habits, serum cholesterol, and mortality from coronary heart disease (CHD) were recorded in men of Japanese ancestry living either in Japan, Honolulu, or San Francisco. As dietary habits changed toward those of the host country, the intake of saturated fat rose from 7% of calories in Japan to 12% in Honolulu and 14% in San Francisco. This was associated with similar increases in dietary cholesterol and resulted in increases in serum cholesterol, mean body weights, and mortality from CHD. (*Adapted from* Kato *et al.* [4].)

COMMON FATTY ACIDS

CODE	COMMON NAME
Saturated	
12:0	Lauric acid
14:0	Myristic acid
16:0	Palmitic acid
18:0	Stearic acid
Monounsaturated	
16:1n-7 *cis*	Palmitoleic acid
18:1n-9 *cis*	Oleic acid
18:1n-9 *trans*	Elaidic acid
Polyunsaturated	
18:2n-6,9 all *cis*	Linoleic acid
18:3n-3,6,9 all *cis*	α-linolenic acid
18:3n-6,9,12 all *cis*	γ-linolenic acid
20:4n-6,9,12,15 all *cis*	Arachidonic acid
20:5n-3,6,9,12,15 all *cis*	Eicosapentaenoic acid
22:6n-3,6,9,12,15,18 all *cis*	Docosahexaenoic acid

FIGURE 8-7. Common fatty acids found in food and the human body. Saturated fatty acids, monosaturated (*ie*, containing one double bond) and polyunsaturated fatty acids (*ie*, containing two or more double bonds) are shown. Three saturated fatty acids (lauric, myristic, and palmitic) have the most pronounced low-density lipoprotein (LDL) cholesterol–elevating effect, whereas the effect of stearic acid tends to be neutral. Relative to these fatty acids, both monounsaturated and polyunsaturated fats have an LDL-lowering effect.

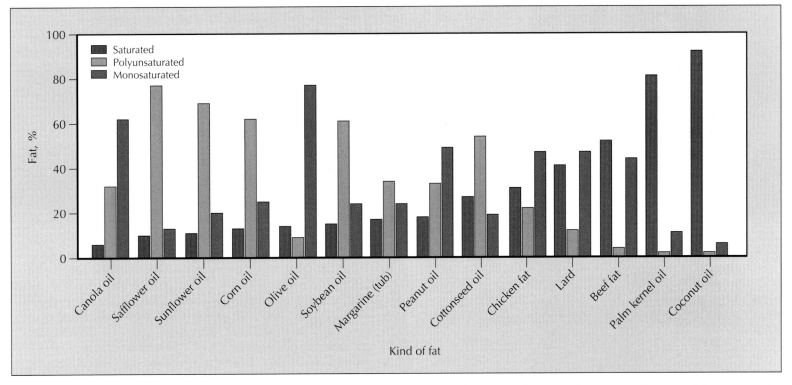

FIGURE 8-8. Common sources of fat in the diet arranged by relative proportion of saturated fat. Diets higher in fats that contain monounsaturated and polyunsaturated fatty acids and lower in those fats that contain saturated fatty acids are associated with a lower risk of developing cardiovascular heart disease [5].

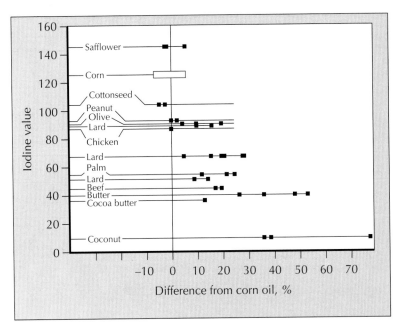

FIGURE 8-9. Serum cholesterol–elevating effects of dietary fats compared with those of corn oil. Saturated fats such as those found in chicken fat, lard, palm oil, beef fat, cocoa butter, butter, and coconut oil increased serum cholesterol levels relative to corn oil–enriched diets. There is an inverse relationship between iodine value, which represents the degree of unsaturation of the fat, and the increase in serum cholesterol relative to the corn oil–enriched diet. Fats that consist largely of saturated fatty acids thus tend to increase serum cholesterol significantly more than unsaturated fatty acids such as canola oil, soybean oil, olive oil, peanut oil, cottonseed oil, and safflower oil. Serum cholesterol generally increases approximately 2 to 3 mg/dL for every 1% of calories that are consumed as saturated fatty acids (see Fig. 8-17). (*Adapted from* Ahrens *et al.* [6].)

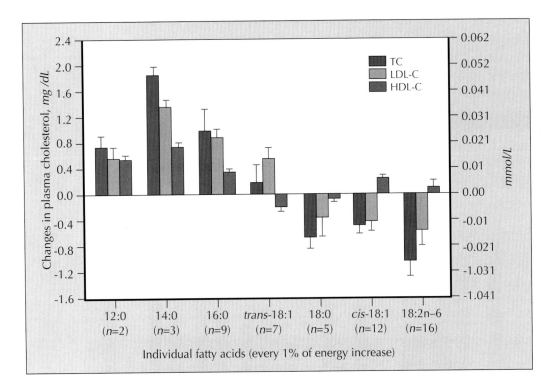

FIGURE 8-10. Individual saturated, monounsaturated, and polyunsaturated fatty acids and plasma cholesterol levels. The effect of oleic acid (18:1) on total cholesterol (TC), low-density lipoprotein (LDL) cholesterol (LDL-C) and high-density lipoprotein (HDL) cholesterol (HDL-C) levels was calculated by comparing the response reported for carbohydrate (assumed to be a neutral reference point). The effects of other fatty acids were estimated by making comparisons with oleic acid (18:1). Saturated fatty acids (with the exception of stearic acid) and *trans* fatty acids tend to raise LDL and HDL cholesterol levels, whereas unsaturated fatty acids tend to lower both. (*Adapted from* Kris-Etherton and Yu [7].)

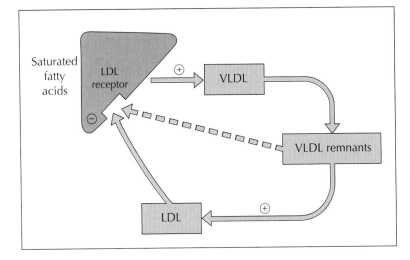

FIGURE 8-11. Proposed mechanism by which dietary saturated fatty acids raise serum cholesterol. low-density lipoprotein (LDL) is derived from very low-density lipoprotein (VLDL), which enters plasma from the liver. LDL is removed from plasma after binding to LDL receptors, predominantly in the liver. A mechanism by which dietary saturated fatty acids elevate the LDL cholesterol level appears to be downregulation of expression of hepatic LDL receptors. Dietary saturated fatty acids have been shown to inhibit LDL receptor activity, although the mechanism of action remains unclear. Serum cholesterol–raising saturated fatty acids also appear to increase LDL production rates.

FOODS LOW IN SATURATED FAT

Fruits and vegetables
Grains and cereals
Nonfat and low-fat dairy products
Fish, lean meat, and poultry without skin
Vegetable oils (except palm, palm kernal, and coconut oils)

FIGURE 8-12. Foods low in saturated fat. Foods low in saturated fat include fruits and vegetables; grains and cereals; nonfat and low-fat dairy products such as nonfat (skim) milk and yogurt; fish, lean meat, and poultry without skin; and vegetable oils (except palm, palm kernel, and coconut oils). When fats are partially hydrogenated, their content of *trans* fatty acids increases and intake should be limited, as should products made from them (*ie*, baked goods, prepared fried foods) (see Fig. 8-21).

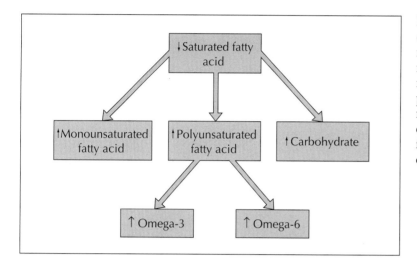

FIGURE 8-13. Replacement of saturated fatty acids in the diet. A decrease in the amount of saturated fatty acids, without replacement, results in reduced caloric intake. A reduction in the saturated fat content of the diet also can be achieved isocalorically by replacing the saturated fatty acids with either carbohydrates, polyunsaturated fatty acids (either omega-6 or omega-3), or monounsaturated fatty acids. Because saturated fat and cholesterol often are found in the same foods, a reduction in the saturated fatty acid content of the diet is also accompanied by a reduction in dietary cholesterol.

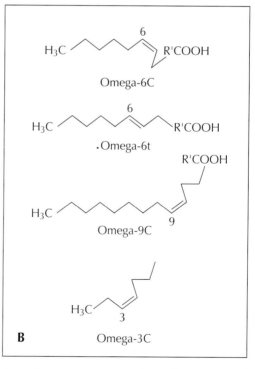

A. NOMENCLATURE OF UNSATURATED FATTY ACIDS

FAMILY	FATTY ACID	DIETARY SOURCES
Omega-6	Linoleic acid (C18:2 ω–6)	Vegetable oils
Omega-9	Oleic acid (C18:1 ω–9)	Vegetable oils, animal fats
Omega-3	Eicosapentaenoic acid (C20:5 ω–3)	Marine oils, fish
trans	Elaidic acid (C)8:1ω9t)	Hydrogenated fat Dairy fat

FIGURE 8-14. Nomenclature (**A**) and structure (**B**) of unsaturated fatty acids. The three major classes of unsaturated fatty acids (omega-3, -6, and -9) derive their names from the number of carbons from the methyl end at which the first double bond appears. For example, linoleic acid (with 18 carbons and two double bonds, the first of which occurs six carbons from the methyl end) is a prototype of an omega-6 fatty acid that is found predominantly in vegetable oils. Elaidic acid is also an omega-3 fatty acid, but has a double bond in the *trans* configuration rather than the more common *cis* configuration. The *trans* fatty acids are found predominantly in hydrogenated fat. Oleic acid (with 18 carbons and one double bond at the ninth carbon from the methyl end) is an omega-9 monounsaturated fatty acid found in certain vegetables and also in animal fats, where it occurs together with saturated fatty acids. Eicosapentaenoic acid (with 20 carbons and five double bonds, the first being at the third carbon from the methyl end) is a classic omega-3 fatty acid found predominantly in marine oils.

DIETARY SOURCES OF POLYUNSATURATED FATTY ACIDS

OMEGA-6 POLYUNSATURATES (LINOLEIC ACID)	OMEGA-3 POLYUNSATURATES
Soybean oil	Fish oils
Safflower oil	
Sunflower seed oil	
Corn oil	

FIGURE 8-15. Dietary sources of polyunsaturated fatty acids. Omega-6 polyunsaturated fatty acids tend to occur mainly in vegetable oils such as those from soybeans, safflowers, sunflower seeds, and corn. Although they all contain a relatively high proportion of linoleic acid (18:2), they also contain other fatty acids, including some saturated fatty acids. Omega-3 polyunsaturated fatty acids, especially eicosapentaenoic acid (20:5) and docosahexaenoic acid (22:6), tend to be found predominantly in fatty fish oils and in blubber from marine mammals. Linoleic acid, also an omega-3 fatty acid, is found predominantly in soybean and canola oils.

FOODS RICH IN MONO-UNSATURATED FATTY ACIDS

Canola (rape seed) oil
Olive oil
Peanut oil
Nuts
Avocados

FIGURE 8-16. Sources of monounsaturated fatty acids (oleic acid). The major oils that contain monounsaturated fatty acids are rape seed (canola), olives, and peanut. All these oils also contain small amounts of saturated and unsaturated fatty acids. Nuts and avocados are also rich dietary sources of monounsaturated fatty acids.

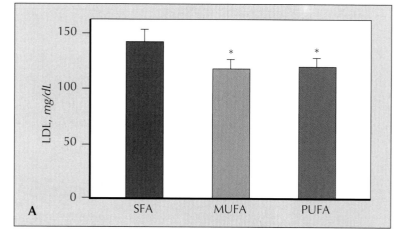

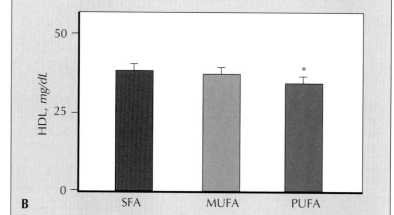

FIGURE 8-17. Effect of dietary fat on plasma lipoproteins. The effect of diets rich in either saturated fatty acids (SFAs), monounsaturated fatty acids (MUFAs), or polyunsaturated fatty acids (PUFAs) on plasma low-density lipoprotein (LDL) and high-density lipoprotein (HDL) cholesterol levels are shown. Both unsaturated fatty acid–rich diets led to a similar degree of reduction of LDL cholesterol levels (**A**). HDL cholesterol level is not significantly different following consumption of either the saturated and monounsaturated fatty acid–rich diets (**B**), although it fell slightly, but significantly, in study subjects consuming polyunsaturated fatty acid–rich diets [8]. Several other studies [8–11], however, have failed to demonstrate a difference in HDL cholesterol levels when comparing diets enriched in PUFAs with MUFAs. Data shown are the mean ± SD from a study of 12 normotriglyceridemic patients. *Asterisks* represent $P < 0.001$ for LDL and $P < 0.02$ for HDL. (*Adapted from* Mattson and Grundy [8].)

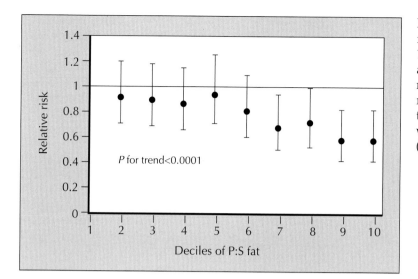

FIGURE 8-18. Multivariate relative risks of coronary heart disease rated by deciles of polyunsaturated (P) to saturated (S) fat (12:0 to 18:0). Diets relatively low in polyunsaturated fatty acids (fats of animal origin) are associated with a high risk of developing coronary heart disease. In contrast, diets relatively high in polyunsaturated fatty acids (fats of vegetable origin) with the exception of tropical oils (palm, palm kernal, and coconut oil) are associated with a lower risk of coronary heart disease. (*Adapted from* Hu *et al.* [12].)

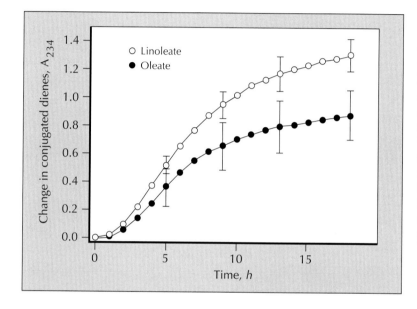

FIGURE 8-19. Dietary effects on the susceptibility of LDL to oxidation. In this study by Reaven *et al.* [13], 13 mildly hypercholesterolemic volunteers consumed either an oleate-enriched diet prepared from an oleate-rich sunflower oil or a linoleate-enriched diet prepared with sunflower oil for 8 weeks. Following isolation of plasma low-density lipoprotein (LDL), the lipoproteins were oxidized. The rate of oxidation was followed by analyzing the formation of conjugated dienes, a measure of lipid peroxidation. The LDL isolated from those study participants who had consumed the linoleate-enriched diet formed conjugated dienes more rapidly and to a greater extent than the corresponding LDL from those who had consumed the oleate-enriched diet. The physiologic significance of this finding with respect to the development of cardiovascular disease continues to be an active area of investigation. (*Adapted from* Reaven *et al.* [13].)

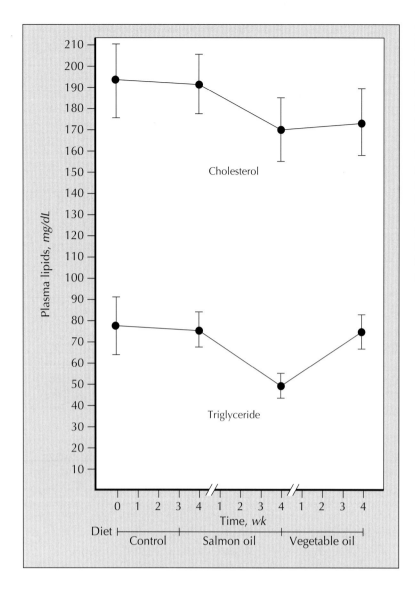

FIGURE 8-20. Effect of fish oils (omega-3 fatty acids) on plasma lipids. In hypertriglyceridemia study subjects, supplements of omega-3 fatty acids primarily lower very low-density lipoprotein (VLDL) levels, which leads to a reduction in both triglycerides and cholesterol. However, low-density lipoprotein (LDL) cholesterol levels do not change (not shown). High-density lipoprotein (HDL) levels tend to increase, as is commonly seen, when triglyceride levels decrease. Several studies in both humans and experimental animals have suggested that omega-3 fatty acids may reduce atherosclerotic artery disease. Several mechanisms may be responsible for this response. Diets rich in fish oils tend to be low in saturated fatty acids. Omega-3 fatty acids may have an antithrombotic effect, both by interfering with platelet aggregation and by modulating prostaglandin and leukotriene metabolism, which in turn may also affect vascular tone. These fatty acids may thus be antithrombotic (see Fig. 8-39), with consequent effects on atherogenesis and thrombosis.

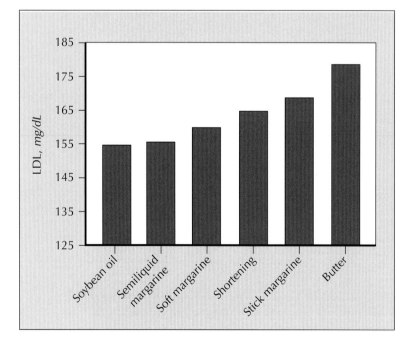

FIGURE 8-21. Effect of hydrogenated fat (*trans* fatty acids) and butter on plasma low-density lipoprotein (LDL) cholesterol levels. In moderately hypercholesterolemic subjects, changing the type of fat in the diet, from soybean oil in the natural state, to ones that have increasing degrees of hydrogenation, hence *trans* fatty acids, results in a progressive increase in LDL cholesterol levels. Likewise, replacing soybean oil with butter results in increased LDL cholesterol levels. This and other similar studies suggest that in addition to recommending restrictions, the saturated fat content of the diet, the restrictions in the *trans* fatty acid content of the diet should also be made.

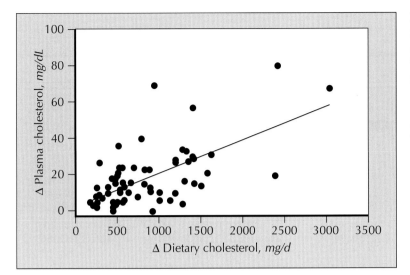

FIGURE 8-22. Relationship between change in dietary cholesterol intake and serum cholesterol levels. The data shown represent 68 clinical studies in 1490 patients summarized by McNamara [15]. There is a positive and significant correlation between the increment in dietary cholesterol intake (in milligrams per day) and the average change in plasma cholesterol levels (in milligrams per deciliter). This change represents an average 1.8 mg/dL change in cholesterol for every 100-mg increment in dietary cholesterol. When the data are normalized per 100 mg/d increment in dietary cholesterol, similar values are obtained, with a mean increase in serum cholesterol of 2.3 mg/dL for every 100 mg/d increase in dietary cholesterol. (*Adapted from* McNamara [15].)

MAJOR SOURCES OF DIETARY CHOLESTEROL

Eggs (yolks)
Dairy fats (milk, cheese, ice cream, butter)
Meat, poultry, fish, shellfish
Organ meats (liver, kidney, sweetbreads, brains)

FIGURE 8-23. Major sources of dietary cholesterol. Dietary cholesterol often occurs in the same foods as saturated fat (*eg*, dairy products, meat, and poultry). The major sources of dietary cholesterol are listed. Egg yolks and dairy products are rich sources of dietary cholesterol, as are all foods rich in mammalian cells. Although eggs and shellfish are a rich source of cholesterol, they are low in saturated fat.

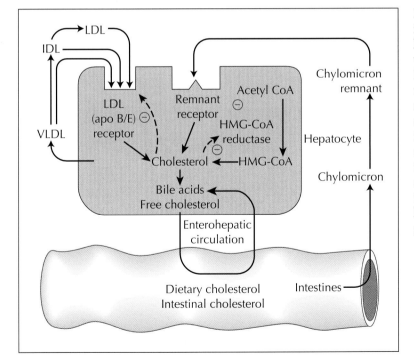

FIGURE 8-24. Proposed mechanisms by which dietary cholesterol influences serum and low-density lipoprotein (LDL) levels. The hepatocyte obtains its cholesterol from chylomicron remnants, very low-density lipoprotein (VLDL), intermediate-density lipoprotein (IDL), and LDL, and endogenous synthesis. The liver uses cholesterol for membrane synthesis, VLDL synthesis, and bile acid synthesis. In addition, it has the capacity to secrete free cholesterol directly into bile. Delivery of exogenous cholesterol to the hepatocyte inhibits the synthesis of new LDL receptors and downregulates hydroxymethyl glutaryl (HMG)-apo B/E reductase, the rate-limiting enzyme in cholesterol synthesis. Thus, dietary cholesterol suppresses the uptake of plasma LDL cholesterol, thereby increasing plasma LDL levels as well as inhibiting hepatic cholesterol synthesis. HMG-CoA—hydroxymethyl glutaryl coenzyme A.

OBESITY

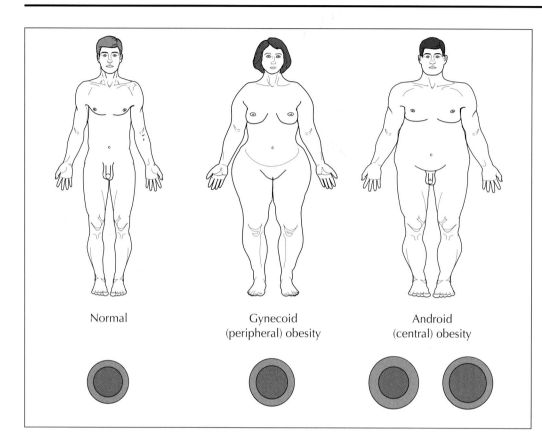

FIGURE 8-25. The two major forms of obesity. In gynecoid obesity, which occurs more frequently in females than males, distribution of excess fat is predominantly around the buttocks and thighs, whereas upper body fat distribution tends to be normal. Android obesity occurs more commonly in males and postmenopausal women than females; although the limbs tend to be normal, most of the fat is deposited around the abdomen and chest. Fat deposition in central obesity can either be predominantly subcutaneous, in which most of the excess fat occurs outside the abdominal cavity (central, subcutaneous obesity) or there can be an increased deposition of adipose tissue around the abdominal viscera (central visceral obesity). Central obesity tends to be associated with several atherogenic disorders (see Fig. 8-27). There is a hierarchy of association of obesity with atherosclerotic complication such that central visceral obesity is more commonly associated than central subcutaneous obesity, which occurs with greater frequency than gynecoid obesity. Although central obesity is more common in men, when it occurs in women it has the same metabolic and atherogenic consequences as in men.

Normal

Gynecoid (peripheral) obesity

Android (central) obesity

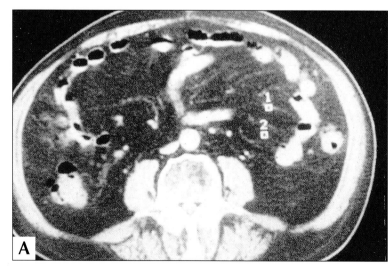

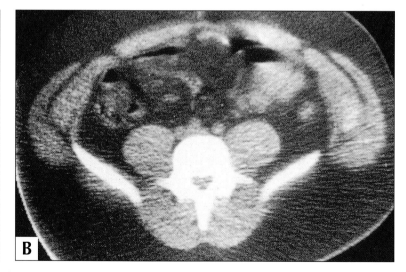

FIGURE 8-26. Computed tomography to demonstrate distribution of abdominal fat. CT across the central abdomen aorta is the best method of distinguishing visceral from subcutaneous fat deposition. The *black areas* represent fat. **A,** This patient clearly has an intra-abdominal (visceral) distribution of his adipose tissue that surrounds the viscera. The amount of subcutaneous fat is normal. **B,** Although having a similar abdominal circumference as the patient in **A,** this subject demonstrates a clearly different distribution of abdominal fat. There is little fat surrounding the viscera; most of the excess fat is deposited subcutaneously and outside the abdominal cavity.

ATHEROGENIC ASSOCIATIONS WITH CENTRAL OBESITY

Insulin resistance
Glucose intolerance and NIDDM
Dyslipidemia
   Hypertriglyceridemia
   Small VLDL and remnants
   Low HDL
   Small, dense LDL
Hypertension

FIGURE 8-27. Atherogenic associations with central obesity. Central, particularly visceral, obesity is associated with several metabolic and other disturbances that may increase the risk of cardiovascular disease (frequently referred to as "metabolic syndrome" or "syndrome X"). These include 1) insulin resistance; 2) glucose intolerance, which sometimes manifests as non–insulin-dependent diabetes mellitus (NIDDM); 3) dyslipidemia; and 4) hypertension. The attendant dyslipidemia reflects one or more of the following abnormalities: hypertriglyceridemia because of the presence of small very low-density lipoprotein (VLDL) particles and their remnants; low levels of high-density lipoprotein (HDL); and the presence of small, dense low-density lipoprotein particles. Often this hypertriglyceridemia and low HDL are not very well marked. However, this combination of risk factors is associated with a markedly increased risk of atherosclerotic complications. The constellation of central obesity and insulin resistance, glucose intolerance or NIDDM (or both), dyslipidemia, and hypertension has been termed the "deadly quartet," syndrome X, or metabolic syndrome. The relationship between obesity and atherosclerosis therefore likely partially results from clustering of cardiovascular risk factors that are associated with central obesity.

CARBOHYDRATES AND FIBER

FOOD SOURCES AND SOLUBILITY OF MAJOR TYPES OF DIETARY FIBERS

SOLUBLE	INSOLUBLE
Pectin	Cellulose
Apples	Whole wheat flour
Citrus fruits	Bran
Strawberries	Cabbage family
Gums	Peas/beans
Oatmeal	Apples
Dried beans	Root vegetables
Other legumes	Lignin
Hemicellulose	Mature vegetables
Bran	Wheat
Cereals	
Whole grains	

FIGURE 8-28. Food sources and solubility of major types of dietary fibers. Dietary fiber, in general, is derived from plant cell walls and consists of both nonstarch structural polysaccharides such as cellulose, hemicellulose, and pectins and the structural nonpolysaccharides, such as lignin. As shown here, fibers can be divided into those that have a high degree of water-holding capacity (the soluble fibers) and those with little water-holding capacity (the insoluble fibers). In addition to their capacity for reducing stool transit time and constipation, dietary fibers may also play a role in inhibiting some forms of intestinal cancers and with respect to soluble fiber, in reducing plasma lipids and, thus, cardiovascular disease. (*Adapted from* Slavin [16].)

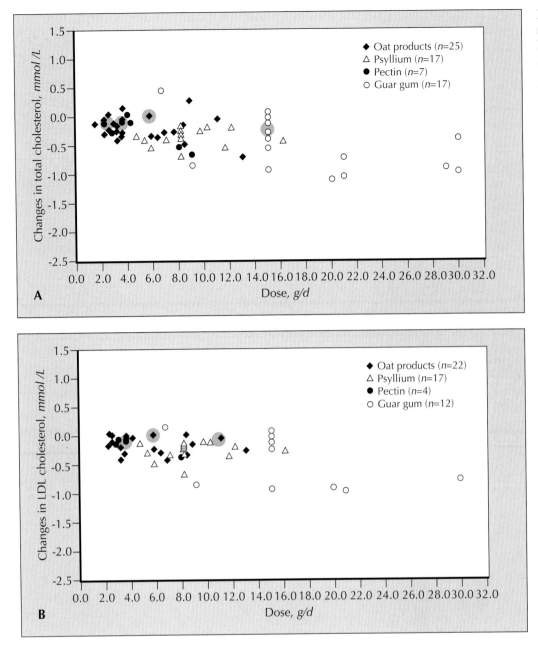

FIGURE 8-29. Relation between dose of soluble fiber and mean lipid changes. Higher levels of soluble fiber intake are associated with lower levels of total and low-density lipoprotein (LDL) cholesterol. Within the range of practical intakes, the effect is modest. However, diets high in foods containing soluble fiber may be low in other foods associated with increased total (**A**) and LDL cholesterol (**B**) levels. (*Adapted from* Brown *et al.* [17].)

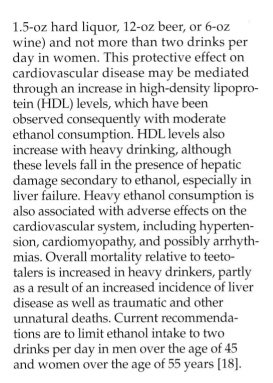

ALCOHOL, CARDIOVASCULAR DISEASE, AND MORTALITY

	TEETOTALER	MILD TO MODERATE INTAKE	HEAVY INTAKE
Impact on risk factors	—	↑HDL	↑HDL ↑Blood pressure ? Arrhythmias
Cardiovascular disease	—	Beneficial	±
Total mortality	—	Beneficial	Detrimental (↑traumatic death and liver disease)

FIGURE 8-30. Ethanol, cardiovascular disease, and mortality. Studies from a wide variety of populations with different genetic and environmental backgrounds have demonstrated a consistent beneficial effect on cardiovascular disease and total mortality of mild to moderate alcohol consumption. The beneficial effect on mortality appears to peak at about two to three drinks in men (a "drink" is generally defined as 1.5-oz hard liquor, 12-oz beer, or 6-oz wine) and not more than two drinks per day in women. This protective effect on cardiovascular disease may be mediated through an increase in high-density lipoprotein (HDL) levels, which have been observed consequently with moderate ethanol consumption. HDL levels also increase with heavy drinking, although these levels fall in the presence of hepatic damage secondary to ethanol, especially in liver failure. Heavy ethanol consumption is also associated with adverse effects on the cardiovascular system, including hypertension, cardiomyopathy, and possibly arrhythmias. Overall mortality relative to teetotalers is increased in heavy drinkers, partly as a result of an increased incidence of liver disease as well as traumatic and other unnatural deaths. Current recommendations are to limit ethanol intake to two drinks per day in men over the age of 45 and women over the age of 55 years [18].

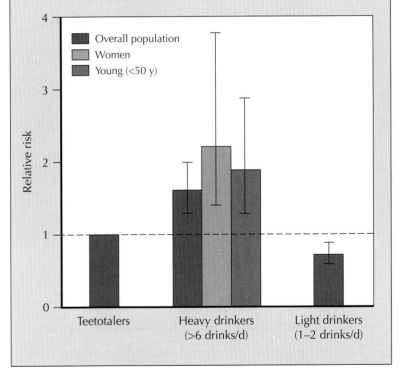

FIGURE 8-31. Effect of ethanol consumption on mortality in the United States. In a study that evaluated the relationship between ethanol intake and mortality in a large ambulatory population, heavy drinkers were found to be at greater risk of death from noncardiovascular causes, especially cirrhosis, unnatural death, and tobacco-related cancers, than nondrinkers. This was particularly true for women and younger people (*ie*, 50 years or younger) in whom the relative risk was higher than the population of heavy drinkers. Light drinkers (one or two drinks per day) had a reduced risk of cardiovascular death, especially coronary heart disease (CHD), independent of their baseline risk. *T bars* indicate 95% CI. (*Adapted from* Klatsky *et al.* [18].)

DIETARY EFFECTS ON LDL, HDL, AND LDL OXIDATION

OVERALL EFFECT OF DIET ON LIPIDS AND LIPOPROTEINS

MULTIPLE REGRESSION EQUATIONS USED TO PREDICT THE EFFECTS OF DIET ON SERUM CHOLESTEROL

KEYS EQUATION:

$$\Delta \text{ Cholesterol (mg/dL)} = 2.7\Delta S - 1.3\Delta P + \sqrt{1.5\Delta C} \text{ mg/1000 cal-d}$$

HEGSTED EQUATION:

$$\Delta \text{ Cholesterol (mg/dL)} = 2.16\Delta S - 1.65\Delta P + 0.068\Delta C \text{ mg/d}$$

FIGURE 8-32. Multiple regression equations used to predict the effects of changes in dietary fat on serum cholesterol. The Keys equation was derived from 43 sets of experiments with groups of normocholesterolemic, hospitalized male patients during the late 1950s. The patients were fed a series of mixed diets containing 40% of calories from fats of different origin for periods of 4 weeks. The data showed that serum cholesterol is consistently elevated by saturated fatty acids with 12, 14, and 16 carbons and lowered by polyunsaturated fatty acids [19,20]. Confirmatory results were obtained in a subsequent series by Hegsted *et al.* [21]. Although the basic observations were the same, the study of Hegsted *et al.* revealed a linear relationship between dietary cholesterol and serum cholesterol, a smaller elevating effect of saturated fatty acids, and a larger serum cholesterol-lowering effect of polyunsaturated fatty acids. Δ C—change in the dietary cholesterol (mg/1000 cal-d); Δ cholesterol—change in serum cholesterol; Δ P—change in the percentage of dietary calories derived from polyunsaturated fatty acids; Δ S—change in the percentage of dietary calories derived from saturated fatty acids. (*Adapted from* Keys *et al.* [22] and Zöllner and Tato [23].)

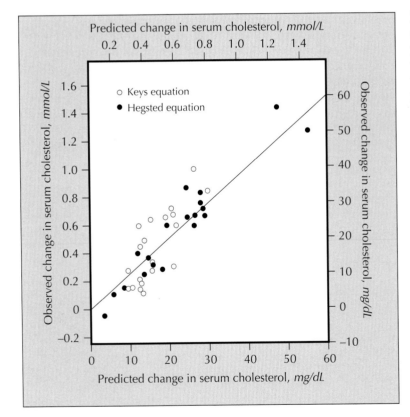

FIGURE 8-33. Predicted versus observed changes in serum cholesterol. When observed changes in serum cholesterol were plotted against predicted changes on the basis of the Keys equation or the Hegsted equation (see Fig. 8-32), a very tight correlation was observed. This correlation is less strong for individual patients, but nonetheless demonstrates the usefulness of these equations designed to predict the response to dietary intervention. It is also conceivable that the correlation would be less tight in free-living individuals in whom dietary compliance may be more difficult to assess.

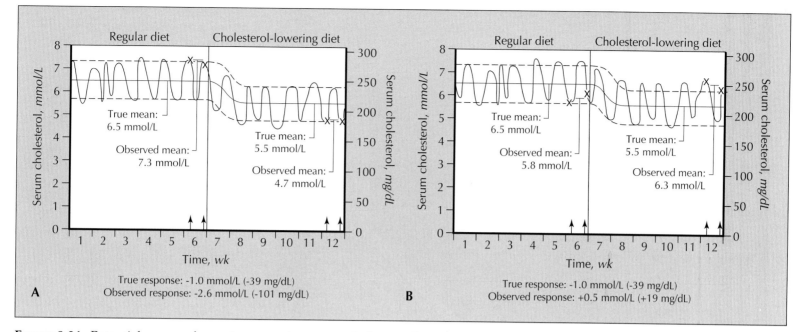

A

True response: -1.0 mmol/L (-39 mg/dL)
Observed response: -2.6 mmol/L (-101 mg/dL)

B

True response: -1.0 mmol/L (-39 mg/dL)
Observed response: +0.5 mmol/L (+19 mg/dL)

FIGURE 8-34. Potential source of error in measuring serum cholesterol response because of natural biologic variation. One source for the variability in response to dietary cholesterol (and fat) in individual patients relates to the finding that serum cholesterol levels are not constant and undergo a biologic fluctuation of up to 10% around a true mean. Timing of the samples can therefore be crucial in evaluating the response of serum cholesterol–lowering diets. **A,** Although the initial blood sample was obtained at a peak of the fluctuation, the sample to evaluate the response to cholesterol-lowering diet was obtained at a trough. This overestimates the true response (1.0 mmol/L; 39 mg/dL) by 1.6 mmol/L (62 mg/dL). **B,** Here, the reverse is true. The initial value was taken at a trough and the follow-up sample at a peak. Although the true response to the diet (a reduction in serum cholesterol of 1 mmol/L; 39 mg/dL) occurred as expected, the apparent response is an increase in serum cholesterol level of 0.5 mmoL (19 mg/dL).

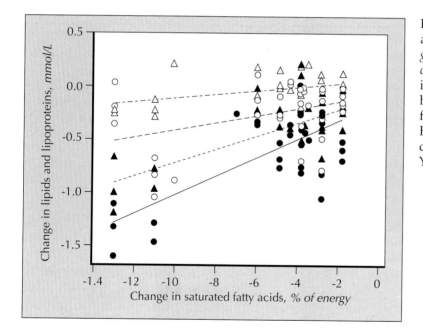

FIGURE 8-35. Relationship between change in the saturated fatty acid content of the diet and total (*closed circles*), LDL (*closed triangles*), and HDL (*open triangles*) cholesterol, and triglyceride (*open circles*) levels. As the relative amount of saturated fat in the diet increases, the smaller the decline in lipid and lipoprotein levels, hence, the higher the absolute level. The correlation is significant for all cholesterol measures, total ($P < 0.001$), LDL ($P < 0.001$), and HDL ($P<0.001$), but not triglyceride levels ($P = 0.06$). HDL—high-density lipoprotein; LDL—low-density lipoprotein. (*Adapted from* Yu Poth *et al.* [24].)

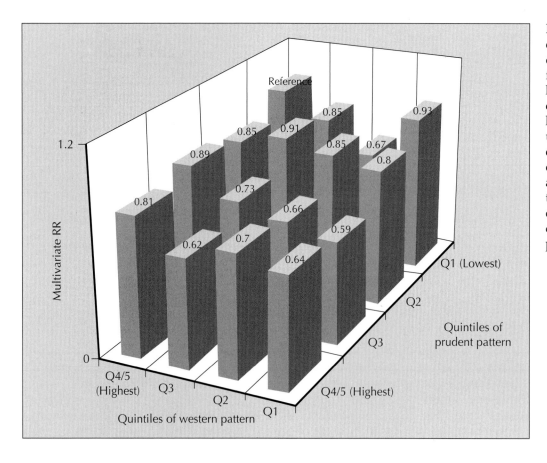

FIGURE 8-36. Multivariate relative risk (RR) of dietary patterns (quintiles of prudent diet) and coronary heart disease, adjusted for age, period, smoking, body mass index, hormone replacement therapy, aspirin use, caloric intake, family history, history of hypertension, multivitamin and vitamin E use, and physical activity. The risk of developing coronary heart disease tends to decrease with increasing quality of the diet as assessed by prudent diet score. Similarly, the risk of developing coronary heart disease tends to increase with decreasing quality of the diet as assessed by western pattern. (*Adapted from* Fung *et al.* [25].)

ANTIOXIDANTS

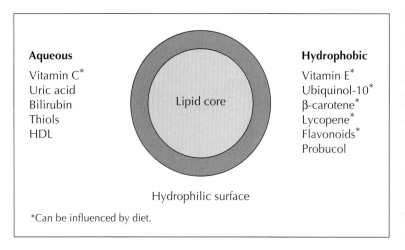

Aqueous

Vitamin C*
Uric acid
Bilirubin
Thiols
HDL

Lipid core

Hydrophobic

Vitamin E*
Ubiquinol-10*
β-carotene*
Lycopene*
Flavonoids*
Probucol

Hydrophilic surface

*Can be influenced by diet.

FIGURE 8-37. Antioxidants and lipoprotein oxidation. Lipoprotein particles consist of a hydrophobic lipid core (containing cholesterol esters, triglycerides, and hydrophobic antioxidants) surrounded by a hydrophilic surface (composed of nonesterified cholesterol, phospholipids, and apolipoproteins). There are two major classes of antioxidants that can affect lipoprotein oxidation. The first includes antioxidants present in the aqueous milieu of the lipoproteins such as vitamin C, uric acid, bilirubin, thiols, and high-density lipoprotein (HDL). The second group of antioxidants, which are hydrophobic, includes vitamin E, ubiquinol-10, β-carotene, lycopene, and flavonoids. These become incorporated into the central lipid core and are transported together with the lipoprotein particle. Antioxidant drugs such as probucol are highly hydrophobic and become incorporated into the lipid core. Other antioxidant drugs can act in the aqueous milieu of the lipoprotein.

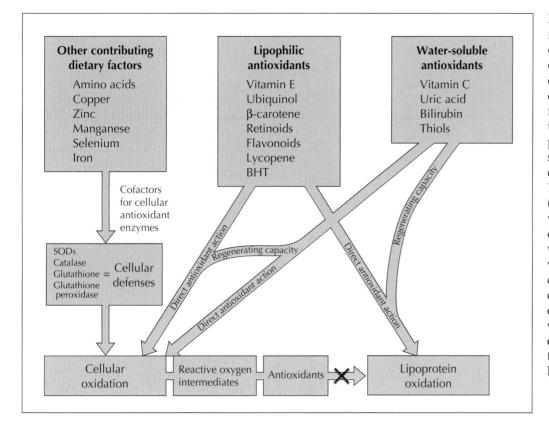

**Other contributing
dietary factors**

Amino acids
Copper
Zinc
Manganese
Selenium
Iron

Cofactors
for cellular
antioxidant
enzymes

SODs
Catalase
Glutathione = **Cellular
Glutathione defenses**
peroxidase

Cellular
oxidation

Reactive oxygen
intermediates

Antioxidants

Lipoprotein
oxidation

Direct antioxidant action
Regenerating capacity
Direct antioxidant action
Direct antioxidant action
Regenerating capacity

**Lipophilic
antioxidants**

Vitamin E
Ubiquinol
β-carotene
Retinoids
Flavonoids
Lycopene
BHT

**Water-soluble
antioxidants**

Vitamin C
Uric acid
Bilirubin
Thiols

FIGURE 8-38. Potential roles of dietary factors in protection against destructive oxidative mechanisms. Normal cellular oxidative mechanisms occur in the mito-chondria or plasma membranes of some cells and contribute to the oxidative modi-fication of lipoproteins by supplying reac-tive oxygen intermediates to initiate lipid peroxidation. This illustration demon-strates how dietary factors could contribute to regulating these processes by 1) acting as chain-breaking antioxidants (*eg*, lipophilic dietary antioxidants such as vitamin E), 2) regenerating the antioxidant capacity of the lipophilic antioxidants (*eg*, water-soluble antioxidants such as vitamin C), or 3) stimulating the normal cellular antioxidant pathways (*eg*, other contributing dietary factors such as copper, zinc, manganese, and selenium, which are cofactors for antioxidant enzymes such as the superoxide dismu-tases [SODs] and glutathione peroxidase). BHT—butylated hydroxytoluene.

Dietary Effects on Nonlipoprotein-Related Risk Factors

DIET AND THROMBOSIS

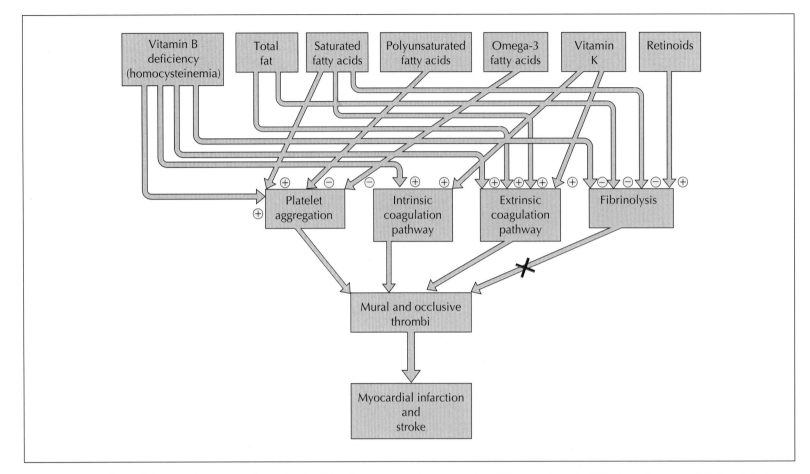

FIGURE 8-39. Effect of dietary factors on thrombosis. The thrombotic process involves four simultaneous, interrelated pathways, each of which may be altered by dietary factors. Initiation of a thrombus involves the adherence and spreading of platelets on an exposed subendothelial matrix followed by the formation of a fibrin clot via stimulation of the extrinsic and intrinsic coagulation pathways. The stabilization of the blood clot involves the balance between the thrombin-induced formation of fibrin and the dissolution of the clot via plasmin-induced fibrinolysis.

The type and amount of dietary fatty acids ingested have been shown to alter platelet adherence and aggregation. Increasing amounts of fat, especially saturated fats, generally stimulate platelet aggregation, whereas increasing polyunsaturated fats (including the omega-3 fatty acids) inhibit platelet aggregation. Current data suggest that these effects may be mediated by changes in the platelet membrane phospholipid composition or the capacity of the platelets to produce the proaggregatory thromboxanes, or both. Increasing total fat also stimulates the tissue factor–induced extrinsic pathway of coagulation potentially by increasing the plasma levels of coagulation factor VII. Both the intrinsic and extrinsic pathways involve several vitamin K–dependent proteins. Dietary vitamin K is therefore an additional factor that could alter the coagulation process.

Dietary factors also appear to alter the anticoagulant properties of the endothelium as well as the fibrinolytic system. For example, diets rich in omega-3 fatty acids reduce the capacity of the endothelium to produce prostacyclin, a potent antiplatelet aggregation factor. Furthermore, increased plasma cholesterol has been shown to inhibit formation of tissue plasminogen activator, which could inhibit the formation of plasmin and the subsequent dissolution of clots. It still remains unclear whether dietary factors impact on the formation of lipoprotein(a). However, in vitro data suggest that increased lipoprotein(a) could also inhibit the formation of plasmin and ultimately reduce the fibrinolytic process.

Finally, an elevation of plasma homocysteine due to dietary deficiencies of folic acid, vitamin B_{12}, or vitamin B_6 can be prothrombotic. For example, data suggest that homocysteine inhibits the expression of thrombomodulin and activation of protein C in endothelial cells and induces the expression of tissue factor. Elevated plasma homocysteine levels also enhance platelet aggregation and impairs fibrinolysis by reducing the binding of tissue plasminogen activator to the endothelium.

DIET AND BLOOD PRESSURE

DIETARY FACTORS AFFECTING BLOOD PRESSURE	
FACTOR	EFFECT
Salt (NaCl)	↑
Ca, Mg, K	↓
Ethanol	↑
Obesity, especially central	↑
Polyunsaturated fatty acids	? ↓

FIGURE 8-40. Dietary factors that affect blood pressure. Several nutritional factors have been shown to affect blood pressure. These include salt (sodium chloride), the intake of which has been demonstrated to be correlated positively with elevated blood pressure in large epidemiologic studies comparing salt intakes in different populations. Within specific populations, the effect is more variable because the hypertensive effect of dietary salt appears to be confined to salt-sensitive patients, who represent a minority of the population. High intakes of calcium, magnesium, and potassium have been associated with a reduction in blood pressure levels. Chronic consumption of large amounts of ethanol also increases blood pressure. The presence of obesity, especially central obesity (see Fig. 8-27), is associated with various cardiovascular risk factors, including hypertension. The central obesity/insulin resistance syndrome probably is causally related to hypertension, because reductions in body weight are associated with lowering blood pressure. Although several studies have suggested that consumption of polyunsaturated fatty acids may reduce blood pressure, this effect is more controversial.

DIET AND HOMOCYSTEINE

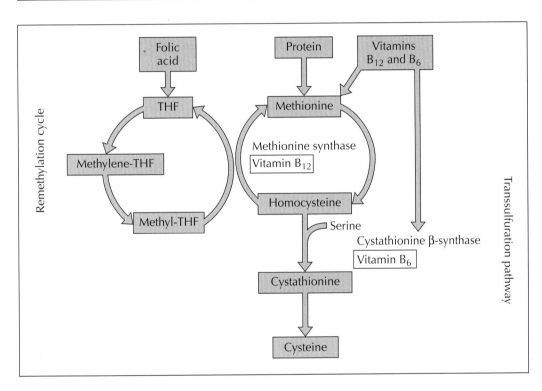

FIGURE 8-41. Role of B vitamins in the metabolism of homocysteine. Elevations of plasma homocysteine can result from a dietary load of methionine coupled with inadequate intake of either folic acid or vitamins B_{12} and B_6. Folic acid and vitamin B_{12} participate in the remethylation cycle and facilitate the conversion of excess homocysteine to methionine through the vitamin B_{12}–dependent enzyme methionine synthase. Homocysteine can also be converted to cysteine through the transsulfuration pathway through formation of the intermediate cystathionine by the vitamin B_6–dependent enzyme cystathionine β-synthase. THF—tetrahydrofolate. (*Adapted from* Welch and Loscalzo [26].)

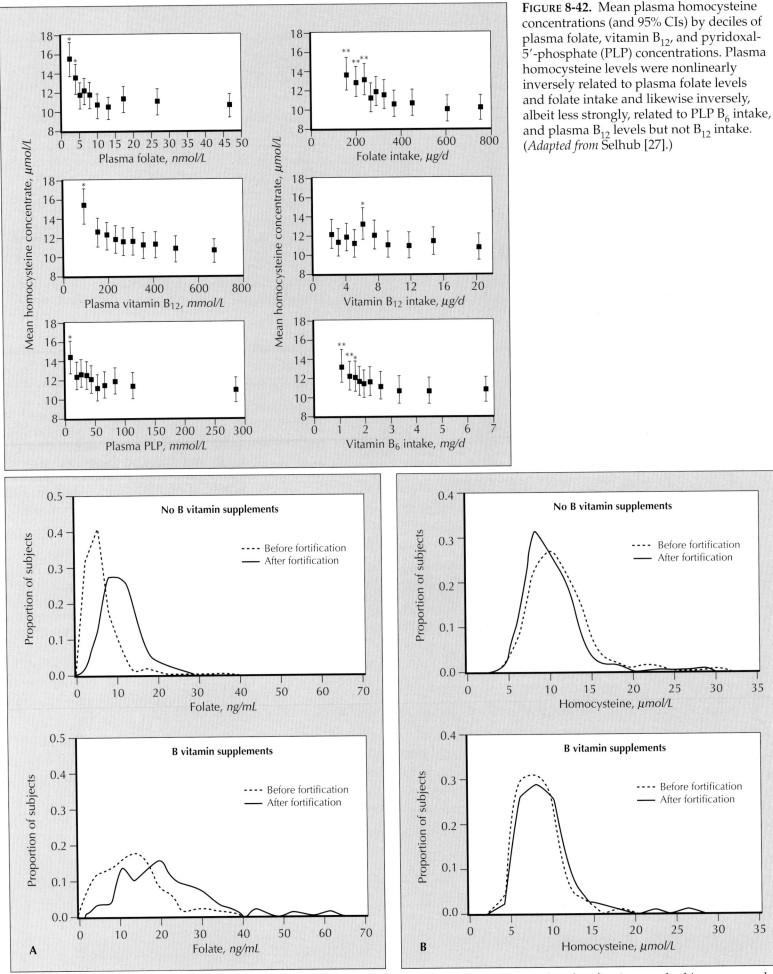

FIGURE 8-42. Mean plasma homocysteine concentrations (and 95% CIs) by deciles of plasma folate, vitamin B_{12}, and pyridoxal-5'-phosphate (PLP) concentrations. Plasma homocysteine levels were nonlinearly inversely related to plasma folate levels and folate intake and likewise inversely, albeit less strongly, related to PLP B_6 intake, and plasma B_{12} levels but not B_{12} intake. (*Adapted from* Selhub [27].)

FIGURE 8-43. Plasma folate concentrations in study group before and after folic acid fortification, according to the use of B vitamin supplements. **A,** Folate fortification resulted in an upward shift in the distribution of plasma folate in both dietary supplement nonusers and users. **B,** Folate fortification resulted in an upward shift in the dietary distribution of plasma homocysteine levels in dietary supplement nonusers but not users. (*Adapted from* Jacques et al. [28].)

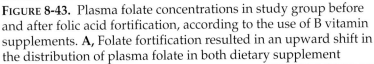

DIET AND BLOOD PRESSURE

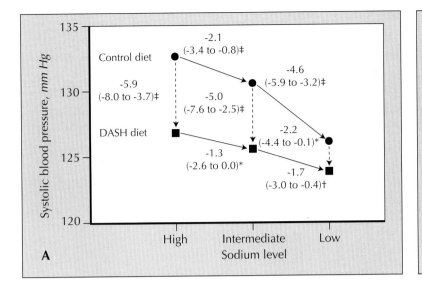

A

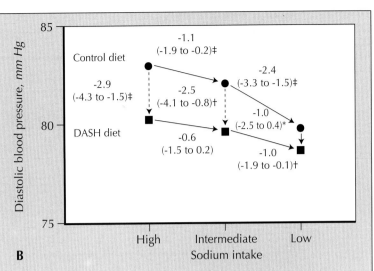

B

FIGURE 8-44. Effect of diet, other than sodium, on blood pressure. This controlled study included 459 adults with systolic blood pressure readings of less than 160 mm Hg and diastolic blood pressures of 80 to 95 mm Hg. Study subjects consumed either a control diet low in fruits, vegetables, and dairy products, with a fat content typical of the average diet in the United States; a diet rich in fruits and vegetables, or a "combination" diet rich in fruits, vegetables,

and low-fat dairy products and with reduced saturated and total fat. The sodium content was similar among these diets. Both the fruit-and-vegetable and "combination" diets reduced systolic (**A**) and diastolic (**B**) blood pressure, with the latter diet resulting in the most efficacious changes observed. The "combination" diet is frequently referred to as the DASH (Dietary Approaches to Stop Hypertension) diet. (*Adapted from* Appel *et al.* [29].)

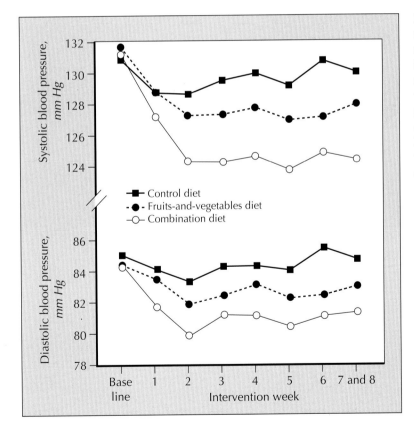

FIGURE 8-45. Effect of diet and sodium on blood pressure. This controlled study included 412 adults who were randomly assigned to eat either a control diet typical of intake in the United States or the DASH (Dietary Approaches to Stop Hypertension) diet. Within the assigned diet, patients were provided with food with a high (*ie*, 3.3 g/d), intermediate (*ie*, 2.5 g/d), and low (*ie*, 1.5 g/d) level of sodium. The DASH diet resulted in lower systolic and diastolic blood pressure readings than the control diet. Reducing the sodium contents of these diets resulted in additional systolic and blood pressure reductions. (*Adapted from* Sacks *et al.* [30].)

CARDIOVASCULAR DISEASE DIETARY PREVENTION TRIALS AND DIETARY RECOMMENDATIONS

PREVENTION TRIALS: CLINICAL ENDPOINTS

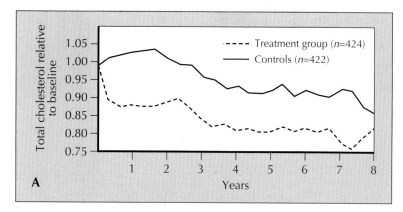

A

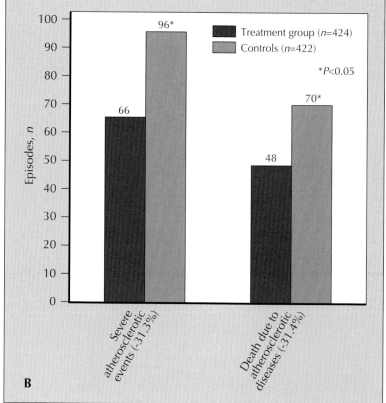

B

FIGURE 8-46. Effect of a cholesterol-lowering fat-modified diet on the incidence of atherosclerotic events and mortality in the Los Angeles Veterans Study [31]. Consumption of a diet in which the content of saturated fat and cholesterol was reduced and the amount of polyunsaturated fat was increased resulted in a lower total cholesterol level in the treatment group relative to findings in the controls (**A**). This was associated with a 31% reduction in both severe atherosclerotic events and deaths due to atherosclerotic disease in the treatment group relative to controls (**B**). These findings suggest that the diet-induced differences in serum cholesterol levels were associated with a reduction in coronary heart disease events and mortality in a study in which male residents of a domiciliary facility received their diets under strictly controlled conditions. *Numbers in parentheses* in **B** are the values for change relative to controls. (*Adapted from* Pyorala [32].)

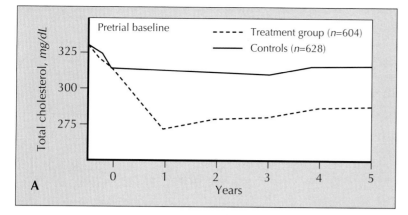

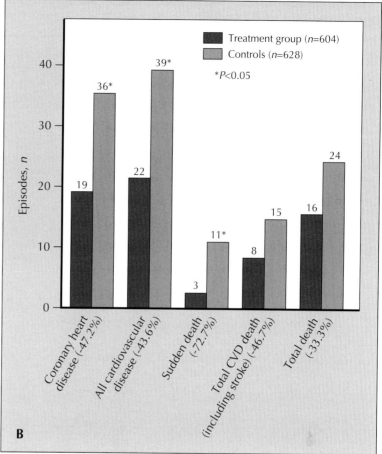

FIGURE 8-47. Effect of a cholesterol-lowering fat-modified diet on the incidence of atherosclerotic events and mortality: Oslo Primary Prevention Study [33]. The diet used in this study mainly reduced the intake of saturated fat and cholesterol, with some increase in the use of polyunsaturated fatty acids. Another major difference between this and the Los Angeles Veterans Study [31] was that smoking cessation was attempted in the treatment group in the Oslo trial. Serum total cholesterol levels were lower in the treatment group throughout the 5 years of this study than in the control subjects (**A**). Various indices of cardiovascular disease and mortality showed approximately 30% to 70% reduction in the treatment group relative to those of controls (**B**). It is estimated that approximately 60% of the total benefit accruing to the intervention group could be attributed to diet-induced changes in the serum cholesterol levels; the remainder resulted from reductions in cigarette consumption. *Numbers in parentheses* in **B** are the values for change relative to controls. (*Adapted from* Pyorala [32].)

DIETARY INTERVENTION TRIALS ON CORONARY EVENTS

TRIAL*	SUBJECTS IN THE INTERVENTION GROUP	DIETARY INTERVENTION	DIETARY FAT IN THE TREATMENT GROUP, % ENERGY	P:S RATIO IN THE TREATMENT GROUP	DURATION, Y	CHANGE IN SERUM CHOLESTEROL, %[†]	CHANGE IN CHD, %[‡]
MRC low-fat diet	123 MI patients, all men	Reduce total fat	22	NR	3	-5	+4
DART	1015 MI patients, all men	Reduce total fat	32	0.8	2	-3.5	-9
Finnish Mental Hospital	676 men	Unsaturated fat → saturated fat	35	1.5	6	-15	-43
Los Angeles Veterans	424 men, most having no evidence of existing heart disease	Unsaturated fat → saturated fat	40	NR	8	-13	-31
Oslo Diet Heart Study	206 MI patients, all men	Unsaturated fat → saturated fat	39	2.4	5	-14	-25
MRC soy oil	199 MI patients, all men	Unsaturated fat → saturated fat	46	2.0	4	-16	-12
Minnesota Coronary Survey	4393 men and 4664 women	Unsaturated fat → saturated fat	38	1.6	4.5	-14	No change
Indian Experiment of Infarct Survival	204 MI patients, primarily men	High fruits, vegetables, nuts, fish, and pulses	24	1.2	1	-9	-40
Lyon Diet Heart Study	302 MI patients, primarily men	Mediterranean diet	31	0.7	2.3	No change	-73

*References for each trial can be found in Hu *et al.* [34].

[†]Refers to the percentage change in serum cholesterol in the treatment group compared with the change in the control group.

[‡]Refers to the percentage in coronary event rates in the treatment compared with the control group.

FIGURE 8-48. Dietary intervention trials with clinical endpoints. In general, dietary intervention trials support the benefit of replacing saturated fat with polyunsaturated fat (indicated by the *arrows*). DART—Diet and Reinfarction Trial; MI—myocardial infarction; MRC—Medical Research Council; NR—not reported. (*Adapted from* Hu *et al.* [34].)

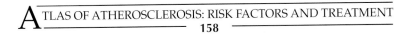

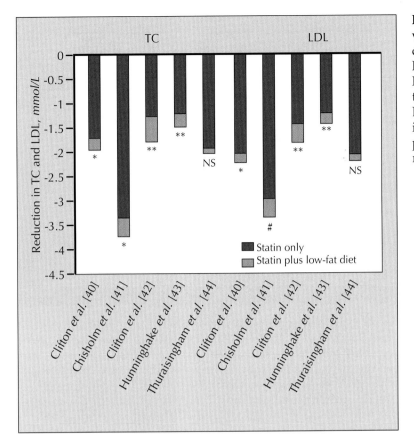

FIGURE 8-49. Added cholesterol-lowering effects by low-fat diets versus high-fat diets in patients on statin therapy. Baseline low-density lipoprotein cholesterol levels were calculated using the Friedewald equation [35] in studies by Clifton *et al.* [36] and Hunninghake *et al.* [37], and were estimated based on the proportion of low-density lipoprotein (LDL) in total cholesterol (TC) (*ie*, LDL is 75.6% of TC) in the Chisholm *et al.* [38] study. The *asterisk* indicates $P < 0.05$; the *pound sign* indicates $P < 0.06$ when statin plus low-fat diet is compared with statin plus high-fat diet response. NS—nonsignificant. (*Adapted from* Clemmer *et al.* [39].)

RECOMMENDED DIET CHANGES

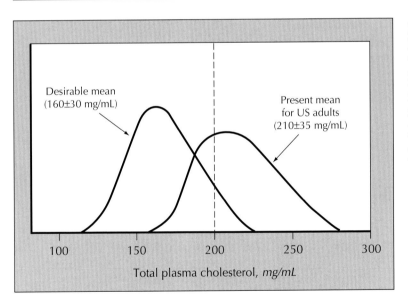

FIGURE 8-50. The population-based approach to cholesterol lowering by diet. The rationale for the population-based approach to the prevention of atherosclerotic disease by dietary change relies on a shift of the distribution of plasma and low-density lipoprotein (LDL) cholesterol levels in the population toward lower levels. A mean reduction of approximately 1% in the population's cholesterol level would be expected to lead to a 2% reduction in coronary heart disease risk. The diet recommended for the population at large is outlined in Figure 8-4.

LDL CHOLESTEROL GOALS AND CUTPOINTS FOR THERAPEUTIC LIFESTYLE CHANGES AND DRUG THERAPY IN DIFFERENT RISK CATEGORIES

RISK CATEGORY	LDL GOAL, *MG/DL*	LDL LEVEL AT WHICH TO INITIATE TLC, *MG/DL*	LDL LEVEL AT WHICH TO CONSIDER DRUG THERAPY, *MG/DL*
CHD or CHD risk equivalents (10-y risk > 20%)	< 100	≥ 100	≥ 130 (100–129: drug optional)*
2+ risk factors (10-y risk ≤ 20%)	< 130	≥ 130	10-y risk 10%–20%: ≥ 130 10-y risk < 10%: ≥160
0–1 risk factor †	< 160	≥ 160	≥ 190 (160–189: LDL-lowering drug optional)

*Some authorities recommend use of LDL-lowering drugs in this category if an LDL cholesterol level of < 100 mg/dL cannot be achieved by therapeutic lifestyle changes. Others prefer use of drugs that primarily modify triglycerides and HDL, *eg*, nicotinic acid or fibrillate. Clinical judgment also may call for deferring drug therapy in this subcategory.

†Almost all people with 0 to 1 risk factor have a 10-y risk < 10%; thus, 10-y risk assessment in people with 0 to 1 risk factor is not necessary.

FIGURE 8-51. The high-risk approach to diet therapy. A complementary approach is the so-called "high-risk approach," which identifies those patients whose cardiovascular risk is markedly increased as a result of increased serum and low-density lipoprotein (LDL) cholesterol levels, often in conjunction with other cardiovascular risk factors. The approach is to identify such high-risk individuals and to lower their cholesterol level initially by dietary means. If diet alone fails to lead to adequate target levels, drug therapy may need to be added to the diet regimen. The Adult Treatment Panel (ATP) III of the National Cholesterol Education Program recommends that formal diet therapy be initiated at the following LDL cholesterol levels: 1) in the absence of, or in the presence of one, other cardiovascular risk factor(s), diet therapy should commence when LDL levels are equal to or greater than 160 mg/dL; 2) when two or more net risk factors are present, a lower threshold (*ie*, LDL cholesterol 130 mg/dL or more) is recommended; and 3) in the presence of established coronary heart disease (CHD), diet therapy or coronary heart disease risk equivalents (see the ATP II Report) should be used when LDL cholesterol levels are equal to or greater than 100 mg/dL. TLC—therapeutic lifestyle changes. (*Adapted from* the Expert Panel on Detection, Evaluation, and Treatment of High Blood Cholesterol in Adults [45].)

NUTRIENT COMPOSITION OF THE THERAPEUTIC LIFESTYLE CHANGES DIET

NUTRIENT	RECOMMENDED INTAKE
Saturated fat*	< 7% of total calories
Polyunsaturated fat	Up to 10% of total calories
Monounsaturated fat	Up to 20% of total calories
Total fat	25%–35% of total calories
Carbohydrate†	50%–60% of total calories
Fiber	20–30 g/d
Protein	Approximately 15% of total calories
Cholesterol	< 200 mg/d
Total calories‡	Balance energy intake and expenditure to maintain desirable body weight/prevent weight gain

* *Trans* fatty acids are another LDL-raising fat that should be kept at a low intake.

†Carbohydrates should be derived predominantly from foods rich in complex carbohydrates including grains, especially whole grains, fruits, and vegetables.

‡Daily energy expenditure should include at least moderate physical activity (contributing approximately 200 kcal/d).

FIGURE 8-52. Dietary and lifestyle therapy for high blood cholesterol. The National Cholesterol Education Program Adult Treatment Panel III has recommended the use of a multifaceted lifestyle approach to reduce risk of developing cardiovascular disease. The key components are to reduce intake of saturated fat to less than 7% of total calories (energy) and cholesterol to less than 200 mg per day. Other specific details of the diets are included in the table. Additional recommendations are weight reduction, increased physical activity, and other therapeutic options such as increasing the intake of soluble fiber and plant sterols and stanols. LDL—low-density lipoprotein. (*Adapted from* the Expert Panel on Detection, Evaluation, and Treatment of High Blood Cholesterol in Adults [45].)

REASONS FOR AN INADEQUATE RESPONSE TO DIET THERAPY

Poor compliance with prescribed diet
Insufficient period for adjustment to dietary change
   and weight reduction
Marked hypercholesterolemia
Biological hypo- or nonresponder
Inadequate prescription for dietary change

FIGURE 8-53. Reasons for an inadequate response to diet therapy. There are several possible reasons for failure of diet therapy. The most common is poor compliance with the prescribed diet. Follow-up may not have allowed sufficient time for adjustment to dietary changes or for achievement of weight reduction, which will result in an exaggerated hypocholesterolemic response to a reduction in the consumption of saturated fat and cholesterol. Patients with severe hypercholesterolemia (*eg*, familial forms) are unlikely to respond to diet therapy alone and usually require a combination of diet and drug therapy. It is possible that some individuals have a biologic resistance to diet therapy (*eg*, are biologic hypo- or nonresponders). Evaluation of the patient's current diet before prescription is important to determine an accurate starting point.

STRATEGIES TO IMPROVE COMPLIANCE WITH A CHOLESTEROL-LOWERING DIET

Explain reasons for requiring dietary change
Evaluate baseline (habitual) diet
Set specific dietary goals
   Select nutritious, tasty foods that are low in saturated fat and
      cholesterol
   Develop diet that matches patient's lifestyle
Offer specific recommendations about dietary change
Provide educational materials
Follow-up regularly
   Reinforcement
   Answer questions
   Address problem areas

FIGURE 8-54. Strategies to improve compliance with diet to lower cholesterol levels. To aid compliance, the patient must understand the reason for recommending dietary change. The patient's baseline (habitual) diet should be assessed to determine which specific changes should be made. It is important to set specific dietary goals for the patient. This includes selection of nutritious and tasty foods that are low in saturated fat and cholesterol and provision of sufficient variety to prevent boredom. It is important to develop a diet that matches the patient's lifestyle, from the standpoints of ethnicity, practicality, and taste preferences. Specific recommendations about dietary and lifestyle change need to be made rather than generalizations. This is best done with the help of a qualified dietitian or nutritionist. Provision of educational materials can be helpful in allowing the patient to study aspects of the diet and lifestyle at leisure. Regular follow-up will enhance compliance. Follow-up will allow a reinforcement of the diet, the opportunity for the patient to ask questions related to specific foods, and to address difficulties with compliance.

POPULAR DIETS AND WEIGHT-LOSS PROGRAMS

DIET/WEIGHT-LOSS PROGRAM AND BASIC PREMISE	WHAT TO EXPECT	CONCERNS FOR CERTAIN NUTRIENTS	ADDITIONAL COSTS
Food Guide Pyramid Uses a graphic tool to help healthy Americans achieve a diet composed of 55%–60% carbohydrate, 15% protein, 25%–30% fat Focuses on food groups, daily servings, serving sizes to prevent nutrient inadequacies, excesses, imbalances Food groups include grains, vegetables, fruit, meat/poultry/fish/nuts, milk/yogurt/cheese, fats/oils/sweets Includes ranges for recommended daily servings to meet a variety of calorie needs	A well-mixed variety of proteins and carbohydrates A basic diet focusing on adequate intakes of protein, vitamins, minerals, and dietary fiber, without excessive amounts of calories, fat, saturated fat, cholesterol, sodium, added sugars, and alcohol Requires some planning to include a variety of foods Requires basic nutrition knowledge to interpret the ways combination foods fit the pyramid Typical breakfast varies but usually includes whole-grain breads or cereals, dairy, fruit	Because there is usually great variety, individuals are unlikely to be at great risk for nutritional deficiencies	No additional costs With physician referral, health insurance usually covers a visit to the dietician
Atkins Diet Very-low-carbohydrate diet (5%–15% carbohydrate [20–50 g/dl]; 30%–40% protein; 50%–55% fat) Induces a state of ketosis (from sugar metabolism to fat metabolism)	Diet can become monotonous Long-term physiologic effects are unknown Many people cannot stay on the diet for an extended period of time Typical breakfast is bacon and eggs	Without supplementation, diet is low in vitamins C, B_1, B_3, folic acid, β-carotene, biotin, potassium, fiber Calcium may be inadequate due to limitations in milk consumption	Book(s) Snack bars, drinks, low-carbohydrate bread mixes are now available if desired Dr. Atkins brand of vitamin/mineral supplement is recommended
Ornish Diet Very-low-fat, low-cholesterol, plant-based diet (up to 75% carbohydrate, 15% protein, < 10% fat [20–25 g/dl]) Diet is designed for reversing atherosclerotic heart disease	No meat, fish, or animal products, except nonfat dairy and egg whites; no oils, fats, seeds, or nuts, except flax High-fiber diet with lots of whole grains, vegetables, fruit Time consuming; can be laborious to plan and prepare meals and snacks Typical breakfast is whole-grain pancakes, nonfat yogurt, fruit	Without meat in the diet, iron intake may be low Possible essential fatty acid deficiency Risk of fat-soluble vitamin deficiencies due to diet being extremely low in fat	Book(s) LifeChoice™ frozen dinners are an option Supplements may include vitamin E and flaxseed or flaxseed oil
Pritikin Diet Very-low-fat, low-cholesterol, low-sodium, high-fiber diet, similar to the Ornish diet Diet is 75%–80% carbohydrate, 10%–15% protein, and <10% fat	Excludes processed grains, animal protein, eggs, fat; no meat, fish, or animal products, except nonfat dairy High-fiber diet with lots of whole grains Time consuming; can be laborious to plan and prepare meals and snacks Typical breakfast is dry, whole-grain toast, nonfat dairy, and fresh fruit	Without meat in the diet, iron intake may be low Possible essential fatty acid deficiency Risk of fat-soluble vitamin deficiencies due to diet being extremely low in fat	Book Option to buy food products from the Pritikin online store (Pritikin@home.com) Programs in California and Florida require fee plus hotel and travel expenses

FIGURE 8-55. Several diet and weight loss programs are available in an ever-changing landscape. Summarized is the US Department of Agriculture Food Guide Pyramid recommendations and some of the currently popular diets. Each has advantages and disadvantages. It is important for the patient to meet his or her individual needs and adhere to a dietary pattern, frequently in association with lower calorie (energy) intakes than are necessary to maintain body weight for an extended period. The focus should be on long-term, rather than short-term, outcomes. Efforts to increase physical activity on a daily basis should be coupled with any dietary plan. In terms of fad diets, it is important to recall that, to date, researchers have failed to reach any consensus on the potential benefits of any current diets with respect to weight loss, prevention of loss of lean muscle mass, or sustaining long-term weight loss. (*Adapted from* Saltzman *et al.* [46].)
(*Continued on next page*)

DIET/WEIGHT-LOSS PROGRAM AND BASIC PREMISE	WHAT TO EXPECT	CONCERNS FOR CERTAIN NUTRIENTS	ADDITIONAL COSTS
Zone Diet Focuses on link between diet and the body's production of insulin and eicosanoid levels. Proposes that maintaining insulin levels in "the zone" will prevent weight gain and low energy levels	A confusing diet utilizing a "food block" counting method that requires much planning and preparation Eat 5 to 6 times per day to consume food every 5 or 6 hours (usually 3 meals, 2 snacks) Typical breakfast is 2 scrambled eggs, 1 oz cheese, 1 slice whole-wheat bread, one-half cantaloupe, 1 tsp butter or margarine	Because there is usually great variety, individuals are unlikely to be at great risk for nutritional deficiencies	Book(s) "Quick start kit" "40-30-30" snack bars ZonePerfect™ omega-3 fish oil capsules Food delivery options are available Vitamin E and other antioxidants Fish oils are recommended
Weight Watchers Individually tailored diet recommends 50%–60% carbohydrate, 10%–20% protein, and <30% fat Winning Points System™ and 1-2-3 Success™ programs allow for variety. Foods fit into a point system, and dieters may consume foods totaling a set number of points per day Focuses on behavioral and long-term dietary changes that will enable a person to maintain weight loss	A well-mixed variety of protein and carbohydrate to help the dieter feel satisfied and less hungry Weight-loss goal setting of up to 2 pounds per week Support groups to motivate and educate people Typical breakfast is 1 whole small bagel, 2 tbsp light cream cheese, 1 cup melon	Because there is usually great variety, individuals are unlikely to be at great risk for nutritional deficiencies	Enrollment fee (includes registration fee and fee for 1 weekly meeting) Weekly fee for meetings Prepackaged frozen meals and desserts are available

FIGURE 8-55. *(continued)*

REFERENCES

1. Kennedy ET, Bowman SA, Powell RA: Dietary-fat intake in the US population. *J Am Coll Nutr* 1999, 18:207–212.

2. Keys A: Coronary heart disease in seven countries. *Circulation* 1970, 41 (suppl I):1–211.

3. Keys A, Menotti A, Karvonen MJ, *et al.*: The diet and 15-year death rate in the seven countries study. *Am J Epidemiol* 1986, 124:903–915.

4. Kato H, Tillotson J, Hichaman MZ, *et al.*: Epidemiological studies of coronary heart disease and stroke in Japanese men living in Japan, Hawaii and California. *Am J Epidemiol* 1973, 97:372–385.

5. US Department of Agriculture: *Composition of Food*. Washington, D.C.: US Government Printing Office.

6. Ahrens EH, Jr, Hirsch J, Insull W, Jr, *et al.*: The influences of dietary fats on serum lipid levels in man. *Lancet* 1957, 1:943–953.

7. Kris-Etherton PM, Yu S: Individual fatty acid effects on plasma lipids and lipoproteins: human studies. *Am J Clin Nutr* 1997, 65 (suppl): 1628S–1644S.

8. Mattson FH, Grundy SM: Comparison of effects of dietary saturated, monounsaturated, and polyunsaturated fatty acids on plasma lipids and lipoproteins in man. *J Lipid Res* 1985, 26:194–202.

9. Baggio G, Pagnon A, Muraca M, *et al.*: Olive oil-enriched diet: effect on serum lipoprotein levels and biliary cholesterol saturation. *Am J Clin Nutr* 1988, 47:960–964.

10. Ginsberg HN, Barr SL, Gilbert A, *et al.*: Reduction of plasma cholesterol levels in normal men on an American Heart Association step I diet or a step I diet with added monounsaturated fat. *N Engl J Med* 1990, 322:574–579.

11. Grundy SM, Nix D, Whelan MF, *et al.*: Comparison of three cholesterol-lowering diets in normolipidemic men. *JAMA* 1986, 256:2351–2355.

12. Hu FB, Stampfer MJ, Manson JE, *et al.*: Dietary saturated fats and their food sources in relation to the risk of coronary heart disease in women. *Am J Clin Nutr* 1999, 70:1001–1008.

13. Reaven P, Parthasarathy S, Grasse BJ, *et al.*: Effects of oleate-rich and linoleate-rich diets on the susceptibility of low density lipoprotein to oxidative modification in mildly hypercholesterolemic subjects. *J Clin Invest* 1993, 91:668–676.

14. Lichtenstein AH, Ausman LA, Jalbert S, Schaefer EJ: Comparison of different forms of hydrogenated fats on serum lipid levels in moderately hypercholesterolemic female and male subjects. *N Engl J Med* 1999, 340:1933–1940.

15. McNamara DJ: Relationship between blood and dietary cholesterol. *Adv Meat Sci* 1990, 6:63–87.

16. Slavin JL: Dietary fiber: classification, chemical analyses, and food sources. *J Am Diet Assoc* 1987, 87:1164–1171.

17. Brown L, Rosner B, Willett WW, Sacks FM: Cholesterol-lowering effects of dietary fiber: a meta-analysis. *Am J Clin Nutr* 1999, 69:30–42.

18. Klatsky AL, Armstrong MA, Friedman GD: Alcohol and mortality. *Ann Intern Med* 1992, 117:646–654.

19. Keys A, Anderson JT, Grande F: Prediction of serum cholesterol responses of man to changes in fats in the diet. *Lancet* 1957, 2:959–966.

20. Keys A, Anderson JT, Grande F: Serum cholesterol in man: diet fat and intrinsic responsiveness. *Circulation* 1959, 19:201–214.

21. Hegsted DM, McGandy RB, Myers ML, *et al.*: Quantitative effects of dietary fat on serum cholesterol in man. *Am J Clin Nutr* 1965, 17:281–295.

22. Keys A, Anderson JT, Grande F: Serum cholesterol response to changes in the diet: I. Iodine value of dietary fat versus 25-P. *Metabolism* 1965, 14:747–758.

23. Zöllner N, Tato F: Fatty acid composition of the diet: impact on serum lipids and atherosclerosis. *Clin Invest* 1992, 70:969–1009.

24. Yu-Poth S, Zhao G, Etherton T, *et al.*: Effects of the National Cholesterol Education Program's Step I and Step II dietary intervention programs on cardiovascular disease risk factors: a meta-analysis. *Am J Clin Nutr* 1999, 69:632–646.

25. Fung TT, Willett W, Stampfer MJ, *et al.*: Dietary patterns and the risk of coronary disease in women. *Ann Intern Med* 2001, 161:1857–1862.

26. Welch GN, Loscalzo J: Homocysteine and atherothrombosis. *N Engl J Med* 1998, 338:1042–1050.

27. Selhub J: Homocysteine metabolism. *Annu Rev Nutr* 1999, 19:217–246.

28. Jacques PF, Selhub J, Bostom AG, *et al.*: The effect of folic acid fortification on plasma folate and total homocysteine concentrations. *N Engl J Med* 1999, 340:1449–1454.

29. Appel LJ, Moore TJ, Obarzanek E, *et al.*: A clinical trial of the effects of dietary patterns on blood pressure. *N Engl J Med* 1997, 336:1117–1124.

30. Sacks FM, Svetkey LP, Vollmer WM, *et al.*: Effects on blood pressure of reduced dietary sodium and the dietary approaches to stop hypertension (DASH) diet. *N Engl J Med* 2001, 344:3–10.

31. Dayton S, Pearce ML: Prevention of coronary heart disease and other complications of atherosclerosis by modified diet. *Am J Med* 1969, 46:751–761.

32. Pyorala K: *Clinical Perspectives on Blood Lipids: Clinical Trials of Lipid Lowering*. London: Current Medical Literature; 1988.

33. Leren P: The Oslo Diet-Heart Study: eleven-year report. *Circulation* 1970, 62:935–942.

34. Hu FB, Manson JE, Willett WC: Types of dietary fat and risk of coronary heart disease: a critical review. *J Am Coll Nutr* 2001, 20:5–19.

35. Friedewald WT, Levy RI, Frederickson RD: Estimation of the concentration of low-density lipoprotein cholesterol in plasma, without use of the preparative ultracentrifuge. *Clin Chem* 1972, 18:499–502.

36. Clifton P, Wight M, Nestel P: Is fat restriction needed with HMG CoA reductase inhibitor treatment? *Atherosclerosis* 1992, 93:59–70.

37. Hunninghake D, Stein E, Dujovne C, *et al.*: The efficacy of intensive dietary therapy alone or combined with lovastatin in outpatients with hypercholesterolemia. *N Engl J Med* 1993, 328:1213–1219.

38. Chisholm A, Mann J, Sutherland W, *et al.*: Dietary management of patients with familial hypercholesterolemia treated with simvastatin. *Q J Med* 1992, 85:825–831.

39. Clemmer KF, Binkoski AE, Coval SM: Diet and drug therapy: a dynamic duo for reducing coronary heart disease risk. *Current Atherosclerosis Reports* 2001, 3:507–513.

40. Clifton P, Wight M, Nestel P: Is fat restriction needed with HMG CoA reductase inhibitor treatment? *Atherosclerosis* 1992, 93:59–70.

41. Chisholm A, Mann J, Sutherland W, *et al.*: Dietary management of patients with familial hypercholesterolaemia treated with simvastatin. *Q J Med* 1992, 85:825–831.

42. Clifton P, Noakes M, Nestel P: Gender and diet interactions with simvastatin treatment. *Atherosclerosis* 1994, 110:25–33.

43. Hunninghake D, Stein E, Dujovne C, *et al.*: The efficacy of intensive dietary therapy alone or combined with lovastatin in outpatients with hypercholesterolemia. *N Engl J Med* 1993, 328:1213–1219.

44. Thuraisingham S, Tan K, Chong K, *et al.*: A randomized comparison of simvastatin versus simvastatin and low cholesterol diet in the treatment of hypercholesterolaemia. *Int J Clin Pract* 2000, 54:78–84.

45. Expert Panel on Detection, Evaluation, and Treatment of High Blood Cholesterol in Adults: Executive Summary of the Third Report of the National Cholesterol Education Program (NCEP) Expert Panel on Detection, Evaluation, and Treatment of High Blood Cholesterol in Adults (Adult Treatment Panel III). *JAMA* 2001, 285:2486–2497.

46. Saltzman E, Thomason P, Roberts SB: Fad diets: a review for the primary care provider. *Nutr Clin Care* 2001, 4:235–242.

LIPID-LOWERING DRUGS

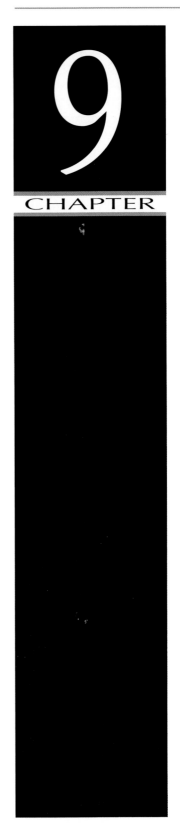

CHAPTER 9

Evan A. Stein

Lipid-lowering drugs are used primarily to reduce the risk of clinical events due to atherosclerotic vascular disease. Their use for both primary prevention (no prior clinical event) and secondary prevention (prior clinical event) of coronary heart disease (CHD) is now firmly established [1–6]. The majority of evidence for clinical benefit exists for the prevention of CHD. However, these drugs are also used in patients with clinical evidence of cerebrovascular or peripheral arterial disease because these patients have a high risk of CHD death and other events, and there is good evidence that the rate of progression of the atherosclerotic process can be delayed in both the carotid and peripheral arteries [3,6,7]. Furthermore, large and statistically significant reductions in stroke in patients with pre-existing CHD have been uniformly achieved in all the recent landmark trials [3,6,8,9].

Hypertriglyceridemia associated with elevated chylomicron levels is associated with the development of pancreatitis. Triglyceride-lowering drugs are occasionally used to reduce the risk of pancreatitis. Also, certain genetic causes of hyperlipoproteinemias are associated with xanthoma formation. Drug therapy that reduces the appropriate lipoprotein concentration reduces the size, cosmetic, and functional problems associated with these xanthomas.

The major impetus to the increased use of lipid-lowering drugs was the Scandinavian Simvastatin Survival Study (4S), published in 1994 [1]. This secondary prevention trial demonstrated that lowering of total and low-density lipoprotein cholesterol (LDL-C) with the drug simvastatin reduced not only the risk of fatal and nonfatal myocardial infarction but also dramatically decreased the all-cause death rate. The landmark 4S trial has been supported, and the clinical benefits of LDL-C lowering extended by other large well-controlled statin trials [2–5]. The population studies have included those with CHD and LDL-C values as low as 115 mg/dL [1–3] and those without pre-existing CHD and LDL-C ranging from about 120 mg/dL [1–5]. Statins used in these trials have been extended to pravastatin and lovastatin. While still limited, there is good evidence from these trials that benefit occurs in all groups evaluated: women, men, elderly, and diabetics [10]. Further stimulation for the use of lipid-lowering agents was the First National Cholesterol Education Program Adult Treatment Panel Guidelines for the Detection, Evaluation, and Treatment of High Blood Cholesterol in Adults in 1988 [11] and updated in 1993, with publication of the full text of these guidelines in 1994 [12]. A third revision was published in 2001 [13].

LDL cholesterol remains the primary target for therapy in the United States, whereas total cholesterol is used in many other countries. Reduction in levels of either have been documented to reduce the risk of CHD. High-density lipoprotein cholesterol (HDL-C) levels are inversely associated with risk of developing CHD. There is more limited clinical trial evidence documenting that increasing HDL-C levels reduces the risk of CHD. The Air Force Coronary Atherosclerosis Prevention Study (AFCAPS) and the recent Veterans Administration High-Density Lipoprotein Intervention Trial (VA-HIT) are the most convincing trials. Low HDL-C cholesterol levels are treated primarily with lifestyle intervention, but drugs including statins and fibrates, to increase HDL-C levels are used in high-risk patients. HDL is generally the second priority for drug treatment. Elevated triglyceride levels are associated with multiple metabolic and lipoprotein abnormalities. There is emerging clinical evidence that suggests that triglyceride lowering is associated with reduced CHD risk [6]. However, triglyceride lowering is currently considered as the third level of consideration for drug therapy in some high-risk patients.

The National Cholesterol Education Program-Adult Treatment Panel III (NCEP-ATP III) guidelines [13] are generally accepted by the medical community for determining treatment in the United States. Guidelines specifi-cally for diabetes and formulated by the American Diabetes Association [14] have also elevated this population to the same risk status as those with CHD. Other countries have developed somewhat different approaches [15]. However, they all focus on lowering LDL-C or total cholesterol with some variation in the level of CHD risk that is required to implement drug therapy. The suggested levels for consideration of drug therapy and target goals for LDL-C in the NCEP and ADA recommendations are contained in Figure 9-1. Appropriate efforts to lower dietary intake of saturated and total fat and cholesterol plus increased physical activity and weight reduction should be done before drug therapy is initiated. Dietary therapy, weight reduction, and increased physical activity are the mainstays of therapy for primary prevention. Efforts should also be made to control all other modifiable risk factors for CHD.

A variety of new clinical trials have demonstrated safety and efficacy of lipid therapy in reducing the risk of initial and recurrent CHD events. Lipid therapy is effective in the setting of acute coronary syndromes to prevent ischemic heart disease over the ensuing months and in diabetic and nondiabetic patients. New agents with greater alterations in lipid levels are now available for the treatment and prevention of vascular disease, and combination therapy has shown to be preventive. The future holds even greater promise as antiatherosclerotic therapy expands further into lipid, glycemic, metabolic, and hematologic domains.

GUIDELINES FOR DRUG TREATMENT

GUIDELINES FOR DRUG TREATMENT OF LDL CHOLESTEROL

	LDL LEVEL FOR DRUG CONSIDERATION, mg/dL (mmol/L)	LDL GOAL OF THERAPY, mg/dL (mmol/L)	NON-LDL GOAL OF THERAPY, mg/dL (mmol/L)
Secondary prevention	≥130 (2.6)		
Clinical evidence of CHD, estimated 10-4 risk > 20.6	≥130 (3.3)	≤100 (2.6)	<130 (3.3)
Or other atherosclerotic disease, diabetes*			
Primary prevention			
With two (or more) other risk factors	≥160 (4.1)	<130 (3.3)	<160 (4.1)
Without two (or more) other risk factors	≥190 (4.9)	<160 (4.1)	<190 (4.9)
*ADA guidelines 1997 with diabetes defined as fasting glucose on two consecutive occasions ≥ 125 mg/dL.			

FIGURE 9-1. Guidelines for drug treatment of low-density lipoprotein cholesterol (LDL-C). Secondary prevention includes all patients with clinical evidence of coronary heart disease (CHD), definite thrombotic stroke or transient ischemic attacks, abdominal aortic aneurysm, or evidence of peripheral arterial disease, including claudication or prior interventional procedures. In primary prevention, an LDL-C level of 220 mg/dL or higher is suggested for initiating drug therapy in men younger than 35 years of age or premenopausal women in the absence of other risk factors [16].

RISK STATUS BASED ON PRESENCE OF CHD RISK FACTORS OTHER THAN LDL CHOLESTEROL (PRIMARY PREVENTION)

POSITIVE RISK FACTORS

Age
  Male ≥45 y
  Female ≥55 y or premature menopause without estrogen replacement therapy
Family history of premature CHD (definite myocardial infarction or sudden death before age
    55 y in male first-degree relative, or before age 65 y in female first-degree relative)
Current cigarette smoking
Hypertension (≥140/90 mm Hg, or on antihypertensive medication)
Low HDL-C (<4.0 mg/dL, 1.0 mmol/L)
Diabetes mellitus*

NEGATIVE RISK FACTOR

High HDL-C (≥60 mg/dL, 1.7 mmol/L)

* Moved to same category of risk as secondary prevention by the American Diabetes Association in 1997 as
  annual risk for CHD in diabetes without CHD is equal to or exceeds that for nondiabetics with CHD [17].

FIGURE 9-2. *High risk*, defined as a net of two or more coronary heart disease (CHD) risk factors, leads to more vigorous intervention. Age (defined differently for men and women) is treated as a risk factor because rates of CHD are higher in the elderly than the young, and in men than women of the same age. Use of antihypertensive medication has not produced the expected reduction in CHD risk and, thus, treated hypertension continues as a risk factor. High-density lipoprotein cholesterol (HDL-C) levels decrease CHD risk and, thus, one risk factor is subtracted. Although obesity is not listed as a risk factor because it operates through other risk factors that are included (hypertension, hyperlipidemia, decreased HDL-C, and diabetes mellitus), it should be considered a target for intervention. Physical inactivity is similarly not listed as a risk factor, but it too should be considered a target for intervention.

DRUG THERAPY FOR HDL CHOLESTEROL AND TRIGLYCERIDES

HDL-C

Secondary target for intervention
Consider if low HDL-C levels persist after lifestyle modification in high-risk patients with
    CHD, multiple risk factors, diabetes mellitus, and chronic renal disease
Use drugs that both lower LDL and increase HDL-C levels
Increase to levels of at least 45 mg/dL (1.2 mmol/L), if possible

TRIGLYCERIDES

Classification of triglycerides
  Normal: <150 mg/dL (1.7 mmol/L)
  Borderline–high: 150–199 mg/dL (1.7–2.2 mmol/L)
  High: 200–499 mg/dL (2.2–5.6 mmol/L)
  Very high: ≥ 500 mg/dL (5.6 mmol/L)

FIGURE 9-3. Drug therapy for high-density lipoprotein cholesterol (HDL-C) and triglycerides. Increasing HDL-C levels appear to be indicated in high-risk patients, but the availability of drug therapy for this purpose is limited. Reducing triglyceride levels for coronary heart disease (CHD) prevention is more controversial. Individuals with triglyceride levels in the range of 200 to 400 mg/dL (2.2 to 4.5 mmol/L) are at greater risk for developing CHD. There is an association of increased risk of pancreatitis in individuals with triglyceride levels exceeding 1000 mg/dL (11.2 mmol/L). LDL—low-density lipoprotein.

ATP III: THE METABOLIC SYNDROME

RISK FACTOR	DEFINITION
Waist circumference	> 102 cm (> 40 in) in men
	> 88 cm (> 35 in) in women
Triglycerides	≥ 150 mg/dL
HDL cholesterol	< 40 mg/dL
	< 50 mg/dL
Blood pressure	≥ 130/ ≥ 95 mm Hg
Fasting glucose	110–125 mg/dL

FIGURE 9-4. The metabolic syndrome. The National Cholesterol Education Program-Adult Treatment Panel III (NCEP-III) recommended a new classification, the metabolic syndrome, for persons thought to be at high risk for vascular disease risk. Persons with three or fewer of the five factors (increased waist circumference, triglycerides, low high-density lipoprotein [HDL] cholesterol, high blood pressure, or impaired fasting glucose) are considered to have the syndrome [13]. (*Adapted from* the Executive Summary of the Third Report of the National Cholesterol Education Program Expert Panel on Detection, Evaluation, and Treatment of High Blood Cholesterol in Adults [Adult Treatment Panel III] [13]).

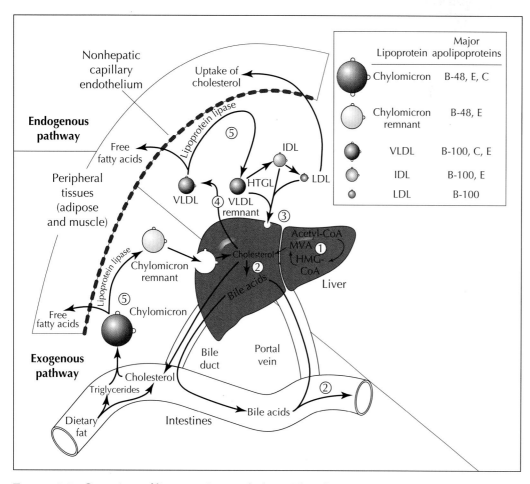

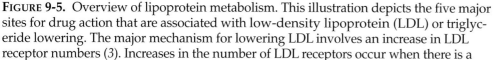

decrease in the cholesterol content of hepatic and other cells. This can occur either by decreasing the rate-limiting enzyme in cholesterol synthesis (hydroxymethyl glutaryl-coenzyme A [HMG-CoA] reductase) (1) or increasing the fecal excretion of bile acids with the resulting decrease in the bile acid pool (2). Enhanced receptor activity (3) increases the removal of LDL plus the precursors of LDL, very low-density lipoprotein (VLDL) remnants, and intermediate-density lipoprotein (IDL). Thus, the formation of LDL can also be decreased. VLDL remnants and IDL also contain triglycerides and thus a modest decrease
in triglycerides may be observed. Inhibition of lipoprotein synthesis (4) decreases the synthesis or secretion of VLDL, the major triglyceride-carrying lipoprotein. Secondarily, the formation of VLDL remnants, IDL, and LDL are decreased and both LDL cholesterol and triglyceride levels are reduced. Increased lipoprotein lipase activity (5) facilitates the removal of triglycerides from both chylomicrons and VLDL. These smaller particles must then be removed from the circulation by the remnant receptor. Moreover, the VLDL remnants can proceed to the formation of IDL and LDL, which can be removed by the LDL receptor. Acetyl-CoA—acetyl coenzyme A; HTGL—hepatic triglyceride lipase; MVA—mevalonate.

FIGURE 9-5. Overview of lipoprotein metabolism. This illustration depicts the five major sites for drug action that are associated with low-density lipoprotein (LDL) or triglyceride lowering. The major mechanism for lowering LDL involves an increase in LDL receptor numbers (3). Increases in the number of LDL receptors occur when there is a

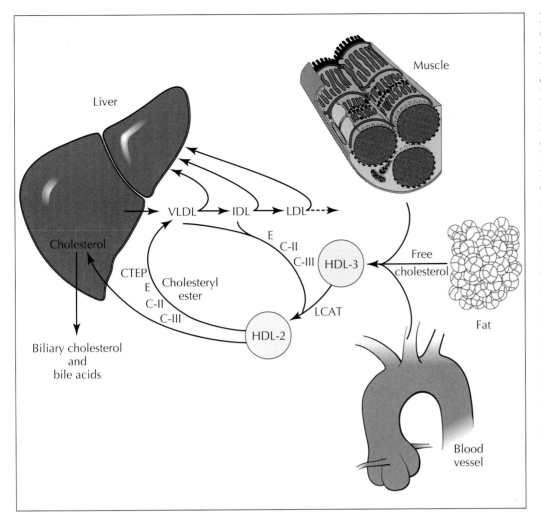

FIGURE 9-6. High-density lipoprotein (HDL) metabolism. The formation and metabolism of HDL are very complex and the mechanism of action of drugs that either increase or decrease HDL have not been well established [11,12]. Apolipoprotein (apo) A-1 is the major protein in HDL, and apo A-1 levels appear to correlate best with changes in HDL levels. Thus, drugs that either increase the synthesis or decrease the catabolism of apo A-1 would be expected to increase HDL levels. However, the origins of the various components of HDL are diffuse and there is an extensive exchange of protein, phospholipid, cholesterol (free and esterified), and triglycerides between HDL and other lipoproteins. Drugs have the potential for influencing HDL levels and function by multiple mechanisms. Because of the complexity and poor understanding, no further discussion of the effects of individual drugs on HDL metabolism is included in this chapter. CETP—cholesteryl ester transfer protein; IDL—intermediate-density lipoprotein; LCAT—lecithin-cholesterol acyltransferase; LDL—low-density lipoprotein; VLDL—very low-density lipoprotein.

AVAILABLE DRUGS

CLASSES OF DRUGS

<u>MAJOR CLASSES</u>

Bile acid sequestrants
  CholestaGel*, Cholestyramine, colestipol
HMG-CoA reductase inhibitors (statins)
  Lovastatin, pravastatin, simvastatin, fluvastatin, atorvastatin, rosuvastatin
Nicotinic acid (niacin)
  Immediate release (crystalline, rapid release)
  Sustained-release (slow, modified release)

<u>OTHER CLASSES</u>

Fibric acid derivatives
  Gemfibrozil, clofibrate, fenofibrate, bezafibrate†

<u>HORMONES</u>

Estrogen replacement in women
Serum estrogen receptor modulators

*Awaiting approval.
†Not yet approved.

FIGURE 9-7. The drugs listed have been approved for use in the United States with the exceptions noted. The major classes of drugs are those that are considered more effective in lowering low-density lipoprotein cholesterol (LDL-C) levels. The fibric acids are less effective for lowering LDL-C levels, generally in the range of 5% to 15%. Fenofibrate is more effective in lowering LDL-C levels, but only patients with normal triglycerides. Estrogen replacement therapy in postmenopausal women can be considered as an alternative therapy for lowering LDL-C levels, but estrogen therapy in women with existing coronary artery disease remains controversial [18].

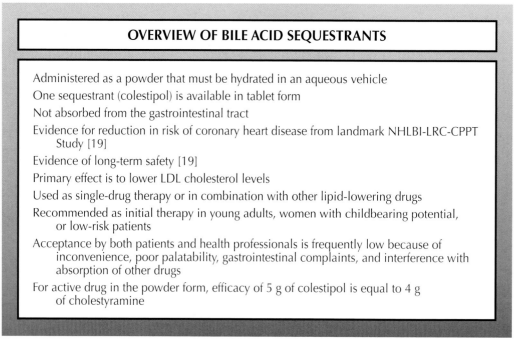

OVERVIEW OF BILE ACID SEQUESTRANTS

Administered as a powder that must be hydrated in an aqueous vehicle

One sequestrant (colestipol) is available in tablet form

Not absorbed from the gastrointestinal tract

Evidence for reduction in risk of coronary heart disease from landmark NHLBI-LRC-CPPT Study [19]

Evidence of long-term safety [19]

Primary effect is to lower LDL cholesterol levels

Used as single-drug therapy or in combination with other lipid-lowering drugs

Recommended as initial therapy in young adults, women with childbearing potential, or low-risk patients

Acceptance by both patients and health professionals is frequently low because of inconvenience, poor palatability, gastrointestinal complaints, and interference with absorption of other drugs

For active drug in the powder form, efficacy of 5 g of colestipol is equal to 4 g of cholestyramine

FIGURE 9-8. Overview of bile acid sequestrants. Bile acid sequestrants are effective in lowering low-density lipoprotein (LDL) cholesterol levels but patient acceptance, especially of higher doses, is frequently low. They are ideal drugs for initial therapy in low-risk patients with moderate elevations of LDL cholesterol or in patients in whom long-term safety considerations are of major importance.

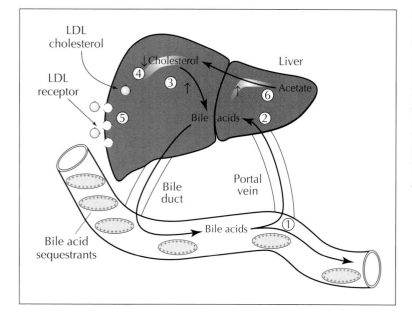

FIGURE 9-9. Mechanism of action of bile acid sequestrants. The bile acid sequestrants are highly charged resins that are not absorbed. They form insoluble complexes with bile acids in the gut and increase their fecal excretion (*1*). There is a decrease in the recirculation and pool of bile acids (*2*) resulting in a compensatory increase in the conversion of cholesterol to bile acids (*3*). Hepatic cholesterol content is decreased (*4*) with an increase in low-density lipoprotein (LDL) receptor numbers (*5*) and an increased rate of removal of LDL from the circulation. However, there is also a compensatory increase in cholesterol synthesis (*6*), which limits the increase in LDL receptors and the decrease in plasma LDL receptors that can be achieved and may also raise triglycerides.

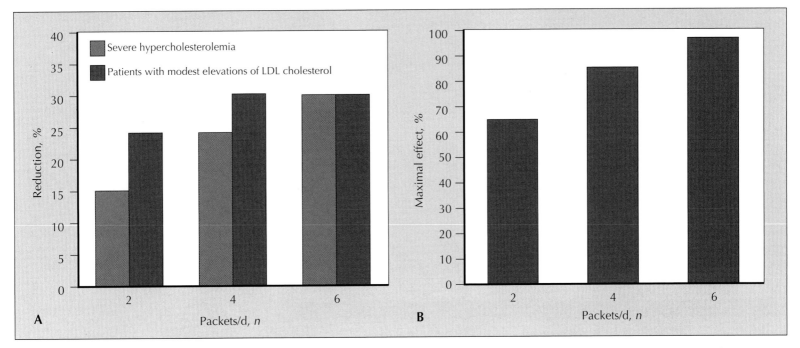

FIGURE 9-10. Effects of bile acid sequestrants on low-density lipoprotein cholesterol (LDL-C) levels [20–23]. **A,** The usual reported dose-response effects of the bile acid sequestrants on LDL-C levels. The maximum reduction in LDL-C is generally in the range of 27% to 30% with daily doses of 24 g of cholestyramine or 30 g of colestipol (six packets). With smaller doses, the percent reduction in LDL-C is inversely related to baseline LDL-C levels [22]. **B,** The percent maximum reduction in LDL-C that is generally reported in dose-response studies. Frequently, 60% to 65% of the maximal effect can be achieved with only two packets per day (8 g cholestyramine or 10 g colestipol) and 80% to 90% with four packets per day. The side effects are also dose-dependent. Patients frequently tolerate two packets per day (8 g of cholestyramine; 10 g of colestipol), others will tolerate up to four packets per day, but very few will tolerate more than that. Thus, smaller doses are usually recommended to maximize the amount of LDL-C lowering that can be achieved while minimizing the side effects.

MAJOR CLINICAL TRIALS WITH BILE ACID SEQUESTRANTS

PRIMARY PREVENTION

Lipid Research Clinics Coronary Primary Prevention Trial (LRC–CPPT) [18]
  Decreased risk for fatal and nonfatal myocardial infarction

SECONDARY PREVENTION

Angiographic trials show reduced rate of progression or increased regression of
  atherosclerosis in the coronary arteries
NHLBI Type II Coronary Intervention Study [24]
St. Thomas Atherosclerosis Regression Study (STARS) [25]
Cholesterol Lowering Atherosclerosis Study (CLAS) [26] (nicotinic acid)
Familial Atherosclerosis Treatment Study (FATS) [27] (lovastatin)

FIGURE 9-11. Clinical trials with bile acid sequestrants. The major clinical trial was the Lipid Research Clinics Coronary Primary Prevention Trial (LRC–CPPT), which demonstrated that lowering of low-density lipoprotein cholesterol (LDL-C) with cholestyramine reduced the risk of fatal and nonfatal myocardial infarction. Several trials have shown angiographic evidence of improvement in the coronary arteries either with cholestyramine as single-drug therapy (NHLBI and STARS) or with colestipol in combination with either nicotinic acid or lovastatin (CLAS, FATS).

SIDE EFFECTS OF BILE ACID SEQUESTRANTS

Palatability
   Taste and grittiness of powder formulations
Difficulty in administration
   Need to mix powder formulation in liquid vehicle
   Need to take large number of tablets or capsules
Gastrointestinal complaints
   Constipation, nausea, vomiting, heartburn, belching, and abdominal pain
Drug–drug interactions
   Coadministration shown to decrease absorption of thiazide, warfarin, statins,
      exogenous thyroxine, β-blockers, and cardiac glycosides
Hypertriglyceridemia
   Contraindicated as single-drug therapy in patients with dysbetalipoproteinemia
      and triglycerides >400 mg/dL

FIGURE 9-12. Side effects of bile acid sequestrants. The sandy or gritty consistency, the need for mixing with a vehicle, and achieving a uniform consistency make administration difficult for some patients. Gastrointestinal complaints are frequent. Also, the time of administration must be considered. Generally, these drugs are used in patients with triglyceride levels below 200 to 250 mg/dL. Marked increases in both serum cholesterol and triglyceride levels are observed when these drugs are used in patients with marked hypertriglyceridemia, whereas some increase in triglycerides is usually noted in patients with triglycerides exceeding 250 mg/dL.

ADMINISTRATION OF BILE ACID SEQUESTRANTS

Generally mixed with water or juice. There are a number of new flavored branded
   generic forms of cholestyramine
Tablet form (colestipol) is available in 1-g tablets, but the total number of tablets that must
   be administered will be considered excessive by many patients
Usually administered once or twice daily within 1 h of meals
Single dose is preferably administered with the major (evening) meal. This is the most
   effective time for administration and avoids drug interactions with drugs taken in the
   morning or at bedtime
Administer other drugs either 1 h before or 4 h after
A single dose of 8 g of cholestyramine (2 packets) or 10 g of colestipol administered
   within 1 h of the evening meal is a popular and practical regimen

FIGURE 9-13. Administration of bile acid sequestrants. The tablet forms may make it easier for some patients to take these drugs. The type and amount of vehicle may make the powder form more acceptable to some patients. Single-dose administration is especially useful for patients who take multiple drugs throughout the day.

STATINS

OVERVIEW OF STATINS

Most effective class of drugs for lowering LDL cholesterol
Lower triglycerides 5% to 35%, depending on baseline
   triglyceride level. Also increases HDL-C 4% to 10%, with
   more HDL-C elevation occurring the higher the baseline
   triglycerides.
Easy to administer
Very few drug–drug interactions
Well tolerated by patients, including older patients
Most widely prescribed class of lipid-altering drugs

FIGURE 9-14. Overview of statins. The statins have made the use of drugs for lowering low-density lipoprotein (LDL) cholesterol an achievable goal because of their effectiveness, ease of administration, and wide acceptance by both patients and health care professionals. HDL-C—high-density lipoprotein (HDL-C).

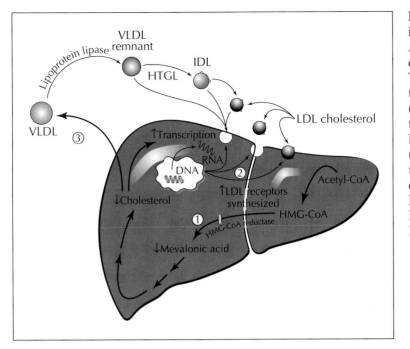

FIGURE 9-15. Mechanism of action of statins [23,24]. The statins inhibit the rate-limiting enzyme, hydroxymethyl glutaryl-coenzyme A (HMG-CoA) reductase, in cholesterol biosynthesis (1). The major organs for cholesterol biosynthesis are the small intestine and liver. The associated decrease in hepatic and cellular cholesterol concentration stimulates the production of low-density lipoprotein (LDL) receptors, which increase the rate of removal of LDL from the plasma (2). There is also increased removal of very low-density lipoprotein (VLDL) remnants and intermediate-density lipoprotein (IDL), which are precursors to LDL formation. In some patients, there may also be a decrease in lipoprotein synthesis (3). The enhanced removal of VLDL remnants and IDL and the inhibition of lipoprotein synthesis may contribute to the modest triglyceride-lowering effect of the statins. Acetyl-CoA—acetyl coenzyme A; HTGL—hepatic triglyceride lipase.

A: LDL-C REDUCTION

	DOSE, MG	% DECREASE
Fluvastatin*	20	20
	40	26
	80	34
Pravastatin*	10	21
	20	27
	40	33
Lovastatin*	10	22
	20	28
	40	34
	80	40
Simvastatin*	20	34
	40	40
	80	47
Atorvastatin*†	10	39
	20	43
	40	50
	80	60
Rosuvastatin	10	51
	20	57
	40	63

*Dosed in evening or bedtime.

†*Data from* Jones [30] and Hunninghake D, Insull W, Knopp R, *et al.*: Comparison of the efficacy of atorvastatin versus cerivastatin in primary hypercholesterolemia. *Am J Cardiol* 2001, 88:635–639.

B: TRIGLYCERIDE REDUCTION

Dependent on baseline triglycerides

< 150 mg/dl; minimal triglyceride reduction

150–250 mg/dL; % triglyceride reduction = 50% of %LDL-C reduction

> 250 mg/dL; % triglyceride reduction = % LDL-C reduction

Note that in subjects with triglyceride > 250 mg/dL, the LDL-C decrease for all statins is 3% to 6% less than that shown here for any dose

C: HDL-C ELEVATION

Also dependent on baseline triglycerides

< 150 mg/dL; HDL-C increase of 2%–5%

150–250 mg/dL; HDL-C increase of 4%–8%

> 250 mg/dL; HDL-C increase of 8%–14%

FIGURE 9-16. Lipid and lipoprotein effects of the statins [28–32]. **A,** Low-density lipoprotein cholesterol (LDL-C) reduction. **B,** Triglyceride (TG) reduction. **C,** High-density lipoprotein cholesterol (HDL-C) elevation. The reduction in LDL-C with the statins tends to be a log–linear relationship rather than linear. After the initial dose of statin, the additional reduction in LDL-C is generally only 6% to 8% each time the dose is doubled. The approximate dose response for each statin is depicted. Approximately equivalent reductions in LDL-C are produced by 0.04 mg of cervistatin, 1 mg of atovastatin, 2 mg of simvastatin, 4 mg of lovastatin, 5 mg of pravastatin, and 8 mg of fluvastatin up to their maximal approved doses. HDL-C increases of 5% to 10% are generally observed, and the increases are only slightly dose-dependent. Greater increases may be obtained in patients with low HDL-C and elevated TG levels. The reduction in TGs in subjects with TGs lower than 250 mg/dL is in the range of 5% to 12% with only a very slight dose-response effect. Greater decreases in TGs in the 20% to 40% range are seen in hypertriglyceridemic (> 250 mg/dL) patients, together with a dose-response curve. In hypertriglyceridemic subjects, the percent TG reduction is equal to the LDL-C reduction (TG:LDL-C ratio = 1:1), and thus in these subjects there is a log–linear dose response for TG reductions. Each doubling of statin results in a further 6% to 7% TG decrease.

PHARMACOLOGIC PROPERTIES OF STATINS

	ADMINISTERED FORM	SOLUBILITY	EXCRETION	PLASMA HALF-LIFE, *h*
Lovastatin	Prodrug	Lipophilic	Hepatic	3
Simvastatin	Prodrug	Lipophilic	Hepatic	—
Pravastatin	Parent	Hydrophilic	Renal and hepatic	3
Fluvastatin	Parent	Hydrophilic	Hepatic	<1
Atorvastatin	Parent	Hydrophilic	Hepatic	15
Rosuvastatin	Parent	Hydrophilic	Hepatic (90%) Renal (10%)	20

FIGURE 9-17. Pharmacologic properties of statins. There are several pharmacologic differences among the statins, some of which are described in this table. Lovastatin and simvastatin are administered as the prodrug that is converted to the active drug; they are also very lipophilic. There have been occasional reports of enhanced anticoagulant effect with highly protein-bound drugs such as lovastatin and simvastatin. Despite many pharmacologic differences, no definite clinical evidence for differing toxicities has been demonstrated. Lovastatin is administered with food to enhance its bioavailability. Pravastatin, atorvastatin, simvastatin, cerivastatin, and fluvastatin are best administered at bedtime; food has no effect on simvastatin bioavailability. Differences in bioavailability may not be directly correlated with overall effect on low-density lipoprotein cholesterol levels and timing relative to meals is a minor issue.

CLINICAL TRIALS WITH STATINS

ANGIOGRAPHIC TRIALS

Clinical evidence of a beneficial effect on the atherosclerotic process:

Reduced rates of progression/increased regression in the coronary arteries

Preliminary evidence of reduced progression in the carotid and peripheral arteries (angiographic or ultrasound studies)

Some studies also show a reduced number of CHD events

Representative studies include:

Monitored Atherosclerosis Regression Study (MARS) [33]

Canadian Coronary Artery Intervention Trial (CCAIT) [34]

Pravastatin Limitation of Atherosclerosis in Coronary Arteries (PLAC–1) [35]

Pravastatin, Lipids, and Atherosclerosis in the Carotid Arteries (PLAC–2) [36]

Asymptomatic Carotid Artery Plaque Study (ACAPS) [37]

Post CABG [38]

CLINICAL ENDPOINT TRIALS

Even with completion of a number of major endpoint trials, additional primary and secondary trials are still in progress

Secondary prevention trials

Scandinavian Simvastatin Survival Study

Most definitive trial to date involving 4444 participants with evidence of CHD who were followed for 5.4 y

Simvastatin administration was associated with a 30%–44% reduction in total mortality and major CHD events

Cholesterol and Recurrent Events in patients (CARE)

A secondary prevention trial using pravastatin in subjects with mildly elevated cholesterol levels

Lipid [3]

The largest (9000 subjects) secondary prevention trial in a very broad range of patients (cholesterol 150–250 mg/dL). Also used pravastatin

Primary Prevention Trials

West of Scotland Coronary Prevention Study (WOSCOPS)

The first primary prevention trial using a statin (pravastatin) conducted in 6595 men with high LDL-C (mean total cholesterol 272 mg/dL)

Significant reduction in CAD morbidity

Air Force/Texas Coronary Artery Prevention Study (AF/TexCAPS)

Primary prevention trial in men and women with fairly normal LDL-C levels (115 mg/dL–175 mg/dL) and low HDL-C (< 45 mg/dL in men and < 48 mg/dL in women) using lovastatin

Significant reduction in CAD end points that included unstable angina

FIGURE 9-18. Clinical trials with statins. The Scandinavian Simvastatin Survival Study conclusively demonstrated the benefits of low-density lipoprotein cholesterol (LDL-C) lowering in patients with coronary heart disease (CHD). The smaller angiographic trials demonstrated reduced rates of progression in the coronary arteries. A reduction in clinical events has also been demonstrated in meta-analyses of these trials and also in some individual trials. CAD—coronary artery disease; HDL-C—high-density lipoprotein cholesterol.

CAUSES OF DEATH IN THE SCANDINAVIAN SIMVASTATIN SURVIVAL STUDY		
TRIAL	PLACEBO (*n* = 2223)	SIMVASTATIN (*n* = 2221)
Cancer	35	33
Suicide	4	5
Trauma	3	1
Other	7	7
All non-CVD	49 (2.2%)	46 (2.1%)
All CVD	207 (9.3%)	136 (6.1%)

FIGURE 9-19. Statin in secondary prevention: impact on cardiovascular disease (CVD) and non-CVD death. Shown here are the causes of death in the Scandinavian Simvastatin Survival Study (4S). Median follow-up was 5.4 years. (*Adapted from* the Scandinavian Simvastatin Survival Group [1].)

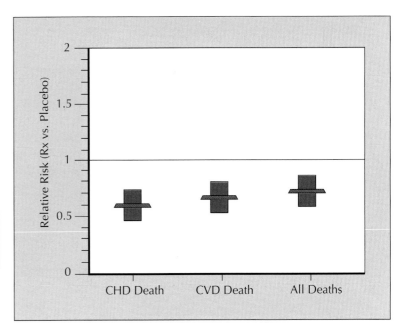

FIGURE 9-20. Benefit of statin therapy in secondary prevention. Shown here is the relative risk for death in 4444 patients with coronary heart disease (CHD) in the Scandinavian Simvastatin Survival Study (4S). Median follow-up was 5.4 years. CVD—cardiovascular disease. (*Adapted from* the Scandinavian Simvastatin Survival Group [1].)

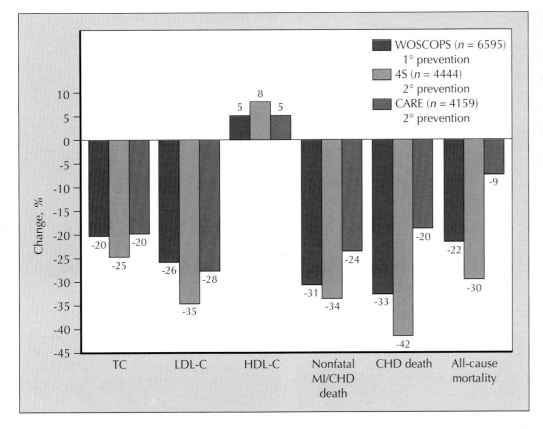

FIGURE 9-21. Summary of effects of lipid lowering on lipids and clinical events in recent statin trials. The average change in the levels of total cholesterol (TC), LDL cholesterol (LDL-C), and HDL cholesterol (HDL-C) are shown for three clinical trials that used statin medications for primary prevention (West of Scotland Coronary Prevention Study [WOSCOPS]; 40 mg/d pravastatin) [39] and secondary prevention (Scandinavian Simvastatin Survival Study [4S]; 10 to 40 mg/d simvastatin [40], and Cholesterol and Recurrent Events [CARE]; 40 mg/d pravastatin [41]). Alongside are the differences in event rates between active therapy and placebo for nonfatal myocardial infarction (MI)/coronary heart disease (CHD) death, CHD death alone, and all-cause mortality.

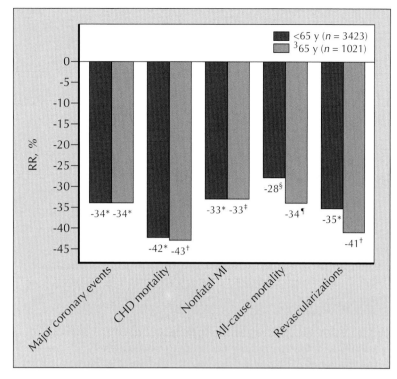

FIGURE 9-22. Reduction in coronary events and revascularizations in older adults with established coronary heart disease (CHD). Similar decrements in event rates were observed in the active treatment group (simvastatin 10 to 40 mg/d) for younger (< 65 years of age) and older (≥ 65 years of age) participants in the 4S trial [42]. The endpoints included major coronary events, CHD mortality, nonfatal myocardial infarction (MI), all-cause mortality, and revascularizations. All *P* values represent within-group differences (treatment vs placebo). *P<0.001; †P=0.003; ‡P=0.004; §P=0.007; ¶P=0.009. RR—relative risk. (*Data from* Miettinen *et al.* [42].)

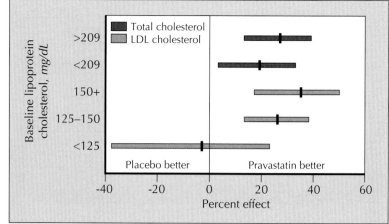

FIGURE 9-23. Effect of 40 mg of pravastatin on major coronary events: CARE subgroup analysis. The reduction of coronary events in the CARE study was related to the baseline cholesterol level [41]. Persons with baseline low-density lipoprotein cholesterol (LDL-C) of 125 to 150 mg/dL or greater than 150 mg/dL who took pravastatin 40 mg/d experienced lower risk for major coronary events during follow-up in comparisons with persons on placebo. Persons with LDL-C lower than 125 mg/dL at baseline did not benefit from active therapy. (*Adapted from* Sacks *et al.* [41].)

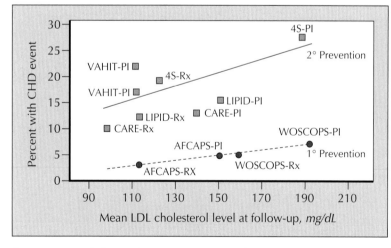

FIGURE 9-24. Relation between coronary heart disease (CHD) events and low-density lipoprotein (LDL) cholesterol in recent lipid trials. The relation between mean LDL cholesterol on therapy and the percent of clinical trial participants developing a CHD event were related and separate slopes were observed for primary prevention trials and secondary prevention studies. Data were derived from a variety of trials [39,51,43–46]. Pl—placebo; Rx—treatment. LIPID—Long-Term Intervention with Pravastatin in Ischaemic Disease; VAHIT—Veterans Administration High-density Lipoprotein Intervention Trial.

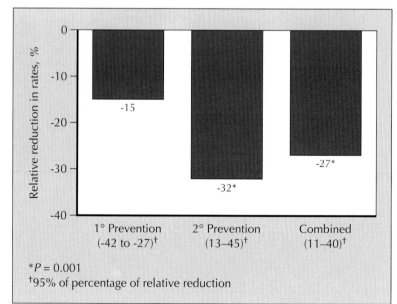

FIGURE 9-25. Statins and stroke events: meta-analysis of primary and secondary prevention trials. Lipid lowering was related to reduced risk for stroke in a meta-analysis of statin trials that targeted primary and secondary prevention of coronary heart disease. (*Adapted from* Crouse *et al.* [47].)

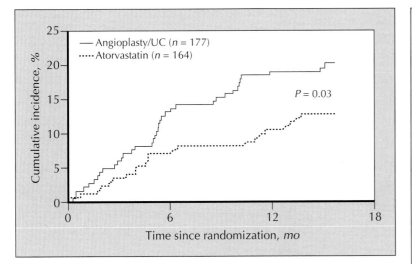

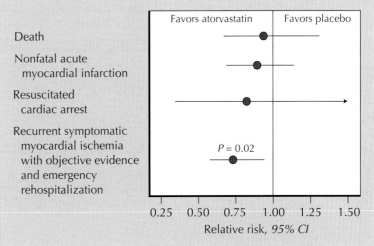

FIGURE 9-26. Atorvastatin versus placebo therapy in the setting of acute coronary syndromes. The time to first event (recurrent symptomatic myocardial ischemia with objective evidence and requiring urgent rehospitalization) was significantly reduced in the treatment group compared with the placebo group (relative risk, 0.74; 95% CI, 0.57–0.95 in the Atorvastatin Versus Revascularization Treatment (AVERT) trial [48]. (*Adapted from* Pitt *et al.* [48].)

FIGURE 9-27. Effects of atorvastatin on early recurrent ischemic events in acute coronary syndromes in the Myocardial Ischemia Reduction with Aggressive Cholesterol Lowering (MIRACL) trial. In this trial, 3086 persons with an acute coronary syndrome were randomly assigned within 96 hours to 80 mg/d of atorvastatin or placebo and followed for 16 weeks. The primary endpoint event defined as death, nonfatal acute myocardial infarction, cardiac arrest with resuscitation, or recurrent symptomatic myocardial ischemia with objective evidence and requiring emergency rehospitalization was 14.8% in the atorvastatin group and 17.4% in the placebo group, for a relative risk of 0.84 (*P* = 0.048). There were no significant differences in risk of death, nonfatal myocardial infarction, or cardiac arrest [49]. (*Adapted from* Schwartz *et al.* [49].)

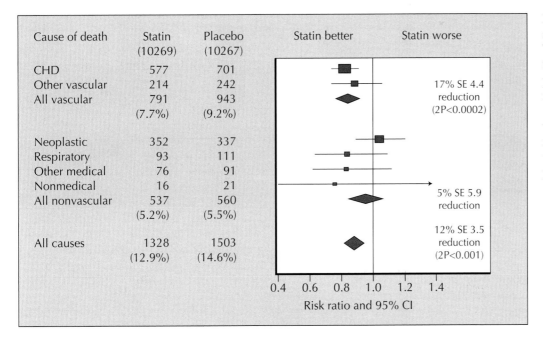

FIGURE 9-28. Simvastatin and cause-specific mortality heart protection study. The recently reported Heart Protection Study, a primary prevention study of persons 40 to 80 years of age who were at increased risk of coronary heart disease (CHD) death due to prior disease and with total cholesterol greater than 135 mg/dL at baseline, demonstrated a reduction in death rates for vascular disease in persons taking 40 mg simvastatin/d (Unpublished data).

SIDE EFFECTS OF HMG CoA REDUCTASE INHIBITORS

INCREASED TRANSAMINASE LEVELS

0.1%–2.5% of treated patients develop increases of > 3 × upper-normal limit, especially at higher doses
Rapidly reversible, no evidence of chronic liver disease

MYOPATHY

Diffuse muscle pain and CPK > 10 × upper-normal limit
Primarily seen when higher doses of statins are used in combination with cyclosporine, gemfibrozil, and occasionally erythromycin and niacin

MISCELLANEOUS

Gastrointestinal complaints, arthralgias, and headaches

FIGURE 9-29. Side effects of reductase inhibitors. The side effect profile of the statins is very favorable, considering their efficacy in lowering low-density lipoprotein cholesterol levels. Initial monitoring of transaminase levels is indicated, but abnormalities are rapidly reversible with a reduction in dosage, and discontinuance of drug is rarely required to prevent rhabdomyolysis and renal failure. The incidence of all side effects is low. If side effects do occur, use of another statin may be tried. CPK—creatinine phosphokinase; HMG-CoA—hydroxymethyl-glutaryl coenzyme A.

FATAL RHABDOMYOLYSIS AND STATINS IN THE UNITED STATES

VARIABLE	LOVASTATIN	PRAVASTATIN	SIMVASTATIN	FLUVASTATIN	ATORVASTATIN	CERIVASTATIN	TOTAL
Year approved	1987	1991	1991	1993	1996	1997	—
Fatal cases of rhabdomyolysis	19	3	14	0	6	31	73
Prescriptions, $n \times 10^6$	99.2	81.4	116.1	37.4	140.4	9.8	484.3
Reporting rate (per 10^6 prescriptions)	0.19	0.04	0.12	0	0.04	3.16	0.15

FIGURE 9-30. Fatal rhabdomyolysis and statins in the United States. Reports of fatal rhabdomyolysis were tracked since the first release of statin medications in 1987. Rates were consistently low across the different types of statins except for cerivastatin, which was subsequently withdrawn from the market in 2001 [50].

ADMINISTRATION OF STATINS

TIME

Single-dose administration is always more effective in the evening
Lovastatin is administered with evening meal; all others are usually administered at bedtime
Fluvastatin is administered as 40 mg twice a day at maximal dose

FREQUENCY

Generally administered as a single dose
At higher doses, twice-daily administration can be considered for slightly greater efficacy, although the cost is also greater, and compliance may decrease

USUAL DAILY-DOSE RANGE, *mg*

Lovastatin, 10–80
Simvastatin, 20–80
Pravastatin, 10–40
Fluvastatin, 20–80
Atorvastatin, 10–80
Rosuvastatin, 10–80

FIGURE 9-31. Administration of statins. The statins are usually administered at bedtime as a single evening dose. A slightly greater low-density lipoprotein cholesterol lowering effect may be observed with twice-daily administration, but the cost of two lower dosage tablets is considerably greater than that of a single higher dosage tablet.

GENERAL FEATURES OF NICOTINIC ACID

Favorably affects all lipid and lipoprotein levels in the direction that should decrease risk for CHD. Moderately lowers Lp(a) levels. Lowers total and LDL-C and triglycerides; increases HDL-C [38]

The immediate release formulations have more triglyceride lowering and HDL-C–raising effect, even at lower doses (1500–3000 mg/d), while LDL-C reduction often requires higher doses (3000–5000 mg/d). Sustained release niacin has more initial effect on LDL-C with slightly less impact on triglyceride and HDL-C (doses should not exceed 2000 mg/d) [51]

Two formulations used: immediate (rapid, crystalline) niacin (IR) or sustained-release (slow, modified) niacin (S-R). both formulations are available without prescription and are inexpensive, but great caution is needed in their use as quality and potential toxicity vary widely. There are FDA-approved and regulated immediate and sustained-release niacin formulations that, although more expensive, are reliable and have fewer side effects [52,53]

Side-effect frequency is quite high, especially at higher doses when hepatic toxicity is the most common, most notably with sustained-release formulations

Often increases blood glucose and uric acid; should be used with caution in diabetics and those with gout

Difficult drug to administer and achieve compliance

FIGURE 9-32. Overview of nicotinic acid. Nicotinic acid is primarily considered for use because of cost considerations or to increase HDL-C levels. However, acceptance by both patients and health care professionals is extremely limited because of the high frequency of side effects. CHD—coronary heart disease; FDA—US Food and Drug Administration; HDL-C—high-density lipoprotein cholesterol; LDL-C—low-density lipoprotein cholesterol; Lp(a)—lipoprotein a.

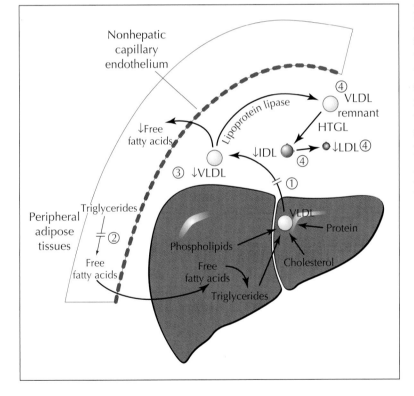

FIGURE 9-33. Mechanism of action of nicotinic acid. Inhibition of lipoprotein synthesis is generally considered to be the major effect of nicotinic acid (1). Inhibition of lipolysis of the stored fat in adipose tissue (2) with the resultant decrease in free fatty acids delivered to the liver could also indirectly decrease lipoprotein synthesis. The clinical significance of this mechanism has not been well documented in humans. Inhibition of lipoprotein (possibly apolipoprotein B) synthesis decreases very low-density lipoprotein (VLDL) secretion or synthesis (3), and all subsequent lipoproteins in this pathway (VLDL remnants, intermediate-density lipoprotein [IDL] and low-density lipoprotein [LDL]) are also decreased (4). Nicotinic acid may also modestly lower lipoprotein (a) levels by unknown mechanism(s). HTGL—hepatic triglyceride lipase.

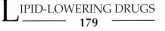

NICOTINIC ACID PREPARATIONS

Nicotinamide

No lipid-altering effects

Nicotinic acid; immediate-release (IR), crystalline, or rapid

Most effective drug for increasing HDL-C; also effective in reducing triglyceride [38]

Large doses are required to achieve significant decreases in LDL-C

More initial skin reaction (flushing), which decreases rapidly with dose escalation. Less hepatotoxicity, even at higher doses than slow release (SR)

Niacor*

Available by prescription

Administered with meals twice or three times a day

Usual dose 1500–4500 mg/d

Flushing decreased by coadministration with food, low-dose aspirin (81 mg), and rapid escalation of initial dose from 250 mg to 1500 mg over 14 days

Large increases in HDL-C, decreases triglyceride, Lp(a), and LDL-C (at higher doses)

Nicotinic acid; (SR) sustained or modified

Used primarily for lowering LDL-C but less effective for HDL-C raising and triglyceride lowering

More effective than IR preparations for lowering LDL-C, but less effective for HDL-C raising and triglyceride lowering

Risk of severe hepatotoxicity is greater than for IR preparations and occurs at much lower doses

Niaspan†, Advicor (combination with lovastatin)

Available by prescription

Administered as a single bedtime dose

Usual dose 1000–2000 mg/d; starting doses 375 mg, 500 mg, 750 mg for 1 week each

May be better tolerated than IR niacin

Increases HDL-C, lowers total and LDL-C and triglycerides

* Upsher-Smith Laboratories, Inc., Minneapolis MN.
†KOS Pharmaceuticals, Inc., Miami, FL.

FIGURE 9-34. Nicotinic acid preparations [19,38,51]. Because these preparations are available without a prescription, patients must be instructed to take nicotinic acid or niacin only and be aware of inconsistencies and variabilities between non-FDA–regulated preparations. The use of slow-release preparations is still contro- versial, although a new less hepatotoxic FDA-approved formula- tion is now available. FDA—US Food and Drug Administration; HDL-C—high-density lipoprotein cholesterol; LDL-C—low- density lipoprotein cholesterol; Lp(a)—lipoprotein (a).

LIPID AND LIPOPROTEIN EFFECTS OF NICOTINIC ACID

DOSE, mg/d	LDL-C, % CHANGE			HDL-C, % CHANGE			TRIGLYCERIDE, % CHANGE		
	IR*	IR†	SR†	IR*	IR†	SR†	IR*	IR†	SR†
500	—	-2	-6	—	9	-2	—	-11	-7
1000	—	-6	-12	—	25	2	—	-30	-7
1500	-5	-14	-22	20	30	12	-22	-30	-25
2000	—	-18	-33	—	31	17	—	-39	-30
3000	-16	-21	0	29	35	‡	-29	-41	‡
4500	-21	—	0	33	—	‡	-34	—	‡

*Data from Illingworth et al. [38].
†Data from McKenney et al. [51].
‡Dose should not be used.

FIGURE 9-35. Lipid and lipoprotein effects of nicotinic acid. There have not been controlled clinical trials to document the dose-response effects of nicotinic acid. Although there is some variance in results in two recent studies [38,51], the major findings are shown. Relatively large dose of crystalline niacin (immediate-release [IR]) are required to achieve reductions of 20% or more in low-density lipoprotein cholesterol (LDL-C). The slow-release (SR) forms are more effective in lowering LDL-C. Significant increases in high-density lipoprotein cholesterol (HDL-C) can be achieved with IR of 1.5 g or less. The SR form was less effective in increasing HDL-C.

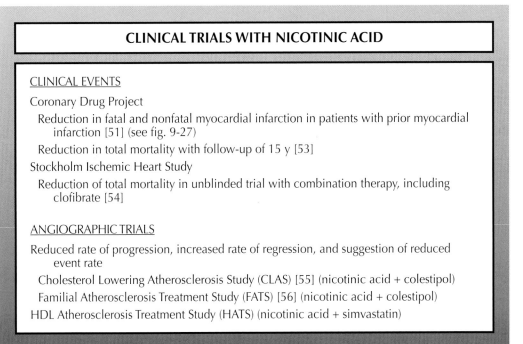

CLINICAL TRIALS WITH NICOTINIC ACID

<u>CLINICAL EVENTS</u>

Coronary Drug Project

    Reduction in fatal and nonfatal myocardial infarction in patients with prior myocardial
        infarction [51] (see fig. 9-27)

    Reduction in total mortality with follow-up of 15 y [53]

Stockholm Ischemic Heart Study

    Reduction of total mortality in unblinded trial with combination therapy, including
        clofibrate [54]

<u>ANGIOGRAPHIC TRIALS</u>

Reduced rate of progression, increased rate of regression, and suggestion of reduced
       event rate

    Cholesterol Lowering Atherosclerosis Study (CLAS) [55] (nicotinic acid + colestipol)

    Familial Atherosclerosis Treatment Study (FATS) [56] (nicotinic acid + colestipol)

HDL Atherosclerosis Treatment Study (HATS) (nicotinic acid + simvastatin)

FIGURE 9-36. Clinical trials with nicotinic acid. The only major trial with nicotinic acid as single-drug therapy is the Coronary Drug Project. There are no reports of major reported primary prevention trials.

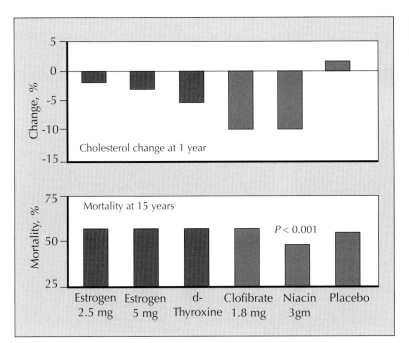

FIGURE 9-37. Nonfibrate, nonresin therapies in secondary prevention. Shown here are results from the Coronary Drug Project: lipid changes and mortality. (*Adapted from* Canner *et al.* [53].)

HDL ATHEROSCLEROSIS TREATMENT STUDY (HATS) CLINICAL RESULTS: PRIMARY PREVENTION OF CHD WITH LIPID THERAPY AND ANTIOXIDANTS

FIRST COMPARISON GROUP	EVENT RATE, %	SECOND COMPARISON GROUP	EVENT RATE, %	RELATIVE RISK	P VALUE
Simvastatin-niacin (*n* = 38)	3	Placebo (*n* = 38)	24	0.10	0.03
Simvastatin-niacin plus antioxidants (*n* = 42)	14	Antioxidants (*n* = 42)	21	0.64	0.40
Simvastatin-niacin (*n* = 80)	9	No simvastatin-niacin (*n* = 80)	22	0.64	0.02
No antioxidants (*n* = 76)	13	Antioxidants (*n* = 84)	18	1.38	0.38

FIGURE 9-38. Clinical results of the HDL Atherosclerosis Treatment Study (HATS). The results showed that combined therapy with simvastatin-niacin, but not with antioxidants (800 IU vitamin E, 1000 mg vitamin C, 25 mg β-carotene, 100 μg sele-nium) was related to lower risk for composite clinical coronary heart disease events (death from coronary causes, confirmed myocardial infarction or stroke, or revascularization for wors-ening ischemic symptoms) [58].

SIDE EFFECTS OF NICOTINIC ACID

Flushing and vasomotor symptoms
  Affects almost all patients with initial doses of IR preparations
  Most common cause for discontinuance
  Can be markedly reduced or eliminated by coadministration of low-dose aspirin (81 mg) taken with food; rapid increase in dose from 250 mg to 1500 mg in 2 weeks. Frequency is less with SR preparations and Niaspan
Upper gastrointestinal complaints
  Heartburn, nausea, vomiting, abdominal pain, gastrointestinal bleeding, and activation of peptic ulcer
Dose-dependent hepatotoxicity
  Most common with SR preparations even at low doses of 1500–2000 mg. Uncommon with IR until dose exceeds 4500 mg
Dose-dependent hyperglycemia
  Generally not used or used with caution in non–insulin-dependent diabetes mellitus; on average, causes a 10–30 mg/dL increase in fasting glucose level
Dose-dependent hyperuricemia or gout
  If history of gout or elevated uric acid, pretreat with allopurinol
Miscellaneous
  Myriad infrequent side effects, including acanthosis nigricans, retinal edema, increase in supraventricular arrhythmias
  Needs to be used with caution in conjunction with statins, as at least one case of rhabdomyolysis has been reported [57].

FIGURE 9-39. Side effects of nicotinic acid [26]. There are multiple side effects, and some can be quite severe. Careful clinical and biochemical monitoring is required until the final dose has been determined. IR—immediate release; SR—sustained release.

FIBRIC ACIDS

GENERAL FEATURES OF FIBRIC ACIDS

Gemfibrozil and fenofibrate are available in the United States
Primarily used to decrease triglyceride levels
Modest increases in HDL-C and decreases in LDL-C if hypertriglyceridemia is not present
Easy to administer
Relatively few side effects and drug–drug interactions
Evidence for reduction in risk for CHD in primary [59,60] and secondary prevention [6]
Generally not used as first drug for reducing CHD risk

FIGURE 9-40. General features of fibric acids. The popularity of the fibric acids has decreased since the introduction of the statins, which are also easy to administer. Concerns about long-term safety and valuable effect on low-density lipoprotein cholesterol (LDL-C) of fibric acids limit their use. CHD—coronary heart disease; HDL-C—high-density lipoprotein cholesterol.

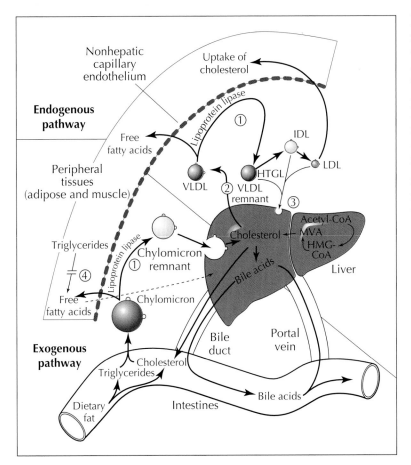

Figure 9-41. Mechanism of action of fibric acids [21,61–63]. The mechanism of action of the fibric acids has not been completely established and may also be dependent upon the specific fibric acid used. All fibric acids increase lipoprotein lipase activity (*1*), which results in decreased very low-density lipoprotein (VLDL) and triglyceride levels. Other reported mechanisms that have been less well documented include decreased lipoprotein synthesis (*2*), increased low-density lipoprotein (LDL) receptor activity (*3*), and decreased lipolysis within adipose tissue (*4*), which could indirectly decrease lipoprotein synthesis. Acetyl-CoA—acetyl coenzyme A; HMG-CoA—hydroxymethyl glutaryl-coenzyme A; HTGL—hepatic triglyceride lipase; IDL—intermediate-density lipoprotein; MVA—mevalonate.

LIPID AND LIPOPROTEIN EFFECTS OF FIBRIC ACIDS

LDL CHOLESTEROL

The reduction in LDL-C is inversely related to baseline triglyceride levels

Patients with triglyceride levels <200 mg/dL generally achieve 10%–12% reductions in LDL-C. Conversely, patients with triglyceride levels of >400 mg/dL may have an increase in LDL-C levels. This is due to compositional changes in LDL such that when triglyceride levels are decreased, the cholesterol ester content of LDL increases.

Greater decreases may be seen with fenofibrate, which is now available in the United States

HDL CHOLESTEROL

Increases of about 10%–15% are usually observed

Greater increases are seen in patients with low HDL-C levels or with hypertriglyceridemia

TRIGLYCERIDES

Reductions are usually in the range of 25%–50%

Greater decreases are seen in patients who have higher triglyceride values

Figure 9-42. Lipid and lipoprotein effects of the fibric acid study [21,64,65]. The fibric acids are usually the most effective class of drugs for lowering triglycerides. Many patients with hypertriglyceridemia also have hyperglycemia and hyperuricemia. Thus, the fibric acids would be preferred to nicotinic acid in these patients. The effects on low-density lipoprotein cholesterol (LDL-C) and high-density lipoprotein (HDL-C) are modest.

CLINICAL TRIALS WITH FIBRIC ACIDS

<u>MAJOR PRIMARY PREVENTION TRIALS</u>

WHO Clofibrate Study
  Decrease in fatal and nonfatal myocardial infarction
  Increase in non-CHD mortality both during the trial and for entire duration of
    follow-up [60,66]
Helsinki Heart Study (gemfibrozil) [60,64]
  34% reduction in fatal and nonfatal myocardial infarction [60]
  Reduction in risk due to both the increase in HDL-C and the decrease in LDL-C
  Increase in non-CHD death rate, especially during posttrial observation [64]
Bezafibrate Infarction Prevention trial (BIP) [67]
  Secondary prevention trial with bezafibrate
  Nonsignificant reduction in fatal and nonfatal CAD
Veterans Administration—HDL Intervention Trial (VA-HIT) [6] (*see* Figs. 9-33 and 9-34)
  Secondary prevention trial with gemfibrozil
  Patients with low HDL-C and normal LDL-C and triglycerides
  22% reduction in fatal and nonfatal CAD
  No offsetting morbidity or mortality

FIGURE 9-43. Clinical trials with fibric acids. Both of the major primary prevention trials with three different fibrates showed a reduction in coronary heart disease (CHD) events. The enthusiasm for the use of these drugs is diminished by the observations of a lack of uniform benefit across all trials and an increase in non-CHD death rate. No large prevention trial with fenofibrate has been reported. Clofibrate is no longer used in most countries. CAD—coronary artery disease; HDL-C—high-density lipoprotein cholesterol; LDL-C—low-density lipoprotein cholesterol; WHO—World Health Organization.

VETERAN'S ADMINISTRATION HDL INTERVENTION TRIAL

2531 male patients with CHD
  HDL-C < 40 mg/dL
  LDL-C <140 mg/dL
  Triglyerides <300 mg/dL
7-year follow up
  gemfibrozil vs placebo

FIGURE 9-44. Fibrate therapy and secondary prevention. Shown here are the results from the Veterans' Administration HDL Intervention Trial (VA-HIT). CHD—coronary heart disease; HDL-C—high-density lipoprotein cholesterol; LDL-C—low-density lipoprotein cholesterol.

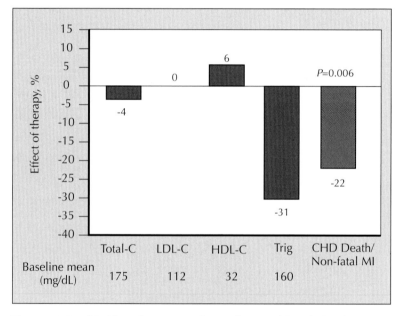

FIGURE 9-45. Lipid and coronary heart disease (CHD) deaths: nonfatal myocardial infarction with fibrate therapy. Shown here are the VA-HIT results: (gemfibrozil vs placebo). HDL-C—high-density lipoprotein cholesterol; LDL-C—low-density lipoprotein cholesterol; MI—myocardial infarction; Total-C—total cholesterol; Trig—triglycerides. (*Adapted from* Rubins *et al.* [6].)

SIDE EFFECTS OF FIBRIC ACID

Primarily gastrointestinal complaints
    Flatulence, abdominal discomfort, change in stools, gallstones
Highly protein-bound drugs
    Potentiate anticoagulant effect of coumarin anticoagulants
Increase lithogenicity of bile and cholelithiasis
Possible increase in non-CHD death rate
    No single cause for this increased mortality is evident, and
        latest two trials, VA-HIT and BIP, raised no safety concerns
Myopathy is rarely reported but can occur in subjects with impaired
    renal function and when coadministered with statins

FIGURE 9-46. Side effects of fibric acid [59,60,64,66]. The fibric acids are generally well tolerated with the more frequent side effects being gastrointestinal in nature. They are highly protein-bound drugs and can increase the free or nonprotein-bound concentration of other highly bound drugs such as the oral anticoagulants, thus potentiating their effect. CHD—coronary heart disease.

ADMINISTRATION OF FIBRIC ACID

Usual dose
  Gemfibrozil, 600 mg twice daily
  Fenofibrate, 100–300 mg daily in single or divided doses for
    original formulation
    New micronized preparations available in either 67-mg or
      200-mg capsules (100 mg of original formulation = 67 mg
      micronized)
    Bezafibrate, 400 mg daily in single dose. Not available in
      United States.
Renal excretion
  Primarily excreted by kidney; dose must be reduced if
    significant reduction in renal function
Highly protein-bound
  Dose must be reduced if used in patients with very low serum
    albumin levels

FIGURE 9-47. Administration of fibric acids. Gemfibrozil and fenofibrate are currently available in the United States. The dose of both drugs should be reduced in patients with significantly impaired renal function because the parent drug and its metabolite are primarily excreted by the kidney. Gemfibrozil is also present in the plasma in high concentrations and is over 95% bound to serum albumin; thus the dose should be reduced if serum albumin concentrations are very low.

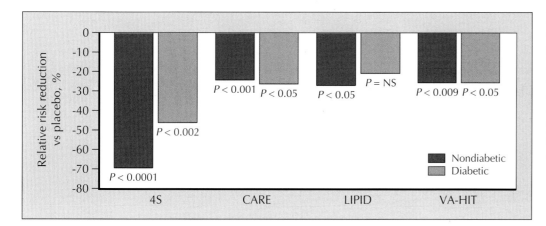

FIGURE 9-48. Reduction in cardiovascular disease (CVD) relative risk: results from secondary prevention trials. A summary of lipid-lowering results has typically shown a similar reduction in CVD risk in diabetics and nondiabetics for simvastatin in 4S (hard coronary heart disease [CHD]) [67], pravastatin in CARE and LIPID (both hard CHD) [41,45], and gemfibrozil in VA-HIT (hard CHD or stroke) [46].

PROBUCOL

SUMMARY OF MAJOR EFFECTS OF PROBUCOL

LDL-C reduction of 5%–15% [68,69]

HDL-C reduction of 20%–25% [68,69]

Major interest has been in potential use as an antioxidant [70]

    Powerful antioxidant in in vitro and animal studies

    In the PQRST femoral angiogram clinical trial, there was no
    evidence of clinical benefit

Lack of large studies to define long-term safety

Side effects

    Variety of gastrointestinal complaints, including loose stools

    Prolongs Q-T interval

    Hypertriglyceridemia may be made worse

Removed from the market in most counties including the
    United States

    Occasional use in patients who do not respond to or tolerate
    other medications

FIGURE 9-49. Summary of major effects of probucol. The current role of probucol as a lipid-lowering drug is not clear. It modestly lowers low-density lipoprotein cholesterol (LDL-C) but also significantly decreases high-density lipoprotein cholesterol (HDL-C) levels. Although there is considerable interest in its antioxidant effect, the Probucol Quantitative Regression Swedish Trial (PQRST) did not demonstrate clinical benefit in terms of atherosclerosis progression.

HORMONAL REPLACEMENT THERAPY

EFFECTS OF ESTROGEN REPLACEMENT ON CHD RISK

Epidemiologic studies indicate that estrogen replacement in postmenopausal women
    reduces CHD risk [72–75]

    50% in primary prevention

    80% in secondary intervention

Conjugated estrogens (0.625 mg) or equivalent dose of other estrogen [76]

    LDL-C reduction of 10%–15%

    HDL-C increase of 10%–15%

Clinical Trial

    Heart and Estrogen/Progestin Replacement Study (HERS) [8]

    Only large randomized, double-blind placebo-controlled trial to date

    Postmenopausal women with a uterus and clinical evidence of CHD

    Daily administration of 0.625 mg of conjugated equine estrogen and 2.5 mg of medrox-
    yprogesterone acetate for 4+ years

    No significant reduction in fatal and nonfatal MI and increased risk in the first year after
    initiating therapy

Other clinical trials

    Women's Health Initiative (WHI) is currently underway [77]

    Primary prevention

    Evaluating estrogen only and estrogen plus progestin

    Non-CHD events such as breast and colon cancer are being evaluated

SERMS

    No clinical trials to date to evaluate potential effect on CHD risk

FIGURE 9-50. Effects of estrogen replacement on coronary heart disease (CHD) risk. The only large prospective trial with combination therapy of estrogen plus progestin did not show a reduction in CHD risk [18]. The results of ongoing trials are anxiously awaited. HDL-C—high-density lipoprotein cholesterol; LDL-C—low-density lipoprotein cholesterol; MI—myocardial infarction.

HORMONAL REPLACEMENT THERAPY AND CHD RISK

Combination of estrogen and progestin used in postmenopausal women with a uterus
  Addition of progestin does reduce risk of endometrial hyperplasia and cancer
  Long-term effects on incidence of breast cancer has not been definitely established
  Requires regular monitoring with mammograms and pelvic examinations
  Interest in potential effect of different progestin preparation on CHD risk when used in combination with estrogen
Estrogen only used in women without a uterus
  No large completed clinical trials to define effect on CHD risk
  Long-term effects on incidence of breast cancer have not been established
  Requires regular monitoring with mammograms
  Less epidemiologic information on combination therapy than estrogen only
  Not known if progestin alters risk reduction produced by estrogen only
  Addition of progestin does reduce risk of endometrial hyperplasia and cancer
Long-term effects of estrogen alone or estrogen/progestin on incidence of breast cancer have not been definitely established
Estrogen or estrogen/progestin replacement therapy does require regular monitoring with mammograms and pelvic examinations
Oral estrogen can cause severe hypertriglyceridemia and pancreatitis. Check fasting lipids prior to start of therapy and 4–8 wk after starting
Transdermal hormone replacement therapy: less risk of hypertriglyceridemia

FIGURE 9-51. Hormonal replacement therapy and coronary heart disease (CHD) risk [11,74]. The results of large multicenter trials are required to accurately define the comparative effects of estrogen alone or estrogen/progestin combinations for risk of CHD and breast cancer. In women with a uterus, the increased risk of endometrial hyperplasia and carcinoma associated with estrogen only are markedly reduced by estrogen/progestin combinations. Regular clinical monitoring is required for all women on any type of hormonal replacement therapy.

USE OF HORMONAL REPLACEMENT THERAPY

Can be used as an alternative or in combination with lipid-lowering drugs in postmenopausal women with elevated low-density lipoprotein cholesterol level [11,75] but avoid in those with hypertriglyceridemia
Other benefits
  Maintains bone density (↓ risk of osteoporosis and its complications)
  Relieves vasomotor symptoms
  Decreases some urinary tract symptoms
  Alleviates other perimenopausal and postmenopausal symptoms
Individualized decision involving both patient and health care professional

FIGURE 9-52. Use of hormonal replacement therapy [11,74]. Maintenance of bone density and decreased incidence of the complications of osteoporosis is a documented, long-term benefit of hormonal replacement therapy. Hormonal replacement therapy is often used for short-term alleviation of a multiplicity of symptoms associated with perimenopausal and postmenopausal states. The final decision to use hormonal replacement therapy requires an assessment of the benefits versus the risks; unfortunately, these have not been clearly defined in controlled clinical trials.

COMBINATION THERAPY

INDICATIONS FOR COMBINATION THERAPY

Greater effect on a single lipoprotein abnormality
Control multiple lipid and lipoprotein abnormalities
Achieve target lipid and lipoprotein goals at reduced cost
Reduce the likelihood of side effects due to smaller doses of individual drug that are administered

FIGURE 9-53. Indications for combination therapy [11,78–81]. Combination therapy is under utilized. The dose-response for most drugs is log-linear, which means that the major portion of the effect of an individual drug can be achieved with lower doses. Combination therapy is especially useful to control multiple lipoprotein abnormalities, and the use of smaller doses of individual drugs in combination therapy frequently reduces cost and side effects.

RECOMMENDED COMBINATION THERAPY OF ELEVATED LDL CHOLESTEROL AND NORMAL TRIGLYCERIDES

Statin + bile-acid sequestrant
  Both drugs increase LDL-C receptor numbers by differing mechanisms
  Effect is greater than can be achieved by either drug alone; overall effect is additive or synergistic [78]
Statin + nicotinic acid [38]
  Statin increases LDL receptor number; niacin inhibits lipoprotein synthesis
  Useful if both LDL-C lowering and HDL-C raising are desired
Bile acid sequestrant + nicotinic acid
  Efficacy in lowering LDL-C is additive
  Combination is frequently not tolerated because of frequency of side effects with both drugs

FIGURE 9-54. Combination therapy for elevated low-density lipoprotein cholesterol (LDL-C) levels and normal triglycerides [11]. Statin plus a bile acid sequestrant is the most effective combination for lowering LDL-C. The combination of statin plus nicotinic acid is the ideal combination for both lowering LDL-C and increasing high-density lipoprotein cholesterol (HDL-C) levels.

RECOMMENDED COMBINATION THERAPY OF ELEVATED LDL CHOLESTEROL AND TRIGLYCERIDES

Statin + nicotinic acid
  Effect of two drugs is additive
  Both drugs decrease LDL-C and triglyceride in dose-dependent manner. Low HDL-C is common, and both drugs increase HDL-C levels
  Risk of myopathy small
Statin + fibric acid derivative
  If nicotinic acid is not tolerated and baseline triglyceride level is ±500 mg/dL or higher
  Fibric acid has little effect on LDL-C levels, but decreases triglycerides and increases HDL-C
  Fibric acid generally produce greater triglyceride decreases than niacin
  Risk of myopathy greater
  Useful in non–insulin-dependent diabetes mellitus
Fibric acid + nicotinic acid
  Dose of nicotinic acid that is tolerated is usually insufficient to control LDL-C levels
  Both drugs decrease triglycerides and increase HDL-C levels

FIGURE 9-55. Drug combinations for patients with elevations of both low-density lipoprotein cholesteral (LDL-C) and triglycerides (200 to 500 mg/dL) [11]. HDL-C—high density lipoprotein cholesterol.

COMPLIANCE WITH DRUG REGIMENS

Proper education of patient
  Lifelong need for treatment
  Indications for drug use
  Expected effects of drug use
  Expected benefit on CAD, PVD, and stroke
  Possible side effects
  Mechanism for dealing with side effects
  Written materials are helpful, especially for drugs that are difficult to administer
Periodic monitoring with regularly scheduled visits and feedback of lipid levels and interim telephone contacts initially
Need for chronic therapy
Cost may be an obstacle

FIGURE 9-56. Compliance with drug regimens. Adequate instruction and appropriate monitoring of the patient is essential for good compliance. CAD—coronary artery disease; PVD—peripheral vascular disease.

REFERENCES

1. The Scandinavian Simvastatin Survival Group: Randomised trial of cholesterol lowering in 4444 patients with coronary heart disease: the Scandinavian Simvastatin Survival Study (4S). *Lancet* 1994, 344:1383–1389.

2. Sacks FM, Pfeffer MA, Moye L, *et al.*: The effect of pravastatin on coronary events after myocardial infarction in patients with average cholesterol levels. *N Engl J Med* 1996, 335:1001–1009.

3. The Long-Term Intervention with Pravastatin in Ischaemic Disease (LIPID) Study Group: Prevention of cardiovascular events and death with pravastatin in patients with coronary heart disease and a broad range of initial cholesterol levels. *N Engl J Med* 1998, 339:1349–1357.

4. Shepherd J, Cobbe SM, Ford I, *et al.*: Prevention of coronary heart disease with pravastatin in men with hypercholesterolemia. *N Engl J Med* 1995, 333:1301–1307.

5. Downs GR, Clearfield M, Weiss S, *et al.*: Primary prevention of acute coronary events with lovastatin in men and women with average cholesterol levels: results of AFCAPS/TexCAPS. Air Force/Texas Coronary Study. *JAMA* 1998, 279:1615–1622.

6. Rubins HB, Robins SJ, Collins D, *et al.*: Gemfibrozil for the secondary prevention of coronary heart disease in men with low levels of high-density-lipoprotein cholesterol. *N Engl J Med* 1999, 341:410–418.

7. Pedersen TR, Kjekshus J, Pyörälä K, *et al.*: Effect of simvasatin on ischemic signs and symtoms in the Scandinavian Simvastatin Survival Study (4S). *Am J Cardiol* 1998, 81:333–335.

8. Crouse 3rd JR, Byington RP, Hoen HM, Furberg CD: Reductase inhibitor monotherapy and stroke prevention. *Arch Intern Med* 1997, 157:1305–1310.

9. Herbert PR, Gaziano JM, Chan KS, Hennekens CH: Cholesterol lowering with statin drugs, risk of stroke and total mortality. An overview of randomized trials. *JAMA* 1997, 278:313–321.

10. Pyörälä K, Pedersen TR, Kjekshus J, *et al.*: Cholesterol lowering with simvastatin improves prognosis of diabetic patients with coronary heart disease. *Diabetes Care* 1997, 20:614–620.

11. Expert Panel: Report of the National Cholesterol Education Program expert panel on detection, evaluation and treatment of high blood cholesterol in adults. *Arch Intern Med* 1988, 148:36–69.

12. National Cholesterol Education Program Second Report of the National Cholesterol Education Program (NCEP) Expert Panel on Detection, Evaluation and Treatment of High Blood Cholesterol in Adults (Adult Treatment Panel II). *Circulation* 1994, 89:1329–1445.

13. Executive Summary of The Third Report of The National Cholesterol Education Program (NCEP) Expert Panel on Detection, Evaluation, And Treatment of High Blood Cholesterol In Adults (Adult Treatment Panel III). *JAMA* 2001, 285:2486–2497.

14. The Expert Committee on the Diagnosis and Classification of Diabetes Mellitus. Report of the Expert Committee on the diagnosis and classification of diabetes mellitus. *Diabetes Care* 1997, 20:1183–1197.

15. Wood D, DeBacker G, Faergeman O, *et al.*: Prevention of coronary heart disease in clinical practice: Recommendations of the Second Joint Task Force of European and other Societies on Coronary Prevention. *Eur Heart J* 1998, 19:1434–1503.

16. National Cholesterol Education Program: Report of the Expert Panel on Blood Cholesterol Levels in Children and Adolescents. Bethesda, MD: National Heart, Lung and Blood Institute; 1991: NIH publication 91-2732.

17. Haffner SM, Miettinen H: Insulin resistance implications for type II diabetes mellitus and coronary heart disease. *Am J Med* 1997, 103:152–162.

18. Hulley S, Grady D, Bush T: Randomized trial of estrogen plus progestin for secondary prevention of coronary heart disease in post menopausal women. *JAMA* 1998, 280:605–613.

19. Lipid Research Clinics Program: The Lipid Research Clinics Coronary Primary Prevention Trial results. I. Reduction in incidence of coronary heart disease. *JAMA* 1984, 251:351–364.

20. Sirtori CR, Manzoni C, Lovati MR: Mechanisms of lipid-lowering agents. *Cardiology* 1991, 78:226–235.

21. Hunninghake DB: Drug treatment of dyslipoproteinemia. *Endocrinol Metab Clin North Am* 1990,19:345–360.

22. Superko HR, Greenland P, Manchester RA, *et al.*: Effectiveness of low-dose colestipol therapy in patients with moderate hypercholesterolemia. *Am J Cardiol* 1992, 70:135–140.

23. LaRosa J: Review of clinical studies of bile acid sequestrants for lowering plasma lipid levels. *Cardiology* 1989, 76(suppl 1):55–64.

24. Bernsike JF, Levy RI, Kelsey SF, *et al.*: Effects of therapy with cholestyramine on progression of coronary arteriosclerosis: results of the NHLBI Type II Coronary Intervention Study (STARS). *Lancet* 1992, 339:563–569.

25. Watts GF, Lewis B, Brunt JNH, *et al.*: Effects on coronary artery disease of lipid-lowering diet, or diet plus cholestyramine, in the St. Thomas Atherosclerosis Regression Study (STARS). *Lancet* 1992, 339:563–569.

26. Blankenhorn DH, Nessim SA, Johnson RL, *et al.*: Beneficial effects of combined colestipol-niacin therapy on coronary atherosclerosis and coronary venous bypass grafts. *JAMA* 1987, 257:3233–3240.

27. Brown G, Albers JJ, Fisher LD, *et al.*: Regression of coronary artery disease as a result of intensive lipid-lowering therapy in men with high levels of apolipoprotein B. *N Engl J Med* 1990, 323:1289–1298.

28. The Simvastatin Pravastatin Study Group: Comparison of the efficacy, safety and tolerability of lovastatin and simvastatin in the management of primary hypercholesterolemia. *Am J Cardiol* 1993, 71:1408.

29. Frolich J, Brun LD, Blank D, *et al.*: Comparison of the short-term efficacy and tolerability of lovastatin and simvastatin in the management of primary hypercholesterolemia. *Can J Cardiol* 1993.

30. Jones P, Kafonek S, Laurora I, Hunninghake D: Comparative dose efficacy study of atorvastatin versus simvastatin, pravastatin, lovastatin, and fluvastatin in patients with hypercholesterolemia (the CURVES study). *Am J Cardiol* 1998, 81:582–587.

31. Stein EA, Lane M, Laskarzewski P: Comparisons of statins in hypertriglyceridemia. *Am J Cardiol* 1998, 81:66B–69B.

32. Bakker-Arkema RG, *et al.*: Efficacy and safety of a new 17 HMG-CoA reductase inhibitor, atorvastatin in patients with hypertriglyceridaemia. *JAMA* 1996, 275:128–133.

33. Blankenhorn DH, Azen SP, Kramsch DM, *et al.*: Coronary angiographic changes with lovastatin therapy. The Monitored Atherosclerosis Regression Study (MARS). *Ann Intern Med* 1993, 119:969–976.

34. Waters D, Higginson L, Gladstone P, *et al.*: Effects of monotherapy with an HMG CoA reductase inhibitor on the progression of coronary atherosclerosis as assessed by serial quantitative arteriography. The Canadian Coronary Atherosclerosis Intervention Trial. *Circulation* 1994, 89:959–968.

35. Pitt B, Mancini GBJ, Elis SG, *et al.*: Pravastatin limitation of athero-sclerosis in the coronary arteries (PLAC I) [abstract]. *J Am Coll Cardiol* 1994, 23(suppl):131A.

36. Crouse JR, Furberg CD, Byington BP, *et al.*: The PLAC-2 Trial: effects of pravastatin on atherosclerosis progression and clinical events [abstract]. *Circulation* 1993, 87:702.

37. Furberg CD, Adams HP, Jr., Applegate WB, *et al.*: Effect of lovas-tatin on early carotid ataherosclerosis and cardiovascular events. *Circulation* 1994, 90:1679–1687.

38. Illingworth DR, Stein EA, Mitchel YB, *et al.*: Comparative effects of lovastatin and niacin in primary hypercholesterolemia, a prospec-tive trial. *Arch Intern Med* 1994, 154:1586–1595.

39. Shepherd J, Cobbe SM, Ford I, *et al.*: Prevention of coronary heart disease with pravastatin in men with hypercholesterolemia. West of Scotland Coronary Prevention Study Group. *N Engl J Med* 1995, 333:1301–1307.

40. The 4S Group: Randomised trial of cholesterol lowering in 4444 patients with coronary heart disease: the Scandinavian Simvastatin Survival Study (4S). *Lancet* 1994, 344:1383–1389.

41. Sacks FM, Pfeffer MA, Moye LA, *et al.*: The effect of pravastatin on coronary events after myocardial infarction in patients with average cholesterol levels. Cholesterol and Recurrent Events Trial investigators. *N Engl J Med* 1996, 335:1001–1009.

42. Miettinen TA, Pyorala K, Olsson AG, *et al.*: Cholesterol-lowering therapy in women and elderly patients with myocardial infarction or angina pectoris: findings from the Scandinavian Simvastatin Survival Study (4S). *Circulation* 1997, 96:4211–4218.

43. The 4S Group: Baseline serum cholesterol and treatment effect in the Scandinavian Simvastatin Survival Study (4S). *Lancet* 1995, 345:1274–1275.

44. Downs JR, Clearfield M, Weis S, *et al.*: Primary prevention of acute coronary events with lovastatin in men and women with average cholesterol levels: results of AFCAPS/TexCAPS. *JAMA* 1998, 279:1615–1622.

45. The Long-Term Intervention with Pravastatin in Ischaemic Disease (LIPID) Study Group: Prevention of cardiovascular events and death with pravastatin in patients with coronary heart disease and a broad range of initial cholesterol levels. *N Engl J Med* 1998, 339:1349–1357.

46. Rubins HB, Robins SJ, Collins D, *et al.*: Gemfibrozil for the secondary prevention of coronary heart disease in men with low levels of high-density lipoprotein cholesterol. Veterans Affairs High-Density Lipoprotein Cholesterol Intervention Trial Study Group. *N Engl J Med* 1999, 341:410–418.

47. Crouse JR III, Byington RP, Hoen HM, Furberg CD: Reductase inhibitor monotherapy and stroke prevention. *Arch Intern Med* 1997, 157:1305–1310.

48. Pitt B, Waters D, Brown WV, *et al.*: Aggressive lipid-lowering therapy compared with angioplasty in stable coronary artery disease. Atorvastatin versus Revascularization Treatment Investigators. *N Engl J Med* 1999, 341:70–76.

49. Schwartz GG, Olsson AG, Ezekowitz MD, *et al.*: Effects of atorvas-tatin on early recurrent ischemic events in acute coronary syndromes: the MIRACL study: a randomized controlled trial. *JAMA* 2001, 285:1711–1718.

50. Staffa JA, Chang J, Green L: Cerivastatin and reports of fatal rhab-domyolysis. *N Engl J Med* 2002, 346:539–540.

51. McKenney JM, Proctor JD, Harris S, *et al.*: A comparison of the effi-cacy and toxic effects of sustained- vs immediate-release niacin in hypercholesterolemic patients. *JAMA* 1994, 271:672–677.

52. Coronary Drug Project Research Group: Clofibrate and niacin in coronary heart disease. *JAMA* 1975, 231:360–381.

53. Canner PL, Berge KG, Wenger NK, *et al.*: Fifteen year mortality in coronary drug project patients: long-term benefit with niacin. *J Am Coll Cardiol* 1986, 8:1245–1255.

54. Carlson LA, Rosenhamer G: Reduction of mortality in the Stockholm ischemic Heart Disease Secondary Prevention Study by combined treatment with clofibrate and nicotinic acid. *Acta Med Scand* 1988, 2223:405–418.

55. Blankenhorn DH, Nessim SA, Johnson RL, *et al.*: Beneficial effects of combined colestipol-niacin therapy on coronary atherosclerosis and coronary venous bypass grafts. *JAMA* 1987, 257:3233–3240.

56. Brown G, Albers JJ, Fisher LD, *et al.*: Regression of coronary artery disease as a result of intensive lipid-lowering therapy in men with high levels of apolipoprotein B. *N Engl J Med* 1990, 323:1289–1298.

57. Reaven P, Witzum JL: Lovastatin, nicotinic acid and rhabdomyol-ysis. *Ann Intern Med* 1988, 109:597–598.

58. Brown BG, Zhao XQ, Chait A, *et al.*: Simvastatin and niacin, antiox-idant vitamins, or the combination for the prevention of coronary disease. *N Engl J Med* 2001, 345:1583–1592.

59. Committee of Principal Investigators: WHO cooperative trial on primary prevention of ischemic heart disease with clofibrate to lower serum cholesterol: final mortality follow-up. *Lancet* 1984, ii(8403):600–604.

60. Frick MH, Elo O, Haapa K, *et al.*: Helsinki Heart Study: primary-prevention trial with gemfibrozil in middle-aged men with dyslipi-demia; safety of treatment, changes in risk factors, and incidence of coronary heart disease. *N Engl J Med* 1987, 317:1237–1245.

61. Stewart JM, Packard CL, Lorimer AR, *et al.*: Effects of bezafibrate on receptor-mediated and receptor-independent low density lipoprotein catabolism in type II hyperlipoproteinaemic subjects. *Atherosclerosis* 1982, 44:355–365.

62. Yuan J, Tsai M, Hunninghake DB: Changes in composition and distribution of LDL subspecies in hypertriglyceridemc and hyper-cholesterolemic patients during gemfibrozil therapy. *Atherosclerosis* 1994, 110:1–11.

63. Fruchart JC, Duriez P, Staels B: Peroxisome-proliferator–activated receptor-alpha activators regulate genes governing lipoprotein metabolism, vascular inflammation and atherosclerosis. *Curr Opin Lipidol* 1999, 10:245–257.

64. Huttunen JK, Heinonen OP, Manninen V, *et al.*: The Helsinki Heart Study: an 8.5-year safety and mortality follow-up. *J Intern Med* 1994, 235:31–39.

65. Goldberg A, Feldman E, Ginsberg H, Hunninghake D, *et al*: Fenofibrate for the treatment of type IV and V hyperlipoproteine-mias: a double-blind, placebo-controlled multicenter US study. *Clinical Therapeutics* 1989, 11:69–82.

66. WHO Monica Project: A cooperative trial in the primary prevention of ischemic heart disease using clofibrate. *Br Heart J* 1978, 40:1069–1118.

67. Pyorala K, Pedersen TR, Kjekshus J, *et al.*: Cholesterol lowering with simvastatin improves prognosis of diabetic patients with coro-nary heart disease: a subgroup analysis of the Scandinavian Simvastatin Survival Study (4S). *Diabetes Care* 1997, 20:614–620.

68. Hunninghake DB, Bell C, Olson L: Effect of probucol on plasma lipids and lipoproteins in type IIb hyperlipoproteinemia. *Atherosclerosis* 1980, 37:469–474.

69. Reaven PD, Parthasarathy S, Beltz WF, *et al.*: Effect of probucol dosage on plasma lipid and lipoprotein levels and on protection of low density lipoprotein against in vitro oxidation in humans. *Arterioscl Thromb* 1992, 12:318–324.

70. Parthasarathy S, Young SG, Witztum JL *et al.*: Probucol inhibits oxidative modification of low density lipoprotein. *J Clin Invest* 1986, 77:641–644.

71. Walldius G, Erikson U, Ander G, *et al.*: The effect of probucol on femoral atherosclerosis: the Probucol Quantitative Regression Swedish Trial (PQRST). *Am J Cardiol* 1994, 74:875–883.

72. Colditz GA, Willett WC, Stanpfer MJ, *et al.*: Menopause and the risk of coronary heart disease in women. *N Engl J Med* 1987, 316:1105–1110.

73. Stampfer MJ, Colditz GA: Estrogen replacement therapy and coronary heart disease: a quantitative assessment of the epidemiologic evidence. *Prev Med* 1991, 20:47–63.

74. Sullivan JM, Vander Zwaag R, Hughes JP: Estrogen replacement and coronary artery disease: effect on survival in postmenopausal women. *Ann Intern Med* 1990, 150:2557–2562.

75. Grady D, Rubin SM, Petitti DB, *et al.*: Hormone therapy to prevent disease and prolong life in postmenopausal women. *Ann Intern Med* 1992, 117:1016–1037.

76. Granfone A, Campos H, McNamara JR, *et al.*: Effects of estrogen replacement on plasma lipoproteins and apolipoproteins in postmenopausal, dyslipidemic women. *Metabolism* 1992, 41:1193–1198.

77. The Women's Health Initiative Study Group: Design of the Women's Health Initiative Clinical Trial and Observational Study. *Controlled Clinical Trials* 1998, 19:61–109.

78. Schrott H, Stein EA, Dujovne CA, *et al.*: Enhanced low-density lipoprotein cholesterol reduction and cost-effectiveness by low-dose colestipol plus lovastatin combination therapy. *Am J Cardiol* 1995, 75:34–39.

79. Larsen ML, Illingworth DR: Drug treatment of dyslipoproteinemia. *Med Clin North Am* 1994, 78:225–245.

80. Heudebert GR, Van Ruiswyk J, Hiatt J, *et al.*: Combination drug therapy for hypercholesterolemia: the trade-off between cost and simplicity. *Arch Intern Med* 1993, 153:1828–1837.

81. Witztum JL: Intensive drug therapy of hypercholesterolemia. *Am Heart J* 1987, 113:603–609.

THE NEWER CORONARY RISK FACTORS

10

CHAPTER

Peter W.F. Wilson

Although traditional coronary risk factors have included elevated blood pressure, cholesterol, and cigarette smoking, several other factors are now being considered. This chapter provides a sampling of some of these "newer" risk factors, particularly those that have a biologic basis. The major categories to be considered are hematologic, newer lipid particles and their metabolic considerations, vitamins and homocysteine, and aspects of glucose metabolism.

Several types of hematologic risk factors have recently been associated with coronary heart disease (CHD); they include leukocyte count, serum ferritin concentration, fibrinogen and factor VII, tissue-type plasminogen activator (t-PA) antigen, plasminogen activator inhibitor (PAI-1), von Willebrand factor (vWF) antigen, and aspects of platelet function. Mild elevations in the leukocyte count have been considered to indicate an "inflammatory" component of atherosclerosis and have been of interest to researchers but less useful to clinicians. Fibrinogen and factor VII are components of the cascade that lead to a fibrin clot. Advanced atherosclerotic lesions appear to undergo fissuring, fibrin deposition, and fibrinolysis, and greater levels of several factors have been associated with greater risk of cardiovascular disease (CVD). Less population-based information is available on aspects of fibrinolysis, but data suggest that higher levels of t-PA antigen and vWF are associated with progression of vascular disease. Both t-PA antigen and PAI-1 appear to be lower when higher levels of estrogen are present (*eg*, younger women and postmenopausal women who take estrogens). A particularly useful inflammatory marker to assess cardiovascular risk is C-reactive protein (CRP). Newer assay types have shown that higher levels are particularly associated with greater risk of heart disease and it also is related to obesity, estrogen use, and inflammation from rheumatologic conditions. Anti-inflammatory and antiplatelet therapies have successfully treated initial and recurrent CVD. Aspirin is the mainstay of care and the latest review data suggest that more than 75 mg/d is adequate for long-term therapy to prevent CVD, although larger amounts may be appropriate for short-term therapy. Various types of antiplatelet adjunctive therapy have been considered in a large number of trials.

Several new lipid particles have been associated with CHD. For example, higher levels of lipoprotein(a) or lip(a) have been associated with increased risk of CHD in several studies.

This factor may be particularly important for those at greater risk of disease, and increased concentrations may adversely affect the fibrinolytic systems and contribute to lipid deposition. Similarly, small, dense low-density lipoprotein (LDL) particles have been associated with increased CHD risk; however, it has been difficult to separate effect of the LDL size from that of the impact of triglyceride concentration because higher concentrations of triglycerides are highly correlated with a greater prevalence of small LDL particles. In addition, lower concentrations of high-density lipoprotein (HDL) subclasses, namely HDL-2 and HDL-3, have been associated with greater risk of CHD in several studies; however, there appears to be little or no advantage in measuring the HDL subfractions after the total HDL cholesterol level is known. Apolipoprotein E alleles have been associated with different levels of LDL cholesterol. Compared with the ancestral $\epsilon3$ allele, the $\epsilon2$ allele has been associated with lower LDL cholesterol and the $\epsilon4$ allele has been associated with higher LDL cholesterol. Both the $\epsilon2$ and $\epsilon4$ alleles have been associated with a tendency toward higher triglyceride levels, either because of hypertriglyceridemia alone or in concert with low HDL cholesterol or elevated cholesterol levels.

Although increased vitamin E intake has been associated with reduced risk of CHD in observational studies, results of a clinical trial of Finnish smokers and the Heart Outcomes Prevention Evaluation (HOPE) study showed no cardiovascular benefit for vitamin E supplementation. Homocysteine concentrations appear to be a marker for increased risk of CHD, as noted in case-control and prospective studies. Recent carotid artery ultrasound data have shown an association between higher homocysteine levels and carotid stenosis. Given that population data suggest that elevated homocysteine levels are common in the elderly and are typically accompanied by a low levels of plasma vitamin B_{12} and folate, supplementation with these vitamins is now being considered in an effort to retard atherosclerosis.

Much interest has been evinced by the impact of insulin resistance on CHD occurrence. Early reports showed that insulin resistance, determined by excessive insulin response to an oral glucose tolerance load, was associated with an increased risk of CHD. More recent data also show that moderate elevations of glycosylated hemoglobin levels are associated with an increased prevalence of CHD in the elderly.

Imaging of atherosclerotic lesions is gaining momentum in the clinical arena and examples of various images and their relation to cardiovascular sequelae are of interest to clinicians and researchers. Lesions in the abdominal aorta using conventional radiographs, intima medial thickness grading by ultrasound, evaluation of the carotid artery by MRI, scanning of the heart with ultrafast CT, and intravascular ultrasound are shown as examples.

HEMATOLOGIC FACTORS

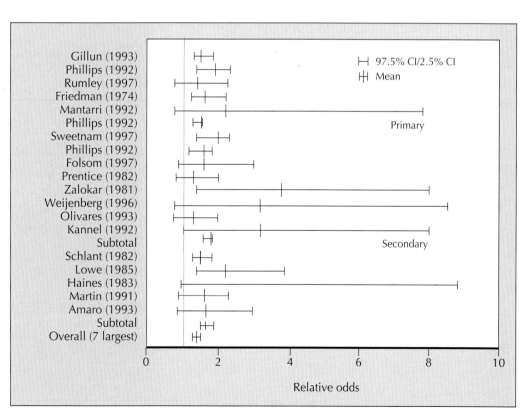

FIGURE 10-1. Leukocyte count and coronary heart disease (CHD) meta-analysis (top vs bottom third). An increased leukocyte count in peripheral blood has been associated with greater risk of myocardial infarction (MI) and CHD in several studies. In most instances, the relative risk of CHD associated with higher leukocyte counts is relatively modest [1].

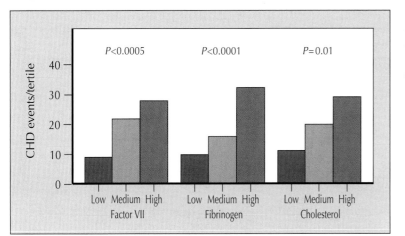

FIGURE 10-2. Higher levels of factor VII, fibrinogen, and cholesterol were associated with later coronary heart disease (CHD) in the Northwick Park Study [2]. In this sample of older men, the degree of statistical significance for the fibrinogen relation with CHD was greater than that for total blood cholesterol.

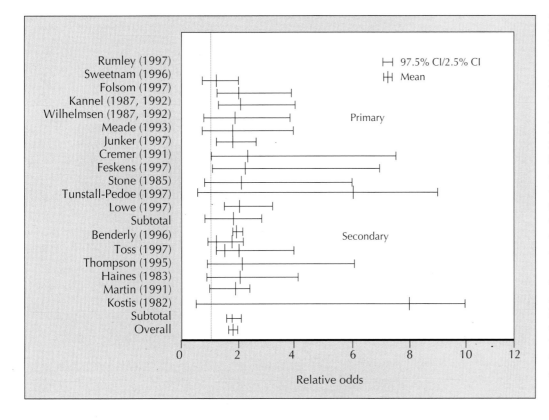

FIGURE 10-3. Fibrinogen and coronary heart disease (CHD): meta-analysis (top vs bottom third). A summary of the effects (mean ± 95% CI) for fibrinogen level and risk for various forms of cardiovascular disease in several prospective studies (Gothenburg, Framingham, Northwick Park, Prospective Coronary Artery Disease in Munster [PROCAM], Caerphilly Speedwell, and Gottingen Risk, Incidence, and Prevalence Study [GRIPS]) shows that a positive association was observed in all studies [1]. The relation was significantly different from 1.0 (a null effect) in all but one study, and the total effect, by meta-analysis, was significant.

Each analysis compares the vascular disease risk for people in the top third of the fibrinogen distribution to the risk for persons in the bottom third of fibrinogen. The overall estimate pools the relative odds associated with the top third fibrinogen compared with the bottom third fibrinogen for several studies. (*Adapted from* Danesh *et al.* [1].)

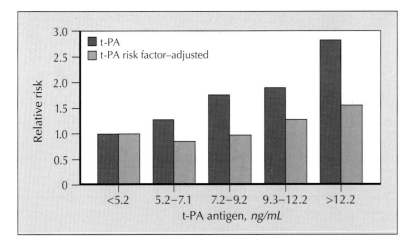

FIGURE 10-4. The relation between tissue-type plasminogen activator (t-PA) and myocardial infarction (MI). Concentration of t-PA was positively associated with a greater risk of MI in the Physician's Health Study. The relation between t-PA concentration and MI was highly statistically significant after adjustment for age and smoking (*P* = 0.0008), but after further adjustment for total cholesterol, high-density lipoprotein (HDL), body mass index, self-reported blood pressure, exercise frequency, parental history of MI before age 60 years, and presence of diabetes, the effect was no longer statistically significant (*P* = 0.14) [3].

HEMOSTATIC FACTORS AND CHD IN PATIENTS WITH ANGINA PECTORIS

VARIABLE	GROUP WITH EVENTS (n=106)	EVENT-FREE GROUP (n=2700)	P VALUE
Fibrinogen, g/L	3.28 (0.74)	3.00 (0.71)	0.01
vWF antigen, %	137.5 (48.8)	124.6 (49.1)	0.05
t-PA antigen, ng/mL	11.9 (4.7)	10.0 (4.2)	0.02
CRP, mg/L	2.15 (1.96)	1.61 (1.38)	0.05

FIGURE 10-5. Hemostatic factors have been associated with a higher 2-year incidence of coronary heart disease (CHD) (later myocardial infarction or sudden death) among patients with angina pectoris who participated in the European Concerted Action on Thrombosis and Disabilities (ECAT) angina pectoris study. The factors considered included fibrinogen, von willebrand factor (vWF) antigen, tissue-type plasminogen activator (t-PA) antigen, and C-reactive protein (CRP) [4]. Entries represent mean ± SD.

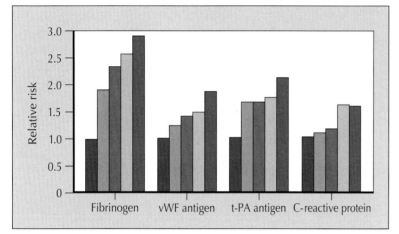

FIGURE 10-6. In the European Concerted Action on Thrombosis and Disabilities (ECAT) study, the relative risk of subsequent coronary heart disease in angina patients was assessed according to quintile of hemostatic factors (fibrinogen, von Willebrand factor [vWF] antigen, tissue-type plasminogen activator [t-PA] antigen, and C-reactive protein). The steepest gradient was observed for fibrinogen level [4].

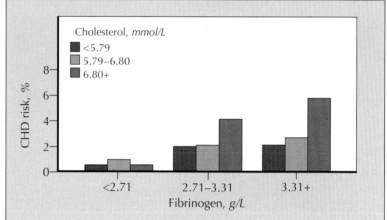

FIGURE 10-7. Synergy between fibrinogen and cholesterol levels (shown in tertiles) was observed for the occurrence of coronary heart disease (CHD) over 2 years among European Concerted Action on Thrombosis and Disabilities (ECAT) study participants with angina pectoris at baseline [4].

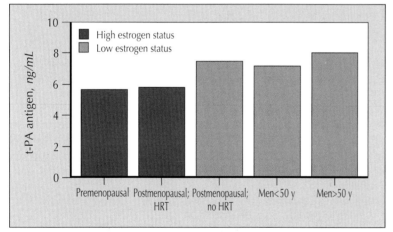

FIGURE 10-8. Tissue-type plasminogen activator (t-pa) antigen levels were lower among patients with high estrogen status (premenopausal women) compared with men younger than 50 years of age (P < 0.001), men 50 years or older (P < 0.001), and postmenopausal women not on estrogen replacement (HRT) (P < 0.001) in a cross-sectional study of 1431 Framingham offspring [5]. Lower t-PA levels accompany higher estrogen states (premenopausal women and postmenopausal women on HRT) and may help to explain the beneficial effects of HRT on coronary heart disease.

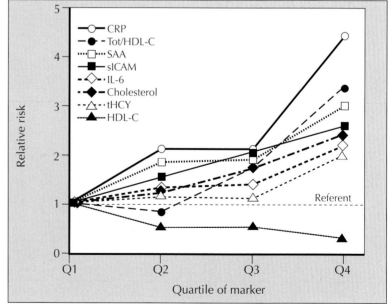

FIGURE 10-9. Inflammation markers and Women's Health Study results. Quartiles of inflammatory markers were related to subsequent cardiovascular disease in the Women's Health Study in a nested case-control study of 122 cases and 244 controls. CRP—C-reactive protein; HDL-C—high-density lipoprotein cholesterol; IL-6—interleukin-6; SAA—serum amyloid A; sICAM—serum intercellular adhesion molecule; tHCY—total homocysteine. (*Adapted from* Ridker *et al.* [6].)

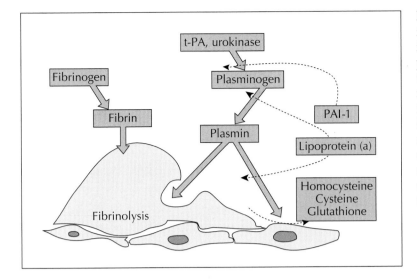

FIGURE 10-10. The fibrin deposition pathway begins with fibrinogen, which is converted to fibrin, a protein that is deposited in atherosclerotic plaques (*left*). Conversely, the fibrinolytic pathway (*right*) follows a cascade with successive activation of tissue-type plasminogen activator (t-PA) or urokinase, plasminogen, and subsequently plasmin. The last protein acts to lyse fibrin deposits. The fibrinolytic sequence can be inhibited (*dashed lines*) at the initial plasminogen activation step by plasminogen activator inhibitor (PAI)-1 and lipoprotein a (lip[a]). The exact role of sulfhydryl-containing amino acids such as homocysteine is less clear. It has been suggested that homocysteine is toxic to the endothelium and the amino acid appears to affect binding of lip(a) to fibrin.

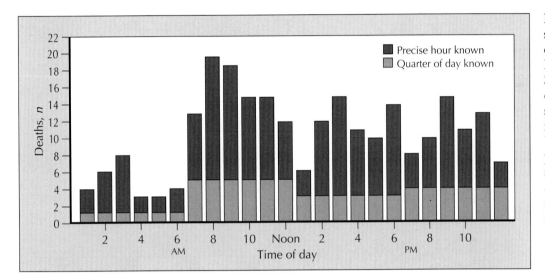

FIGURE 10-11. The frequency of definite sudden cardiac death according to the time of day was plotted for 264 Framingham Heart Study participants who died over a 38-year follow-up interval [7]. Peak incidence occurred from 7 to 9 AM. Similar studies showed an early AM peak for myocardial infarction and stroke. Laboratory studies that complement these projects suggest that a hypercoagulable state, characterized by increased platelet aggregation or coronary vasoconstriction, is more prevalent in the early morning after rising [7,8].

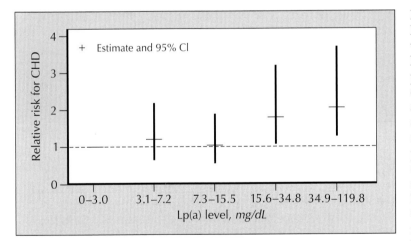

FIGURE 10-12. The concentration of lipoprotein(a) (Lp[a]), a lipoprotein particle with thrombotic properties and homology with plasminogen, was associated with greater risk for coronary heart disease (CHD) in men between 35 and 59 years of age who participated in the Lipid Research Clinic Program and were observed during a 7- to 10-year follow-up [9]. Data are grouped according to quintile of Lp(a) concentration, and the relative risk associated with the top two quintiles (Lp[a] > 15.6 mg/dL) was associated with an increased risk for CHD [9]. Elevated Lp(a), particularly in patients expected to be at high risk for CHD, such as the Lipid Research Clinic Program participants with LDL cholesterol levels above 190 mg/dL in this study, has typically been associated with greater risk of CHD. High Lp(a) and greater CHD risk has not been universal, and no association was reported for Lp(a) level and risk of CHD among US men in the Physician's Health Study [10].

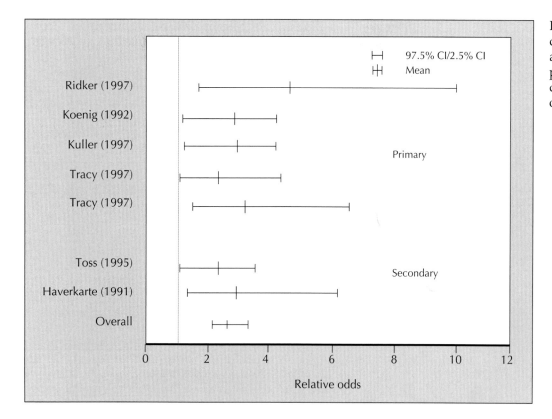

FIGURE 10-13. C-reactive protein (CRP) and coronary heart disease (CHD): meta-analysis for CRP and CHD, comparing participants in the top third of the CRP distribution with those in the bottom third of CRP on a study-by-study basis [1].

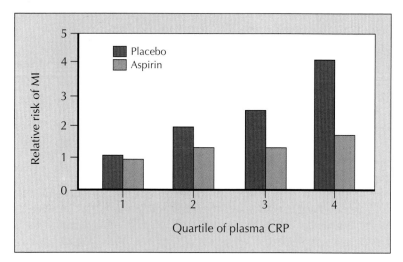

FIGURE 10-14. C-reactive protein (CRP) concentrations obtained at entry into the physicians Health Study. The data were used to determine the relative risk for myocardial infarction (MI) among participants. Participants assigned to aspirin therapy and higher levels of CRP at baseline experienced a lower risk of a first MI during the clinical trial [11].

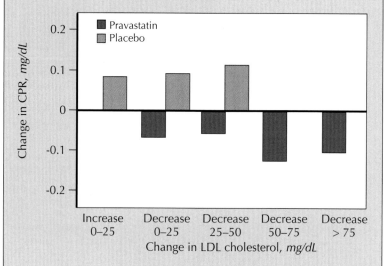

FIGURE 10-15. Relative risk for myocardial infarction (MI) according to C-reactive protein (CRP): aspirin and placebo users. Among MI survivors who participated in the Cholesterol and Recurrent Events (CARE) trial, the CRP levels tended to increase with 5 years of follow-up in the placebo group. Significant reductions in CRP were observed in the pravastatin users, but these changes in CRP were not associated with the degree of low-density lipoprotein (LDL) change [12].

Category of trial	Trials with data, n	Vascular events, n/n (%)		Observed-expected	Variance	Odds ratio (CI) Antiplatelet: Control	Odds reduction, % (SE)
		Allocated antiplatelet	Adjusted control				
Aspirin alone, *mg daily*							
500–1500	34	1621/11215 (14.5)	1930/11236 (17.2)	-147.1	707.8		19 (3)
160–325	19	1526/13240 (11.5)	1963/13273 (14.8)	-219.9	742.6		26 (3)
75–150	12	370/3370 (10.9)	517/3406 (15.2)	-72.0	183.8		32 (6)
<75	3	316/1827 (17.3)	354/1828 (19.4)	-18.9	136.5		13 (8)
Any aspirin*	65	3829/29 652 (12.9)	4764/29 743 (16.0)	-452.3	1717.0		23 (2)
Other antiplatelet drugs							
Dipyridamole	15	392/2696 (14.5)	458/2734 (16.8)	-30.9	173.0		16 (7)
Sulfinpyrazone	19	315/2411 (13.1)	361/2416 (14.9)	-23.8	140.7		16 (8)
Ticlopidine	42	278/3435 (8.1)	385/3475 (11.0)	-50.5	132.3		32 (7)
Suloctidil	6	47/364 (12.9)	59/367 (16.1)	-5.6	20.5		24 (19)
Picotamide	4	41/1583 (2.6)	66/1602 (4.1)	-12.2	25.8		38 (16)
Sulotroban	4	8/406 (2.0)	14/409 (3.4)	-3.2	5.3		45 (33)
Triflusal	2	10/314 (3.2)	19/309 (6.1)	-4.7	6.7		50 (28)
Other†	9	41/647 (6.3)	73/641 (11.4)	-16.1	25.6		47 (15)
Any other single agent	101	1132/11 856 (9.5)	1435/11 953 (12.0)	-147.0	529.9		24 (4)
Aspirin + another antiplatelet drug							
Asp + dipyridamole	46	1036/9703 (10.7)	1393/9738 (14.3)	-172.6	488.7		30 (4)
Asp + sulfinpyrazone	2	38/283 (13.4)	50/278 (18.0)	-6.5	18.5		30 (20)
Any combination	48	1074/9986 (10.8)	1443/10016 (14.4)	-179.1	507.2		30 (4)
All trials	**188**	**6035/51494 (11.7)**	**7644/51736 (14.8)**	**-715.7**	**2449.6**		**25 (2)**

0.0 0.5 1.0 1.5 2.0

Antiplatelet better   Antiplatelet worse

Treatment effect 2P < 0.00001

FIGURE 10-16. Aspirin and prevention of cardiovascular disease. Comprehensive meta-analyses of antiplatelet therapy, considering 287 studies that involved 135,000 patients for prevention of cardiovascular events, have shown that aspirin or other oral therapies are protective in most patients. Even low-dose aspirin (75 to 150 mg/d) is relatively effective, but in the shorter term a loading dose of at least 150 mg is recommended [13].

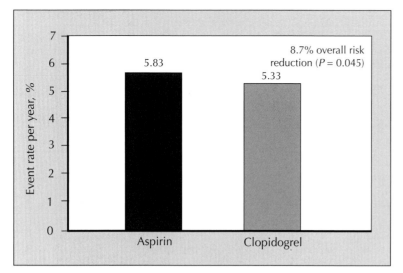

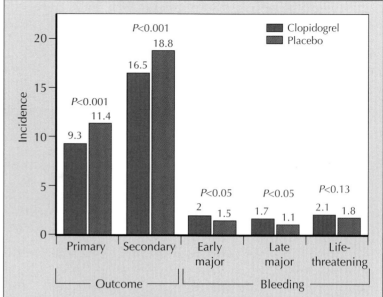

FIGURE 10-17. Aspirin versus clopidogrel bisulfate to prevent recurrent cardiovascular disease (CVD). Newer antiplatelet therapies include agents that selectively inhibit ADP-induced platelet aggregation. In a clinical trial [14] to prevent recurrent CVD that involved 9599 adults taking 75 mg/d of clopidogrel and 9586 adults taking 325 mg/d of aspirin, there were fewer recurrent events in the clopidogrel users (5.83% per year) compared with aspirin users (5.33% per year) over the course of the study. This difference in recurrent disease, based on the composite endpoint of stroke, myocardial infarction, or vascular death, represented an 8.7% reduction in risk ($P = 0.045$). (*Adapted from* the Clopidogrel versus Aspirin in Patients at Risk of Ischaemic Events [CAPRIE] Steering Committee [14].)

FIGURE 10-18. Cerebrovascular disease outcomes were reduced with use of clopidogrel in the Clopidogrel in Unstable angina to prevent Recurrent Events (CURE) trial. Patients with acute coronary syndromes without ST-segment elevation were treated with clopidogrel (300 mg immediately, then 75 mg/d) or placebo within 24 hours after the onset of their symptoms. All participants received aspirin in the dose range of 75 to 325 mg/d. The primary outcome (composite of CVD-cardiovascular disease death, nonfatal MI-myocardial infarction, or stroke) and the secondary outcome (first primary outcome or refractory ischemia) were reduced in the treatment group over a mean duration of 9 months of therapy [15]. Active therapy was associated with more events of major bleeding during early follow-up (onset less than 30 days after starting therapy) and late follow-up (onset more than 30 days after starting therapy), but an increased number of life-threatening bleeding episodes or hemorrhagic stroke were not observed.

NEWER LIPID MEASUREMENTS AND RISK OF CORONARY HEART DISEASE

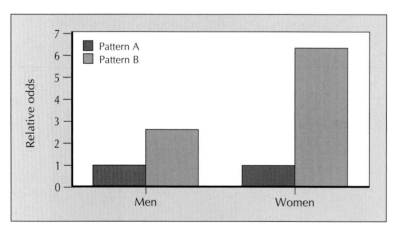

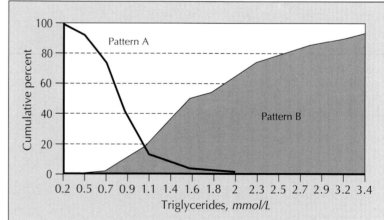

FIGURE 10-19. Low-density lipoprotein (LDL) particles have been classified as exhibiting pattern B (small, dense) or pattern A (large, less dense). Pattern B has been associated with greater odds for coronary heart disease (CHD) among men (92 cases, 98 controls, odds ratio [OR] = 2.7; $P > 0.01$) and women (17 cases, 23 controls, OR = 6.6; $P = 0.08$) in a Boston area case-control study [4]. These data suggest that smaller, denser LDL particles appear to be associated with greater risk for CHD.

FIGURE 10-20. The low-density lipoprotein subclass patterns are strongly associated with triglyceride levels. Pattern A is associated with lower triglyceride levels and pattern B is associated with higher triglyceride levels. For instance, the entire distribution of patients with pattern A is found for patients with triglyceride levels less than 2 mmol/L (approximately 175 mg/dL), and pattern B is almost exclusively confined to triglyceride levels above 0.7 mmol/L (approximately 60 mg/dL) [16].

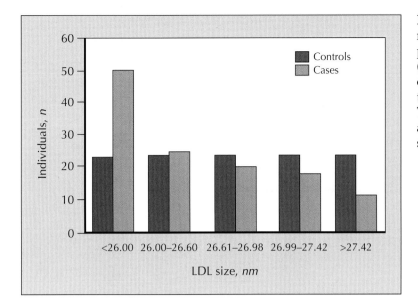

FIGURE 10-21. Low-density lipoprotein (LDL) particle size in coronary heart disease (CHD) cases and controls. Smaller, denser LDL particles were significantly associated with coronary artery disease (CAD) in a prospective, population-based study that used a nested case-control design and included 124 matched pairs. The association with CAD was graded across control quintiles of LDL size. The association of CAD was not statistically significant after adjusting for the total cholesterol per HDL-cholesterol ratio in this study [17].

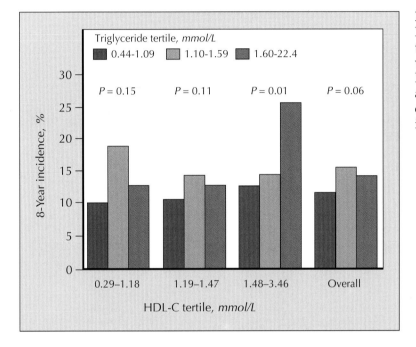

FIGURE 10-22. All-cause mortality and lipids: the Copenhagen Male Study. The association of high-density lipoprotein cholesterol (HDL-C) and triglyceride tertiles with all-cause mortality was investigated during 8 years' follow-up in the Copenhagen Male Study. A high level of fasting triglycerides was found to be an important risk factor for ischemic heart disease; the triglyceride effect was independent of other major risk factors, including HDL-C [18].

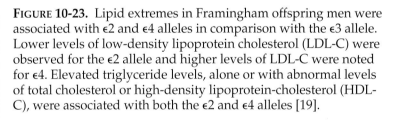

FIGURE 10-23. Lipid extremes in Framingham offspring men were associated with ε2 and ε4 alleles in comparison with the ε3 allele. Lower levels of low-density lipoprotein cholesterol (LDL-C) were observed for the ε2 allele and higher levels of LDL-C were noted for ε4. Elevated triglyceride levels, alone or with abnormal levels of total cholesterol or high-density lipoprotein-cholesterol (HDL-C), were associated with both the ε2 and ε4 alleles [19].

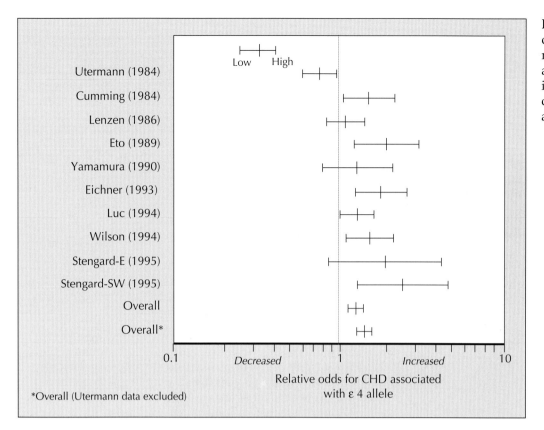

FIGURE 10-24. Alipoprotein ∊4 allele and odds for coronary heart disease (CHD): meta-analysis. Risk for CHD was associated with the ∊4 allele of apolipoprotein E in a variety of observational studies. The overall relative odds associated with the ∊4 allele was approximately 1.5 [20].

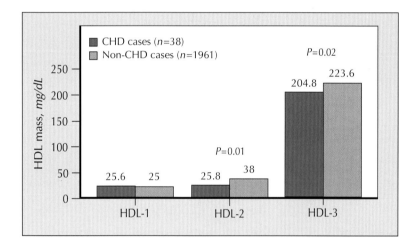

FIGURE 10-25. Associations between high-density lipoprotein (HDL) subfractions and coronary heart disease (CHD) were investigated in a follow-up study of men between 20 and 66 years of age seen at the Donner Laboratories Clinic. Lower concentrations of HDL-2 and HDL-3 by ultracentrifugation were associated with greater risk of CHD [21]. These classic data, determining HDL fractions by ultracentrifugation, suggest that fractionation of HDL may provide information that would improve prediction of CHD.

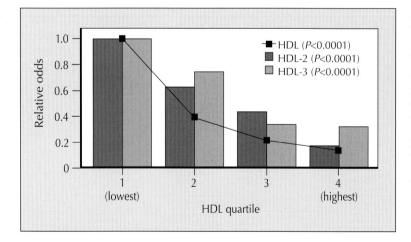

FIGURE 10-26. The relative odds for myocardial infarction (MI) were estimated according to quartile of high-density lipoprotein (HDL)-cholesterol, HDL-2 cholesterol, and HDL-3 cholesterol in a Boston area case-control study [22]. Compared with the lowest quartile for each lipid measure, the relative odds for MI diminished progressively with greater concentrations of HDL cholesterol, HDL-2 cholesterol, or HDL-3 cholesterol. There appeared to be no definite advantage in measuring HDL-2 cholesterol or HDL-3 cholesterol, as the relative odds for MI associated with the highest quartile of HDL-cholesterol or its subfractions were similar [23]. Double precipitation was used to determine HDL subfractions in this study.

VITAMINS AND HOMOCYSTEINE

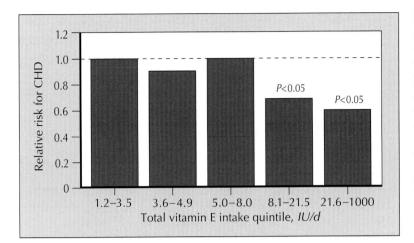

FIGURE 10-27. Vitamin E intake was inversely related to relative risk for coronary heart disease (CHD) in a prospective analysis of the Nurses' Health Study. The relative risk was significantly less than 1.0 for patients in the top two quintiles of vitamin E intake (*ie*, > 8.1 IU/d). These higher intakes of vitamin E were typically not achievable by diet alone and were largely confined to women taking vitamin supplements [25]. It has been hypothesized that the antioxidant nature of vitamin E acts to prevent oxidation of low-density lipoprotein (LDL) cholesterol and retards atherosclerosis. Consumers of vitamins may also be more health conscious generally and manifest other behaviors that tend to reduce coronary heart disease (CHD). Only a clinical trial of vitamin used in this context can answer the issue of vitamin E and cardioprotection.

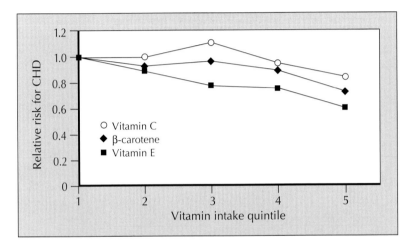

FIGURE 10-28. The quintiles of vitamin intake for β-carotene, vitamin C, and vitamin E were analyzed for a relation with coronary heart disease (CHD) risk for men participating in the Health Professionals Study [24]. Significant inverse trends with CHD were observed for β-carotene ($P = 0.02$) and vitamin E ($P = 0.001$), but not for vitamin C. It has been hypothesized that the antioxidant nature of these vitamins acts to prevent oxidation of low-density lipoprotein cholesterol and retards atherosclerosis [25].

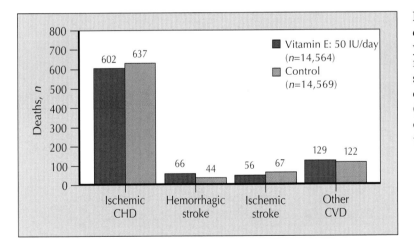

FIGURE 10-29. Vitamin E and death: the Finnish smokers trial. A clinical trial of vitamin E supplementation (50 mg/d for 5 to 8 years) in Finnish smokers ($n = 14,564$) showed no difference in rates of ischemic coronary heart disease (CHD), hemorrhagic stroke, ischemic stroke, or other cardiovascular diseases (CVDs) compared with a similar number of participants receiving placebo ($n = 14,569$). Although vitamin E has been suggested as an antioxidant that might retard CHD and other atherosclerotic diseases, this negative trial suggests no protective effect in smokers [26].

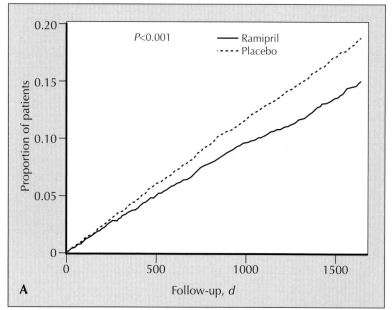

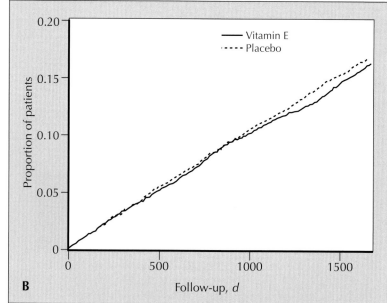

A

Follow-up, *d*

B

Follow-up, *d*

FIGURE 10-30. The angiotensin-converting enzyme inhibitor ramipril and vitamin E were used in a 2 × 2 factorial clinical trial to prevent cardiovascular events in patients at high risk for disease but without evidence of left ventricular dysfunction or heart failure. Treatment with ramipril (10 mg/d) reduced the rates of the primary endpoint (composite of myocardial infarction, stroke, or cardiovascular disease death) as shown in **A** [27], but vitamin E (400 IU/d) had no apparent effect on the outcomes as seen in **B** [28].(**A** *adapted from* Yusuf *et al.* [27]; **B** *adapted from* Yusuf *et al.* [28].)

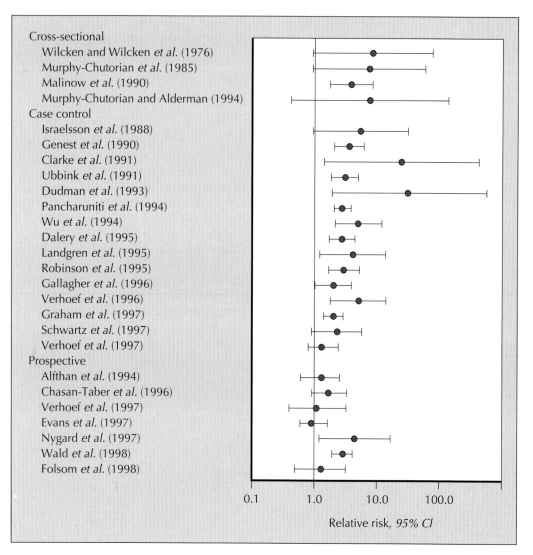

Cross-sectional
  Wilcken and Wilcken *et al.* (1976)
  Murphy-Chutorian *et al.* (1985)
  Malinow *et al.* (1990)
  Murphy-Chutorian and Alderman (1994)
Case control
  Israelsson *et al.* (1988)
  Genest *et al.* (1990)
  Clarke *et al.* (1991)
  Ubbink *et al.* (1991)
  Dudman *et al.* (1993)
  Pancharuniti *et al.* (1994)
  Wu *et al.* (1994)
  Dalery *et al.* (1995)
  Landgren *et al.* (1995)
  Robinson *et al.* (1995)
  Gallagher *et al.* (1996)
  Verhoef *et al.* (1996)
  Graham *et al.* (1997)
  Schwartz *et al.* (1997)
  Verhoef *et al.* (1997)
Prospective
  Alfthan *et al.* (1994)
  Chasan-Taber *et al.* (1996)
  Verhoef *et al.* (1997)
  Evans *et al.* (1997)
  Nygard *et al.* (1997)
  Wald *et al.* (1998)
  Folsom *et al.* (1998)

Relative risk, *95% CI*

FIGURE 10-31. Fasting homocysteine and coronary artery disease (CAD): summary and meta-analysis. This meta-analysis showed that homocysteine levels were highly associated with greater risk for CHD in a variety of studies. The summary odds ratio for a 5-mol/L difference was approximately 1.60 [29].

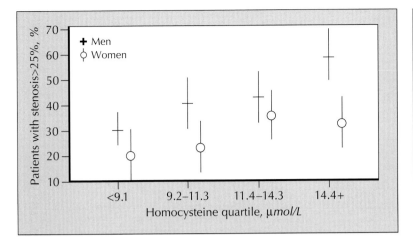

FIGURE 10-32. Greater homocysteine levels in a sample of 1041 older patients were associated with an increased relative odds for carotid stenosis that exceeded 25%. The trend was significant in men ($P<0.001$) and women ($P = 0.03$) [30].

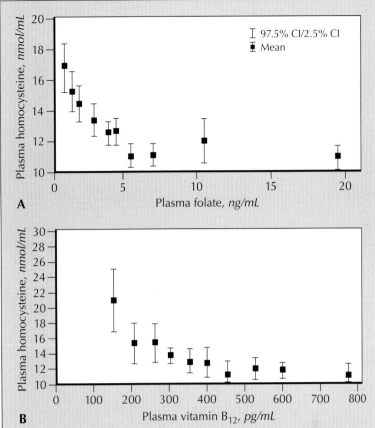

FIGURE 10-33. Plasma folate (**A**) and vitamin B_{12} (**B**) levels were related to concentration of plasma homocysteine in a sample of old Framingham Study participants. Each vertical line represents a decile of folate or vitamin B_{12}. These data suggest that adequate levels of folate, vitamin B_{12}, and pyridoxine (not shown) may be necessary for optimal homocysteine concentrations [31].

GLUCOSE METABOLISM, INSULIN, AND INSULIN RESISTANCE

PLASMA FOLATE AND HOMOCYSTEINE CONCENTRATIONS BEFORE AND AFTER FOLIC ACID FORTIFICATION

PLASMA CHARACTERISTIC	STUDY GROUP	CONTROL GROUP
Mean folate, *ng/mL*		
Baseline	4.6	4.6
Follow-up	10.0	4.8
Folate, *< 3 ng/mL*		
Baseline	22.0%	25.3%
Follow-up	1.7%	20.7%
Mean total homocysteine, *μmol/L*		
Baseline	10.1	10.0
Follow-up	9.4	10.2
Total homocysteine, *> 13 μmol/L*		
Baseline	18.7%	17.6%
Follow-up	9.8%	21.0%

FIGURE 10-34. Plasma folate and homocysteine concentrations before and after folic acid fortification. The impact of folate fortification (140 μg/100 g enriched grains) in the United States was studied. The Framingham cohort participants, who were seen after fortification, were labeled the study group. Controls were study subjects who were seen before fortification. Among those not using vitamin supplements, the mean folate levels increased, the prevalence of low folate decreased, the mean total homocysteine decreased, and the prevalence of high homocysteine decreased significantly (all $P<0.001$) [32].

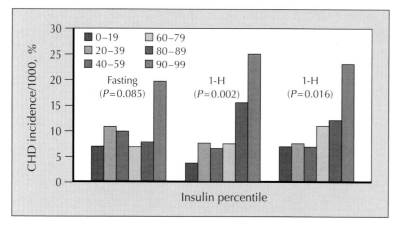

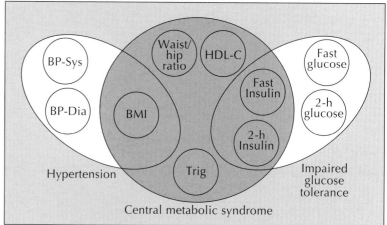

FIGURE 10-35. Glucose tolerance tests (75 g oral load) performed on a Finnish male cohort showed that higher insulin levels (particularly at the 1- or 2-h interval) were associated with an increased incidence of coronary heart disease (CHD) [33]. These data support the concept that abnormal glucose metabolism among nondiabetic patients, exhibited by an excessive insulin response to a glucose challenge, is associated with greater risk of CHD.

FIGURE 10-36. Risk factors for a metabolic syndrome. Metabolic risk factor clustering was studied in the Framingham offspring. When principal components analysis was used, there appeared to be three distinct domains: one related to hypertension that included measurement of blood pressure measures and body mass index (BMI), a second related to glycemia that included fasting and measurement of postprandial glucose and insulin, and a central core with waist/hip ratio, high-density lipoprotein cholesterol (HDL-C), triglycerides (Trig), fasting and postprandial insulin, and BMI. This approach was undertaken to improve understanding of the insulin resistance syndrome, how factors cluster together, and how coronary heart disease (CHD) risk is increased [34]. BP-Dia—diastolic blood pressure; BP-Sys—systolic blood pressure.

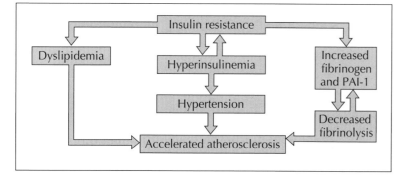

FIGURE 10-37. Schema for insulin resistance syndrome with potential effects on lipids, blood pressure, and fibrinolysis. PAI-1—plasminogen activator inhibitor-1.

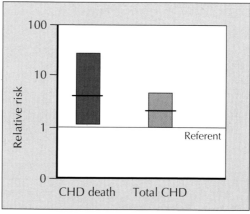

FIGURE 10-38. Relative risk for coronary heart disease (CHD) death in type 2 diabetes mellitus according to levels of hemoglobin A1c (HbA1c) exceeding 7.0 mg/dL. Better glycemic control was associated with lower risk for CHD risk over a 3.5-year follow-up interval of more than 1200 Finnish adults aged 65 to 74 years at baseline. There was a significant increase in the risk of CHD death and all CHD events in type 2 diabetes mellitus study subjects with HbA1c greater than 7.0% compared with diabetic patients who had HbA1c below 7.0 mg/dL [35].

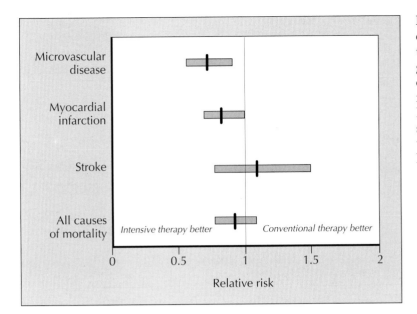

FIGURE 10-39. Relative risk for adverse outcomes: UK Prospective diabetes Study (UKPDS) intensive versus conventional glycemic therapy. This long-term British trial showed that intensive glycemic control with sulfonylureas or insulin compared with conventional therapy was associated with reduced risk for microvascular disease but not for macrovascular disease (border-line significance for myocardial infarction, not significant for stroke and all-cause mortality). Intensive therapy was associated with lower hemoglobin A1c during the trial and greater risk of hypoglycemia [36].

IMAGING

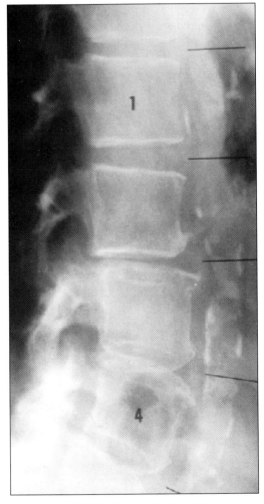

FIGURE 10-40. Radiograph of vertebrae. Calcification of abdominal aorta is greater distally and the prevalence increases greatly during middle age for men and women. Vertebral bodies L1 and L4 are noted on the radiograph. (*From* Wilson *et al.* [37], with permission.)

MULTIVARIATE ADJUSTED RELATIVE RISK ASSOCIATED WITH TERTILES OF AAC VASCULAR EVENTS OVER 22 YEARS OF FOLLOW-UP

EVENT AND TERTILE COMPARISON	MEN, RR (95% CI)	WOMEN, RR (95% CI)	TOTAL, RR (95% CI)
CHD			
2 vs 1	1.31 (0.95–1.80)	1.33 (0.90–1.94)	1.32 (1.03–1.68)
3 vs 1	1.61 (1.13–2.30)	2.41 (1.64–3.55)	1.91 (1.48–2.47)
CVD			
2 vs 1	1.33 (1.02–1.74)	1.25 (0.95–1.65)	1.29 (1.07–1.57)
3 vs 1	1.68–2.27)	1.78 (1.33–2.38)	1.70 (1.38–2.09)
CVD mortality			
2 vs 1	1.74 (1.18–2.59)	1.89 (1.17–3.04)	1.77 (1.30–2.40)
3 vs 1	2.24 (1.48–3.39)	2.42 (1.49–3.92)	2.26 (1.66–3.09)

FIGURE 10-41. Multivariate adjusted relative risk (RR) associated with tertiles of abdominal aorta calcification (AAC) vascular events over 22 years of follow-up. Severity of calcification in the abdominal aorta was related to an increased risk of cardiovascular disease (CVD) over more than 20 years of follow-up in the Framingham Heart Study experience. The calcification effect was statistically significant in men and women after adjustment by factors commonly used to assess cardiovascular risk such as age, cholesterol, high-density lipoprotein cholesterol, blood pressure, smoking, and diabetes mellitus [37]. CHD—coronary heart disease. (*Adapted from* Wilson *et al.* [37].)

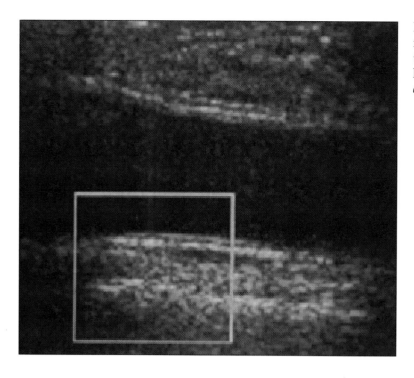

Figure 10-42. Intimal medial thickness (IMT). The IMT can be measured in larger arteries using B-mode ultrasound or other techniques. This image was taken from the abdominal aorta of a healthy 10-year-old boy; the IMT was 0.80 mm [38]. (*From* Jarvisalo *et al.* [38]; with permission.)

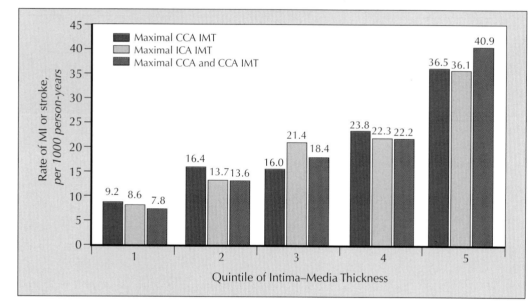

Figure 10-43. Greater carotid intimal medial thickness (IMT) was related to an increased risk of cardiovascular sequelae (myocardial infarction [MI] or stroke) among participants in the Cardiovascular Health Study. This investigation included 5858 study subjects older than 65 years at the onset; the follow-up lasted for a median of 6.2 years. Association between cardiovascular disease events and IMT was significant after adjustment for traditional risk factors. All trends were $P<0.001$ unadjusted and after multivariable adjustment [39]. CCA—common carotid artery; ICA—internal carotid artery. (*Adapted from* O'Leary *et al.* [39].)

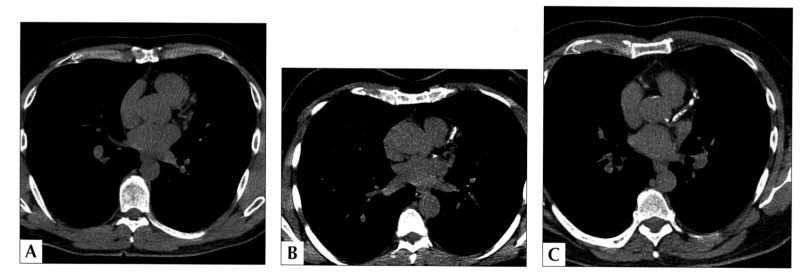

Figure 10-44. Three degrees of coronary artery calcification. **A,** No calcification. **B,** Dense lesion in the lower anterior descending artery with an Agatston score of 257. **C,** Severe multivessel coronary calcification with an Agatston score of 1002. The Agatston score grades the overall severity of the coronary calcification, in which moderate is 100 to 399 and 400 or higher is severe. (*Courtesy of* James Ehrlich, Colorado Heart Imaging, Denver, CO.)

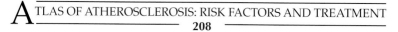

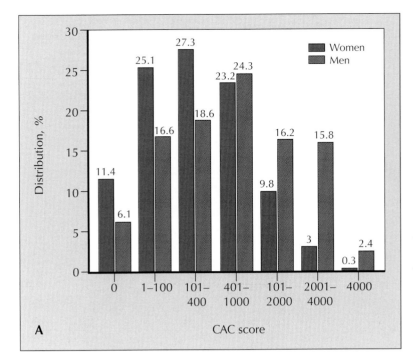

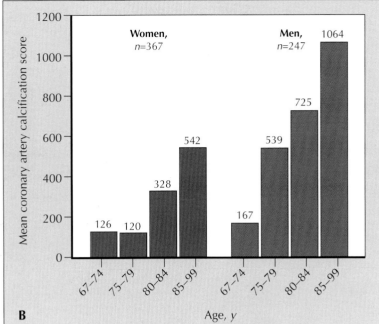

FIGURE 10-45. Coronary artery calcification (CAC) scores. **A,** Distribution of CAC scores in men and women are shown for older adults. The ages ranged from 67 to 99 years (mean, 80 years). **B,** Using electron beam tomography, the median scores were 622 for men and 205 for women, respectively. A history of cardiovascular disease was related to the calcium score and CAC scores in the fourth quartile were related to age, male gender, white race, triglycerides, smoking history, and history of pulmonary disease [40].

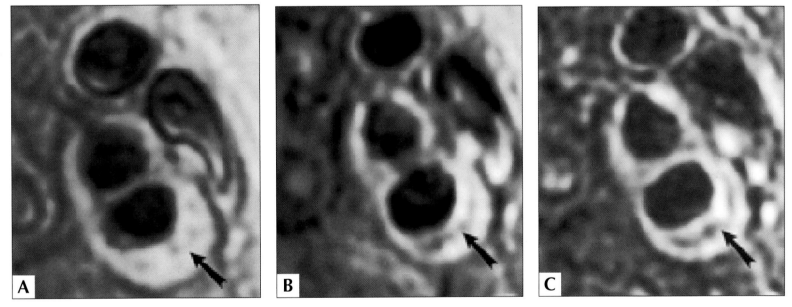

FIGURE 10-46. Diseased left internal carotid artery from a matched control patient. **A,** T1W. **B,** PDW. **C,** T2W. The *arrows* point to the region that has lipid mixed with calcium and appears bright mixed with dark on T1W and very dark on PDW and T2W.

Intensive lipid-lowering therapy in the Familial Atherosclerosis Treatment Study (FATS) was related to improvement in carotid MRIs. This small study highlighted the promise of newer carotid imaging modalities that allow identification of fibrous tissue, calcium, and lipid deposits in the carotid lesions [41]. (*From* Zhao *et al.* [41]; with permission.)

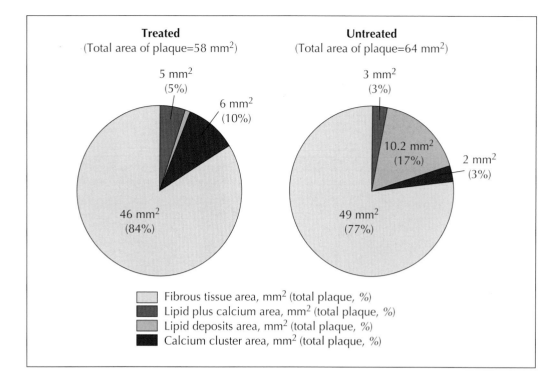

FIGURE 10-47. After lipid-lowering therapy in the Familial Atherosclerosis Treatment Study, the composition of the carotid lesions changed so that less lipid was found than in the untreated plaques. Fibrous tissue, calcium, and calcium plus lipid levels did not differ statistically between the two groups in this small study [41].

Treated
(Total area of plaque=58 mm²)

5 mm²
(5%)

6 mm²
(10%)

46 mm²
(84%)

Untreated
(Total area of plaque=64 mm²)

3 mm²
(3%)

10.2 mm²
(17%)

2 mm²
(3%)

49 mm²
(77%)

☐ Fibrous tissue area, mm² (total plaque, %)
■ Lipid plus calcium area, mm² (total plaque, %)
▨ Lipid deposits area, mm² (total plaque, %)
■ Calcium cluster area, mm² (total plaque, %)

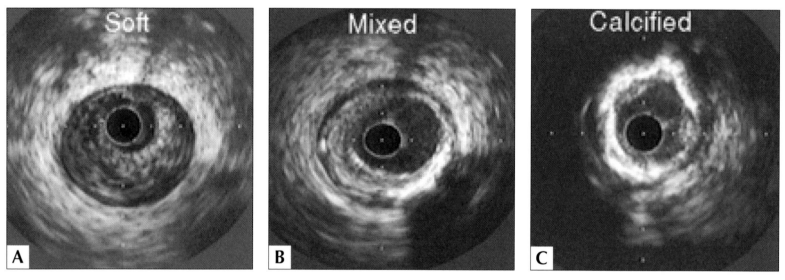

FIGURE 10-48. Atheroma morphology by intravascular ultrasound (IVUS). Soft (**A**), mixed fibrous and calcified (**B**), and heavily calcified (**C**) atheromas. IVUS is a new catheter technique that allows visualization of atherosclerotic lesions within the coronary arteries and study of the remodeling of lesions after specific interventions. The normal intimal thickness is approximately 0.15 mm; this technique allows identification of lipid-laden lesions that have decreased echos, fibromuscular lesions with low-intensity echos, and fibrous or calcified tissues that have stronger echos. (*From* Nissen and Yock [42]; with permission.)

REFERENCES

1. Danesh J, Collins R, Appleby P, Peto R: Association of fibrinogen, C-reactive protein, albumin, or leukocyte count with coronary heart disease: meta-analyses of prospective studies. *JAMA* 1998, 279:1477–1482.

2. Meade TW, Brozovic M, Chakrabarti RR, *et al.*: Haemostatic function and ischaemic heart disease: principal results of the Northwick Park Heart Study. *Lancet* 1986, 2:533–537.

3. Ridker PM, Vaughan DE, Stampfer MJ, *et al.*: Endogenous tissue-type plasminogen activator and risk of myocardial infarction. *Lancet* 1993, 341:1165–1168.

4. Thompson SG, Kienast J, Pyke SD, *et al.*: Hemostatic factors and the risk of myocardial infarction or sudden death in patients with angina pectoris. European Concerted Action on Thrombosis and Disabilities Angina Pectoris Study Group. *N Engl J Med* 1995, 332:635–641.

5. Gebara OCE, Mittleman MA, Sutherland P, *et al.*: Association between increased estrogen status and increased fibrinolytic potential in the Framingham Offspring Study. *Circulation* 1995, 91:1952–1958.

6 Ridker PM, Hennekens CH, Buring JE, Rifai N: C-reactive protein and other markers of inflammation in the prediction of cardiovascular disease in women. *N Engl J Med* 2000, 342:836–843.

7. Willich SN, Levy D, Rocco MB, *et al.*: Circadian variation in the incidence of sudden cardiac death in the Framingham Heart Study population. *Am J Cardiol* 1987, 60:801–806.

8. Muller JE, Tofler GH, Stone PH: Circadian variation and triggers of onset of acute cardiovascular disease. *Circulation* 1989, 79:733–743.

9. Schaefer EJ, Lamon-Fava S, Jenner JL, *et al.*: Lipoprotein(a) levels and risk of coronary heart disease in men: the Lipid Research Clinics Coronary Primary Prevention Trial. *JAMA* 1994, 271:999–1003.

10. Ridker PM, Stampfer MJ, Hennekens CH: Plasma concentration of lipoprotein(a) and the risk of future stroke. *JAMA* 1995, 273:1269–1273.

11. Ridker PM, Cushman M, Stampfer MJ, *et al.*: Inflammation, aspirin, and the risk of cardiovascular disease in apparently healthy men. *N Engl J Med* 1997, 336:973–979.

12. Ridker PM, Rifai N, Pfeffer MA, *et al.*: Long-term effects of pravastatin on plasma concentration of C- reactive protein. The Cholesterol and Recurrent Events (CARE) Investigators. *Circulation* 1999, 100:230–235.

13. Collaboration AT: Collaborative meta-analysis of randomised trials of antiplatelet therapy for prevention of death, myocardial infarction, and stroke in high risk patients . *BMJ* 2002, 324:71–86.

14. CAPRIE Steering Committee: A randomised, blinded, trial of clopidogrel versus aspirin in patients at risk of ischaemic events (CAPRIE). *Lancet* 1996, 348:1329–1339.

15. Yusuf S, Zhao F, Mehta SR, *et al.*: Effects of clopidogrel in addition to aspirin in patients with acute coronary syndromes without ST-segment elevation. *N Engl J Med* 2001, 345:494–502.

16. Austin MA, Breslow JL, Hennekens CH, *et al.*: Low-density lipoprotein subclass patterns and risk of myocardial infarction. *JAMA* 1988, 260:1917–1921.

17. Gardner CD, Fortmann SP, Krauss RM: Association of small low-density lipoprotein particles with the incidence of coronary artery disease in men and women. *JAMA* 1996, 276:875–881.

18. Jeppesen J, Hein HO, Suadicani P, Gyntelberg F: Triglyceride concentration and ischemic heart disease: an eight-year follow-up in the Copenhagen Male Study. *Circulation* 1998, 97:1029–1036.

19. Wilson PW, Myers RH, Larson MG, *et al.*: Apolipoprotein E alleles, dyslipidemia, and coronary heart disease. The Framingham Offspring Study. *JAMA* 1994, 272:1666–1671.

20. Wilson PWF, Schaefer EJ, Larson MG, Ordovas JM: Apolipoprotein E alleles and risk of coronary disease: a meta-analysis. *Arterioscler Thromb Vasc Biol* 1996, 16:1250–1255.

21. Gofman JW, Young W, Tandy R: Ischemic heart disease, atherosclerosis, and longevity. *Circulation* 1966, 34:679–697.

22. Juhan-Vague I, Alessi MC: Plasminogen activator inhibitor 1 and atherothrombosis. *Thromb Haemost* 1993, 70:138–143.

23. Buring JE, O'Connor GT, Goldhaber SZ, *et al.*: Decreased HDL2 and HDL3 Cholesterol, Apo A-I and Apo A-II, and increased risk of myocardial infarction. *Circulation* 1992, 85:22–29.

24. Stampfer MJ, Hennekens CH, Manson JE, *et al.*: Vitamin E consumption and risk of coronary heart disease in women. *N Engl J Med* 1993, 328:1444–1449.

25. Steinberg D: A critical look at the evidence for the oxidation of LDL in atherogenesis. *Atherosclerosis* 1997, 131(suppl):S5–S7.

26. Alpha-tocopherol, Beta Carotene Cancer Prevention Study Group: The effect of vitamin E and beta carotene on the incidence of lung cancer and other cancers in male smokers. *N Engl J Med* 1994, 330:1029–1035.

27. Yusuf S, Sleight P, Pogue J, *et al.*: Effects of an angiotensin-converting-enzyme inhibitor, ramipril, on cardiovascular events in high-risk patients. The Heart Outcomes Prevention Evaluation Study Investigators. *N Engl J Med* 2000, 342:145–153.

28. Yusuf S, Dagenais G, Pogue J, *et al.*: Vitamin E supplementation and cardiovascular events in high-risk patients. The Heart Outcomes Prevention Evaluation Study Investigators. *N Engl J Med* 2000, 342:154–160.

29. Christen WG, Ajani UA, Glynn RJ, Hennekens CH: Blood levels of homocysteine and increased risks of cardiovascular disease: causal or casual? *Arch Intern Med* 2000, 160:422–434.

30. Selhub J, Jacques PF, Bostom AG, *et al.*: Association between plasma homocysteine and extracranial carotid stenosis. *N Engl J Med* 1995, 332:286–291.

31. Selhub J, Jacques PF, Wilson PWF, *et al.*: Vitamin status and intake as primary determinants of homocysteinemia in the elderly. *JAMA* 1993, 270:2693–2698.

32. Jacques PF, Selhub J, Bostom AG, *et al.*: The effect of folic acid fortification on plasma folate and total homocysteine concentrations. *N Engl J Med* 1999, 340:1449–1454.

33. Pyorala K: Relationship of glucose tolerance and plasma insulin to the incidence of coronary heart disease: results from two population studies in Finland. *Diabetes Care* 1979, 2:131–141.

34. Meigs JB, D'Agostino RB, Wilson PWF, *et al.*: Risk variable clustering in the insulin resistance syndrome. *Diabetes* 1997, 46:1594–1600.

35. Kuusisto J, Mykkanen L, Pyorala K, Laakso M: NIDDM and its metabolic control predict coronary heart disease in elderly subjects. *Diabetes* 1994, 43:960–967.

36. UK Prospective Diabetes Study (UKPDS) Group: Intensive blood-glucose control with sulphonylureas or insulin compared with conventional treatment and risk of complications in patients with type 2 diabetes (UKPDS 33). *Lancet* 1998, 352:837–853.

37. Wilson PW, Kauppila LI, O'Donnell CJ, *et al.*: Abdominal aortic calcific deposits are an important predictor of vascular morbidity and mortality. *Circulation* 2001, 103:1529–1534.

38. Jarvisalo MJ, Jartti L, Nanto-Salonen K, *et al.*: Increased aortic intima-media thickness: a marker of preclinical atherosclerosis in high-risk children. *Circulation* 2001, 104:2943–2947.

39. O'Leary DH, Polak JF, Kronmal RA, *et al.*: Carotid-artery intima and media thickness as a risk factor for myocardial infarction and stroke in older adults. Cardiovascular Health Study Collaborative Research Group. *N Engl J Med* 1999, 340:14–22.

40. Newman AB, Naydeck BL, Sutton-Tyrrell K, *et al.*: Coronary artery calcification in older adults to age 99: prevalence and risk factors. *Circulation* 2001, 104:2679–2684.

41. Zhao XQ, Yuan C, Hatsukami TS, *et al.*: Effects of prolonged intensive lipid-lowering therapy on the characteristics of carotid atherosclerotic plaques in vivo by MRI: a case-control study. *Arterioscler Thromb Vasc Biol* 2001, 21:1623–1629.

42. Nissen SE, Yock P: Intravascular ultrasound: novel pathophysiological insights and current clinical applications. *Circulation* 2001, 103:604–616.

DIABETES MELLITUS AND VASCULAR DISEASE RISK

11

CHAPTER

Ira J. Goldberg,
Clay F. Semenkovich,
and Henry N. Ginsberg

Diabetes mellitus is a complex, multifactorial disorder that has an overall prevalence of about 5% in the United States. Whereas approximately 90% of diabetics have type II, or non–insulin-dependent diabetes mellitus (NIDDM), the remainder have type I, or insulin-dependent diabetes mellitus (IDDM). The prevalence of diabetes varies greatly among different ethnic groups, with rates as high as 20% in some Asian-Indian and American-Indian populations. These wide variations in prevalence are accounted for mainly by NIDDM. Although the cause or causes of NIDDM are not known, the environment is clearly very important. The molecular basis for IDDM is better defined, but the primary cause remains unclear. Despite the etiologic and pathogenic differences between NIDDM and IDDM, the chronic sequelae of both forms of diabetes are the same, and vascular disease, particularly coronary heart disease (CHD), is the major cause of morbidity and mortality in diabetic patients.

The increased risk for vascular disease in diabetes is derived from several sources. Clearly, diabetics have a greater prevalence of lipid disorders, particularly hypertriglyceridemia and low levels of high-density lipoprotein (HDL) cholesterol. Hypertension is also increased in diabetic populations. Obesity, which commonly occurs in NIDDM and exacerbates dyslipidemia and hypertension, may be an independent risk factor for CHD. Recent evidence has suggested that the link between obesity and morbidity from CHD occurs only when obesity is abdominal or central. Insulin, or more specifically, hyperinsulinemia, may be an independent risk factor for the development of vascular disease. Hyperinsulinemia is common in the milder forms of NIDDM. All these risk factors may interact and form a syndrome centered around insulin resistance. Finally, some risks specific for diabetes, such as glycosylation of proteins, play important roles in the development of the vascular complications.

The evaluation of risk in the diabetic patient must, therefore, be comprehensive and multifaceted. A full lipid profile, blood pressure, and weight (with a definition of weight distribution) must be obtained together with the usual measures of glucose control. The interaction between these risk factors and insulin resistance provides the physician with nonpharmacologic approaches that can affect several of the risk factors simultaneously. It has become increasingly clear that exercise and weight control are critical components of any therapeutic program for the long-term control of diabetes and its complications. Particularly in the patient with IDDM, tight glucose control must be a central goal of any treatment plan.

Diabetes mellitus cannot be treated solely as a disorder of blood glucose control. It must be approached as a multifaceted disorder whose evaluation and treatment is wide-ranging, and only then will the long-term morbidity and mortality be reduced.

INCIDENCE OF ATHEROSCLEROSIS IN DIABETIC PATIENTS

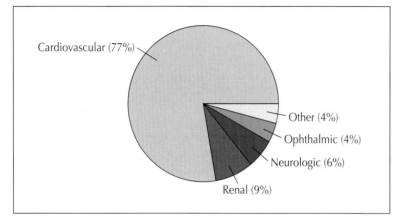

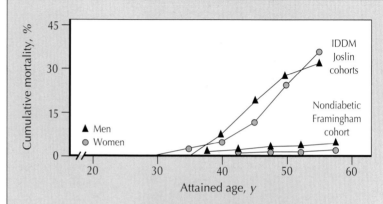

FIGURE 11-1. The chronic complications of diabetes mellitus. These complications are a major cause of hospitalization in the United States. Patients with diabetes mellitus are hospitalized for cardiovascular, renal, neurologic, and ophthalmologic problems at twice the rate of nondiabetics. Statistics from the American Diabetes Association indicate that the average length of hospital stay for these problems is about 9 days; thus, almost six million days of hospital bed use per year can be attributed to the chronic complications of diabetes. Cardiovascular complications account for more than 75% of the hospitalizations arising from the complications of diabetes. (*Adapted from* the American Diabetes Association [1].)

FIGURE 11-2. Although most health care professionals consider cardiovascular diseases a common complication of non–insulin-dependent diabetes mellitus (NIDDM), these problems also arise from longstanding insulin-dependent diabetes mellitus (IDDM). In particular, with prevention and better care of the acute complications of IDDM and the availability of chronic dialysis and renal transplantation, coronary heart disease (CHD) has become a major cause of morbidity and mortality among patients with IDDM. In this study from the Joslin Clinic, a group of 292 individuals with IDDM were followed for 20 to 40 years, and their cumulative mortality over that time period was compared with that of an age-matched group of nondiabetics from the Framingham Study [2,3]. Mortality was similar in the two groups until the age of 30 to 40 years, after which mortality rose sharply in the IDDM group. The rise in CHD cumulative mortality was similar in both the IDDM men and women. (*Adapted from* Krolewski *et al.* [2].)

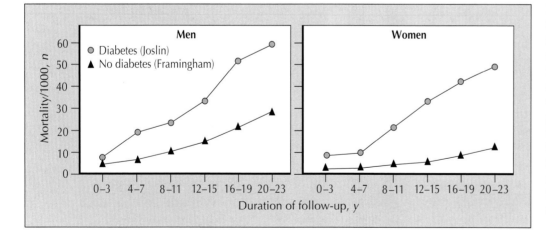

FIGURE 11-3. In a similar study by the Joslin Clinic, patients with NIDDM who were followed for 24 years were compared with an age-matched group of nondiabetics from the Framingham Study. The incidence of coronary heart disease (CHD) mortality with increasing length of follow-up was greater in the NIDDM group, among both the men and the women, compared with the nondiabetics. The relative risk for CHD in the diabetic women versus their nondiabetic counterparts was greater than in the diabetic men. (*Adapted from* Krolewski *et al.* [3].)

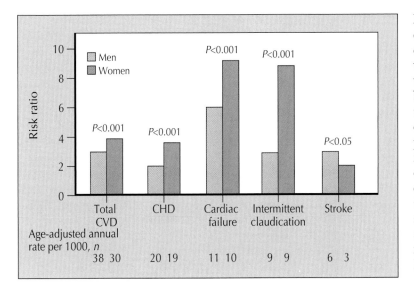

FIGURE 11-4. In the Framingham study, the risk of cardiovascular disease (CVD) was significantly increased in male and female diabetics. The actual age-adjusted rates for cardiovascular events were 38 per 1000 per year for men and 30 per 1000 per year for women. Because nondiabetic women have less CVD than nondiabetic men, the relative risk was greater in diabetic women (3.8%) than in diabetic men (2.4%). If the data are adjusted for total cholesterol, cigarette smoking, systolic blood pressure, and the presence of left ventricular hypertrophy, the relative risks are 2.3% for women and 2.0% for men. When total CVD was broken into categories, increased risk for diabetes was obvious for all types of events. The relatively greater risk in women diabetics was consistently observed, except for stroke. In addition, the Framingham study demonstrated that the presence of diabetes mellitus was associated with a significant increase in all-cause CVD and coronary heart disease (CHD) mortality. (*Adapted from* Wilson and Kannel [4].)

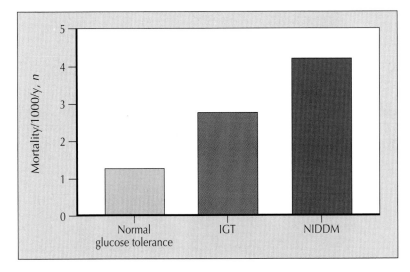

FIGURE 11-5. Stolar [5] found that even impaired glucose tolerance (IGT) was associated with increased mortality from coronary heart disease. NIDDM—non–insulin-dependent diabetes. (*Adapted from* Stolar [5].)

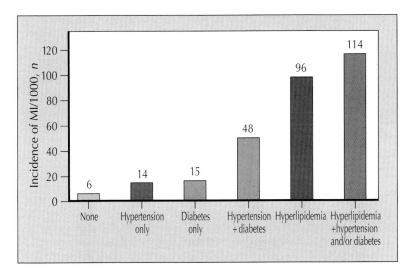

FIGURE 11-6. Similar results have also been reported from a large, prospective study conducted by Assmann and Schulte [6] in Germany. Rates of myocardial infarction (MI) over a 4-year follow-up period in a middle-aged group of men were increased nearly three times in diabetics compared with nondiabetics. When diabetes mellitus and hypertension occurred together, the incidence of MI was eightfold greater than in subjects without any risk factors. If hyperlipidemia was also present, a further twofold increase in risk was observed. These data confirm both the independent risk associated with diabetes mellitus and the synergistic interaction that diabetes has with other common risk factors for coronary heart disease. (*Adapted from* Assmann and Schulte [6].)

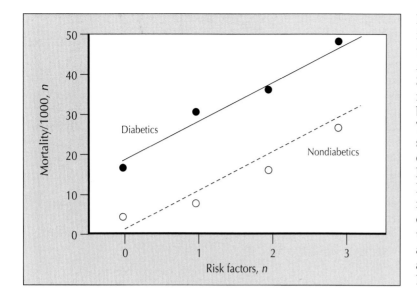

FIGURE 11-7. The interaction of diabetes mellitus and other risk factors for cardiovascular disease. This interaction is most evident in the data from the Multiple Risk Factor Intervention Trial [7]. Approximately 350,000 nondiabetic and 5000 diabetic men, between 35 and 57 years of age, were initially screened during the recruitment phase. These men, who were free of myocardial infarction at baseline, were followed for 6 years and mortality was ascertained. The results indicate that in both groups, major risk factors such as smoking, hypercholesterolemia, and hypertension have additive effects on risk. Moreover, for any number of risk factors, diabetics have two to three times the risk of dying of a cardiovascular event. In fact, a diabetic patient with none of these major risk factors has a risk equivalent to a nondiabetic with two of the three factors. When one considers that approximately 50% of adult diabetics have hypertension and a similar proportion have dyslipidemia, it is evident that an individual with NIDDM generally has five to 10 times the risk of a healthy, nondiabetic individual. (*Adapted from* the American Diabetes Association [8].)

OUTCOME OF DIABETIC PATIENTS WITH ATHEROSCLEROSIS

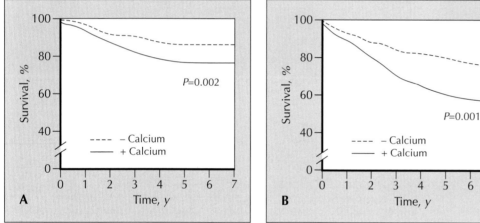

vessels are unlikely to dilate in response to stress so it is not surprising that vascular calcification is a powerful, statistically independent predictor of cardiovascular mortality (**A**) and total mortality (**B**) in diabetes [11]. Lehto *et al.* [11] studied 1059 (478 women and 581 men) Finnish patients with type 2 diabetes. In addition to increasing the risk for death, type 2 diabetics with vascular calcification were at increased risk for fatal and nonfatal myocardial infarction, fatal and nonfatal stroke, and lower-extremity amputation. Duration of diabetes, glycemic control, and older age were associated with vascular calcification, but other traditional risk factors such as hypertension and dyslipidemia were not. Vascular calcification may be one explanation for the decreased myocardial flow reserve detected in patients with type 2 diabetes [12]. (*Adapted from* Lehto *et al.* [11].)

FIGURE 11-8. Vascular calcification predicts accelerated cardiovascular event rates and death in people with diabetes. Compared with nondiabetic vessels, diabetic vascular lesions have increased matrix components such as collagen and fibronectin [9]. They also have more calcium. In a digital subtraction fluoroscopy study of 1461 asymptomatic patients, multivariate logistic regression analysis showed that the major determinants of coronary calcium were diabetes, older age, smoking, and a family history of heart disease [10]. Calcified

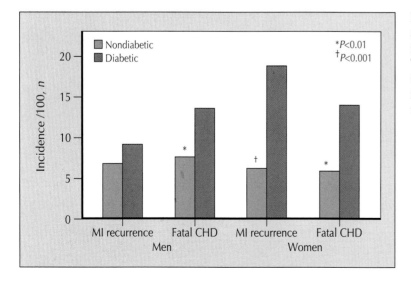

FIGURE 11-9. Diabetics who survive a myocardial infarction (MI) are at significantly greater risk for another cardiovascular event, including death, during the 2 years following their initial event. The relative risk compared with nondiabetics is about twice and this risk appears slightly greater in women than men. Increased incidence of coronary heart disease (CHD) was a major contributor to increased death. (*Adapted from* Abbott *et al.* [13].)

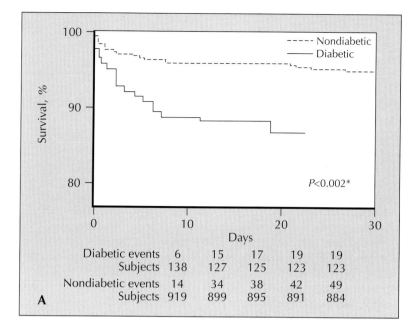

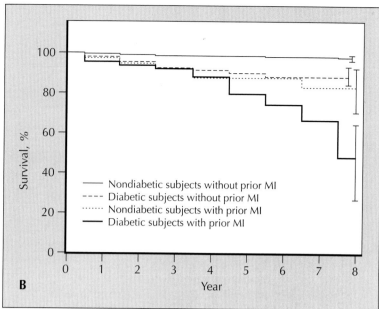

FIGURE 11-10. Patients with diabetes have a much greater mortality after a myocardial infarction (MI) than do nondiabetic patients. **A,** Data from the GUSTO 1 study showing a markedly decreased 30-day survival in diabetics. Similar data showing a decrease in survival by diabetic men and women were obtained in the Minnesota Heart Survey [14]. **B,** Another illustration of the adverse effect of diabetes on cardiovascular outcome. These data were found in a study comparing age-matched diabetics with nondiabetics in Finland. During an 8-year period, the incidence of cardiac events and death were compared. This figure shows only the survival data. Most remarkably, the survival of the diabetic patients with no history of coronary disease was almost identical to that of the control group with known coronary artery disease (CAD); similarly, the incidence of myocardial infarctions was the same in these two groups. As expected, diabetics with a history of CAD had the worst prognosis. It should be noted that the average cholesterol and the number of cigarette smokers in this population exceeded those found in the United States. Nonetheless, these data support the approach that asymptomatic middle-aged diabetic patients should be treated as if they have preexisting cardiovascular disease. (Part A *adapted from* Woodfield *et al.* [15]; part B *adapted from* Haffner *et al.* [16].)

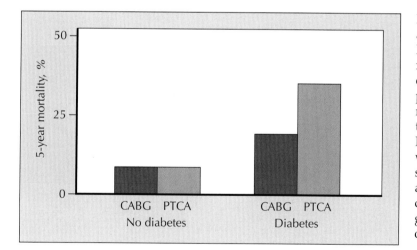

FIGURE 11-11. Patients with diabetes have a less favorable outcome after angioplasty. These data are from the Bypass Angioplasty Revascularization Investigation (BARI) and compare the 5-year mortality of diabetic (*n*=353) and nondiabetic (*n*=1476) patients almost equally divided between percutaneous transluminal coronary angioplasty (PTCA) and coronary artery bypass graft (CABG) surgery. The mortality of the diabetic population was markedly increased, more than twofold for the CABG groups and more than threefold for the PTCA group. Whereas the nondiabetic patients had a similar outcome with the two procedures, the diabetics who had PTCA had a worse survival than those who underwent CABG. The reasons for the more adverse outcome of PTCA are unknown but may reflect clotting or cell-proliferative abnormalities that are more common in the diabetic group. It should be noted that these data pre-date the widespread use of stents in PTCA. (*Adapted from* BARI Investigators [17].)

WHY DOES DIABETES INCREASE ATHEROSCLEROSIS?

POSTULATED REASONS FOR INCREASED ATHEROSCLEROSIS IN DIABETES

Abnormalities of apoprotein and lipoprotein particle distribution ("diabetic dyslipidemia")

Procoagulant state

Insulin resistance and hyperinsulinemia

Glycation and advanced glycation of proteins in plasma and arterial wall

"Glycoxidation" and oxidation

Hormone-, growth factor-, and cytokine-enhanced smooth muscle cell proliferation and foam cell formation

FIGURE 11-12. Postulated reasons for increased atherosclerosis in diabetes. There are multiple postulated explanations for the greater amount of cardiovascular disease in diabetes. Several of these abnormalities are addressed in more detail in subsequent figures. They include increased blood concentrations of lipoproteins and abnormalities in lipoprotein metabolic pathways and changes in blood coagulation leading to accelerated coagulation or decreased fibrinolysis. Patients with non–insulin-dependent diabetes mellitus often have circulating hyperinsulinemia, and even patients with insulin-dependent diabetes mellitus have elevated circulating insulin concentrations after insulin injections. Insulin is a potent growth factor and can accelerate growth of a number of cells, including smooth muscle cells *in vitro*. It has been postulated that stimulation of cell proliferation within the artery may accelerate number of cells and extracellular matrix within the plaque. This hypothesis was tested and at least in cholesterol fed rabbits, exogenous hyperinsulinemia did not alter atherosclerosis progression [18]. Prolonged elevations of plasma glucose lead to glycosylation of blood and arterial wall proteins and creation of advanced glycosylation endproducts (AGEs). These protein changes lead to abnormal protein functioning and could lead to a greater amount of oxidative products. (*Adapted from* Bierman [19].)

A. ANIMAL MODELS OF DIABETES AND ATHEROSCLEROSIS

Alloxan-treated rabbits have less atherosclerosis [19a]

No effect on "most" mouse models of atherosclerosis

FIGURE 11-13. A, Animal models of diabetes and atherosclerosis. Although diabetes is a well-established risk factor in humans, it has been difficult to exacerbate atherosclerosis by making animals diabetic. In 1949, Duff [19a] showed that alloxan diabetes actually decreased atherosclerosis in cholesterol-fed rabbits. This surprising find is thought to be a result of a severe defect in lipolysis and the conversion of atherogenic remnant lipoproteins to larger, triglyceride-rich lipoproteins that are unable to penetrate the vessel wall. The development of a number of mouse models of atherosclerosis has led to expectations that an animal model will be forthcoming in which diabetes accelerates atherosclerosis. Thus far only limited differences in atherosclerosis have been found by crossing mice with diabetogenic strains and by inducing diabetes with streptozotocin. These data suggest that there may be some biologic process that is altered in human, but not rodent, diabetes.

B, Diabetes results in much less cardiovascular disease in a low-cholesterol population. A number of risk factors for the development of coronary artery disease (CAD), including hypertension and cigarette smoking, are much less evident when assessed in populations with a low incidence of CAD. This is thought to be because an essential requirement for atherosclerosis, hypercholesterolemia, is missing. Similarly, if the incidence of CAD is

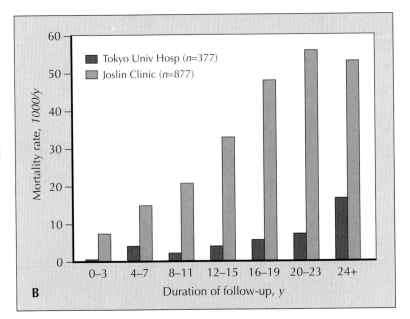

compared in two long-term studies, that from the Joslin Clinic and that from the University of Tokyo, the impact of diabetes can be seen in a lower-risk population. At every year of follow-up, the incidence of CAD was three to five times greater in the Joslin cohort. Other known complications of diabetes, such as renal failure and retinopathy, occurred at similar rates. This suggests that blood sugar control was similar in both groups. Most importantly, these data in conjunction with those from the Scandinavian Simvastatin Survival Study (*see* Fig. 12-29) suggest that reduction of risk due to hyperlipidemia is likely to make more of a major impact in cardiovascular events in diabetic patients. (Part A *adapted from* Kunjathoor *et al.* [20]; part B *adapted from* Matsumoto *et al.* [21].)

QUANTITATIVE CHANGES OF SERUM LIPIDS AND LIPOPROTEINS		
LIPID OR LIPOPROTEIN	IDDM	NIDDM
Serum cholesterol	↑	↑
Serum triglyceride	↑	↑↑
VLDL	↑	↑↑
LDL	↑	↑
HDL	↓	↑

FIGURE 11-14. Typical differences exist between patients with IDDM and NIDDM, as also outlined earlier. These differences may be less obvious when the IDDM patient is poorly controlled, but they are accentuated in well-controlled populations. It is evident from numerous studies that the dyslipidemia of NIDDM is only partially driven by the hyperglycemic state. In contrast, in a typical IDDM patient, abnormalities in lipid metabolism are completely reversed by tight metabolic control of carbohydrate metabolism. These differences in lipid metabolism in the two types of diabetes mellitus are related to the different etiologies of IDDM and NIDDM. In particular, insulin resistance (and obesity) are major factors in the dyslipidemia of NIDDM [22]. VLDL—very low-density lipoprotein.

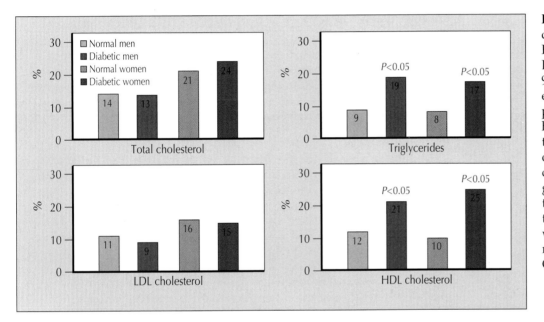

FIGURE 11-15. The typical lipid pattern in diabetic populations. If the diabetics in the Framingham study are categorized using Lipid Research Clinic (LRC) data for the 90th percentiles for total cholesterol, triglycerides, and LDL cholesterol, and the tenth percentile for HDL cholesterol, a pattern of hypertriglyceridemia and low HDL cholesterol becomes apparent [4]. Elevated levels of total and LDL cholesterol are not more common in diabetic patients than in the general population. It should be noted that these data were acquired by superimposing the Framingham data on the LRC data; thus, what is defined as 90th or 10th percentile is not identical for each group. (*Adapted from Garg and Grundy [23].*)

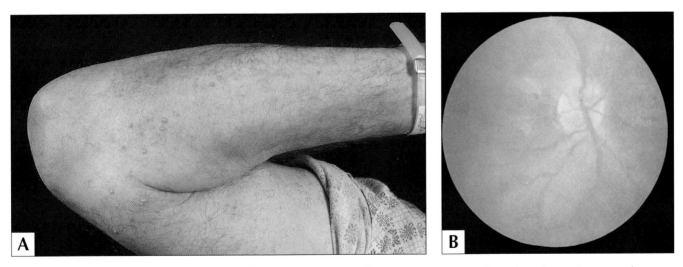

FIGURE 11-16. Lipoprotein disorders are usually asymptomatic. However, a very elevated concentration of triglyceride can present with the "hyperchylomicronemia syndrome." Such patients experience fatigue, abdominal pain, dyspnea, or dementia. The patient's plasma appears hyperlipidemic. The whole blood may have a "cream of tomato" color. **A,** In addition, eruptive xanthomas—small, red papules with a yellow center—are sometimes found on extensor surfaces. Pancreatitis is an infrequent, but very severe, complication of such elevated triglyceride levels. **B,** Fundoscopic examination of an obese man with poorly controlled type II diabetes and hyperchylomicronemia. Hyperlipidemia retinalis, the whitish discoloration of the retina, is observed above the background diabetic retinopathy.

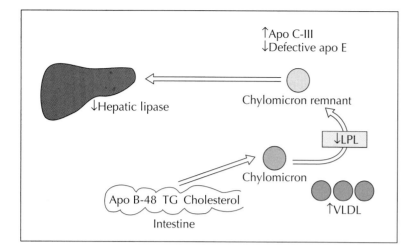

FIGURE 11-17. Potential defects in chylomicron metabolism in diabetes mellitus. After ingestion of fat and cholesterol (and the reabsorption of biliary cholesterol), triglyceride (TG) and cholesteryl esters are synthesized and packaged with apolipoprotein (apo) B-48 in the mucosal cells of the small intestine to produce the chylomicron. After secretion into the circulation from the lymphatic system, the chylomicron interacts with lipoprotein lipase (LPL) at the surface

of endothelial cells in the capillaries of adipose tissue and muscles. Approximately 70% of the TG is hydrolyzed, leading to uptake of fatty acids by fat cells and myocytes. The remaining particle, called the *chylomicron remnant*, travels to the liver where it is internalized, delivering its cholesterol ester and the remaining TG.

The major abnormality in chylomicron metabolism in diabetics may be a deficiency of LPL. In uncontrolled or decompensated IDDM, LPL can be markedly reduced and chylomicron levels can rise significantly, resulting in plasma TG levels exceeding 1000 mg/dL. This abnormality is partially reversible in IDDM patients with insulin treatment. In NIDDM, LPL levels may be slightly to moderately reduced, and this can exacerbate existing problems arising from overproduction of very low-density lipoprotein (VLDL) TG. Reduced LPL in NIDDM may result from insulin resistance and may not be completely reversed by tight diabetic control. Although chylomicron remnants have been reported to be elevated in both IDDM and NIDDM after ingestion of a large fat load, no specific diabetes-induced abnormality in remnant removal has been demonstrated. However, hepatic lipase (HL) can be reduced in diabetes and this has the potential of impacting remnant removal. Apo C-III, an inhibitor of LPL activity and chylomicron removal, may be overproduced in diabetes mellitus and could be the etiology of some cases of hypertriglyceridemia.

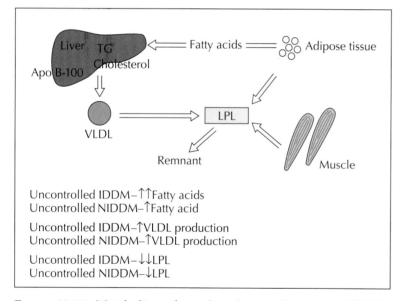

FIGURE 11-18. Metabolism of very low-density lipoprotein (VLDL) metabolism in diabetes mellitus. VLDLs are secreted by the liver after assembly of nascent apolipoprotein (apo) B-100 with triglycerides (TG), cholesterol esters, and phospholipid. Free fatty acid uptake by the liver, which stimulates TG synthesis, is believed to

play a major role in regulating the assembly and secretion of VLDL. Once in the circulation, VLDL behaves very similarly to chylomicrons, interacting with lipoprotein lipase (LPL), losing fatty acids to adipose tissue and muscle, and becoming remnants.

In untreated or decompensated IDDM, plasma fatty acid levels are very high, and uptake by the liver is markedly increased. In all but the most extreme degrees of ketoacidosis, TG synthesis is increased and VLDL secretion rises. The increased VLDL entry into plasma occurs when LPL levels are significantly reduced; therefore, plasma TG levels can increase to levels exceeding 1000 mg/dL. The defect in LPL secondary to insulin deficiency is completely reversible by adequate insulin treatment. Insulin therapy also inhibits lipolysis in adipocytes and reduces plasma fatty acid levels and, therefore, hepatic VLDL production. Tight control of IDDM is associated with normal or better-than-normal plasma TG concentrations. In NIDDM, fatty acid levels in plasma and uptake by the liver are also increased because of insulin resistance or deficiency. LPL levels may be slightly or moderately reduced in individuals with NIDDM; this leads to higher plasma TG concentrations for any level of VLDL production. Treatment of NIDDM with oral agents or insulin can improve TG levels but does not usually normalize them. The inability to attain normal TG concentrations may derive from the underlying insulin resistance or from coexistent obesity.

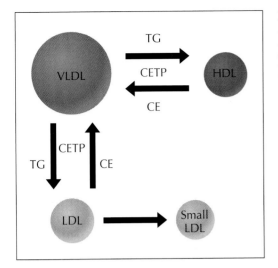

FIGURE 11-19. Plasma lipid exchange. There is a dynamic exchange of plasma lipids that occurs continuously in the plasma. Cholesterol ester transfer protein (CETP) mediates this process. In the setting of increased amounts of triglyceride-rich lipoproteins, either very low-density lipoprotein (VLDL) or chylomicron, triglyceride (TG) is exchanged for cholesterol esters (CE). Both of these lipids are hydrophobic and reside in the core of the lipoproteins. Triglyceride, but not cholesterol ester, is a substrate for the actions of lipoprotein lipase and hepatic lipase, the two most important triglyceride-degrading enzymes in the plasma. Therefore, lipoproteins that become triglyceride enriched can be converted to smaller particles because this core lipid is metabolism to fatty acids. This is the mechanism responsible for the production of smaller dense LDL and HDL3 in hypertriglyceridemia subjects, like those with diabetes. Moreover, because of this metabolic association triglyceride, LDL size and HDL cholesterol are metabolically linked. Thus, individual contributions of each of these factors to cardiovascular risk are confounded by coordinated changes in the other two lipoprotein parameters.

TREATMENT OF LIPID ABNORMALITIES

HYPOLIPIDEMIC DRUG THERAPY

| DRUG | RANGE OF LIPID EFFECTS, % CHANGE | | |
	TRIGLYCERIDE	HDL	LDL
Fibric acid derivatives	↓ 35–50	↑ 10–25	↓ 10–15
HMG-CoA reductase inhibitors	↓ 10—20	↑ 2–10	↓ 20–40
Bile acid resins	↔*	↔ ↑	↓ 15–30
Nicotinic acid	↓ 25–30	↑ 10–25	↓ 10–50

↓—Decrease; ↑—increase; ↔—no change.
*May increase in patients with preexisting hypertriglyceridemia.

FIGURE 11-20. Pharmacologic therapy for diabetic dyslipidemia must be considered if abnormalities in plasma lipid concentrations persist after optimal glycemic control is achieved or, more commonly, when dyslipidemia occurs and glycemic control remains suboptimal. The drugs available to treat dyslipidemia are shown, together with their major effects on plasma lipids. HMG-CoA—hydroxymethyl glutaryl–coenzyme A.

BILE ACID–BINDING RESIN

Action: Increases LDL catabolism, increases very low-density lipoprotein synthesis

Side effects: Decreased absorption of medications, bloating, constipation

Contraindications: Gastrointestinal obstruction, chronic constipation, may exacerbate hypertriglyceridemia

Dose: Colestipol, 20–30 g/d; cholestyramine, 16–26 g/d

FIGURE 11-21. Bile acid–binding resins have been proven safe and effective as LDL-lowering agents over the past two decades. They do not, however, significantly increase HDL cholesterol, and their use is often associated with increases in plasma triglyceride concentrations. The resins do not affect plasma glucose levels, although they cause gastrointestinal side effects, particularly constipation; the latter may be especially problematic in diabetics with autonomic neuropathy. Bile acid–binding resins are often not used as first-line agents for treating diabetic patients with dyslipidemia. They are, however, especially useful in combination with other drugs.

HMG-COA REDUCTASE INHIBITOR

Action: Inhibits HMG-CoA reductase, increases LDL receptors
Side effects: Occasional elevations of liver function tests, myositis
Caution: Cyclosporine, fibric acid drugs, niacin, and erythromycin
Agents: Lovastatin, pravastatin, simvastatin, fluvastatin, atorvastatin

FIGURE 11-22. Hydroxymethyl glutaryl–coenzyme A (HMG-CoA) reductase inhibitors can be useful as single agents to lower isolated elevations of LDL cholesterol, which are at least as common in diabetic patients as in the general population. Many diabetics with existing coronary heart disease require LDL cholesterol levels below 100 mg/dL. This class of drugs has triglyceride-lowering and modest HDL-raising activities. The reductase inhibitors, however, do not affect glycemic control.

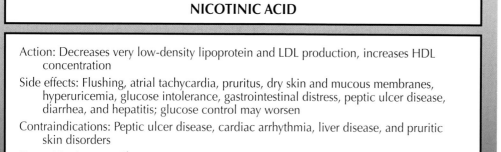

NICOTINIC ACID

Action: Decreases very low-density lipoprotein and LDL production, increases HDL concentration

Side effects: Flushing, atrial tachycardia, pruritus, dry skin and mucous membranes, hyperuricemia, glucose intolerance, gastrointestinal distress, peptic ulcer disease, diarrhea, and hepatitis; glucose control may worsen

Contraindications: Peptic ulcer disease, cardiac arrhythmia, liver disease, and pruritic skin disorders

Dose: Niacin, 1–5 g/d

FIGURE 11-23. Niacin (nicotinic acid) has an activity profile that would be particularly efficacious in patients with diabetes mellitus. It significantly lowers LDL cholesterol and triglyceride levels and increases HDL cholesterol concentrations. Unfortunately, niacin use can result in increased plasma glucose concentrations. Hyperuricemia, which is common in NIDDM patients, can also be made worse. Thus, niacin use is relatively contraindicated in diabetic patients. In a patient already receiving insulin, niacin treatment might be considered with modification of the insulin dose, if necessary. Newer once-a-day niacin preparations are now available and are efficacious.

FIBRIC ACID

Action: Increases triglyceride lipolysis, decreases secretion of very low-density lipoprotein

Side effects: Clofibrate causes cholelithiasis, nausea, abnormal LFTs, and myositis (rare)

Contraindications: hepatic or biliary disease; reduce dose with renal failure

Agents: Clofibrate, gemfibrozil, fenofibrate, bezofibrate

Dose: Gemfibrozil, 600 mg twice daily; clofibrate, 1000 mg twice daily; micronized fenofibrate, 160 mg/d

FIGURE 11-24. Fibrates also have an activity profile that would be effective in most diabetic patients with dyslipidemia. Thus, the major effects of fibrate treatment are lower triglyceride and higher HDL cholesterol levels. Fibrates have only a modest LDL-lowering activity; in fact, when triglyceride levels fall significantly, LDL cholesterol levels may not change or may even increase. The fibrates do not affect plasma glucose levels or diabetic control. LFT—liver function test.

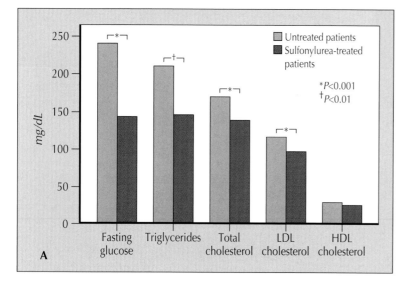

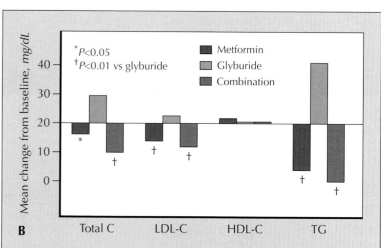

FIGURE 11-25. A, Treatment of NIDDM with oral sulfonylurea agents can also improve plasma lipid levels. In this study by Taskinen *et al.* [22], reductions in plasma triglyceride, total cholesterol, and LDL cholesterol accompanied reductions in plasma glucose levels after 6 weeks of sulfonylurea treatment. Note, however, that HDL cholesterol concentrations did not change. This has been a common finding in studies of this type. **B,** Effect of metformin on plasma lipids. In this study, a group of moderately obese type 2 patients who were receiving glyburide and dietary therapy were randomized for continued therapy or were switched to metformin alone or with continued glyburide. Surprisingly, plasma lipids worsened on the glyburide alone, and triglyceride (TG) and LDL both increased. However, metformin alone or in combination with the glyburide reduced triglyceride and LDL cholesterol levels. Although *A* shows a beneficial effect of a sulfonylurea on plasma lipids, it should be noted that in that study the comparison was with placebo. In the current study, the deterioration might represent a decrease in response to the continued therapy. Thus, metformin alone or when added to a sulfonylurea leads to improvement in lipoprotein proteins. (Part A *adapted from* Taskinen *et al.* [22]; part B *adapted from* DeFronzo and Goodman [24].)

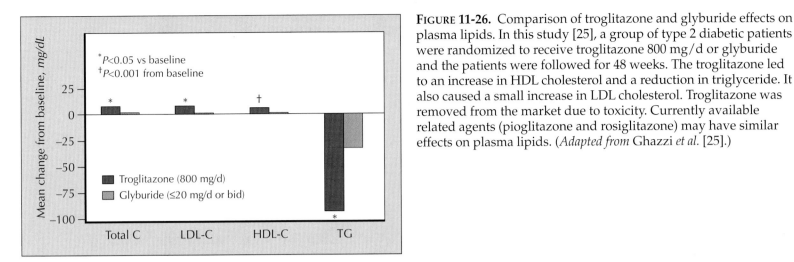

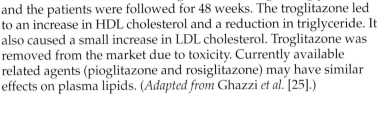

FIGURE 11-26. Comparison of troglitazone and glyburide effects on plasma lipids. In this study [25], a group of type 2 diabetic patients were randomized to receive troglitazone 800 mg/d or glyburide and the patients were followed for 48 weeks. The troglitazone led to an increase in HDL cholesterol and a reduction in triglyceride. It also caused a small increase in LDL cholesterol. Troglitazone was removed from the market due to toxicity. Currently available related agents (pioglitazone and rosiglitazone) may have similar effects on plasma lipids. (*Adapted from* Ghazzi *et al.* [25].)

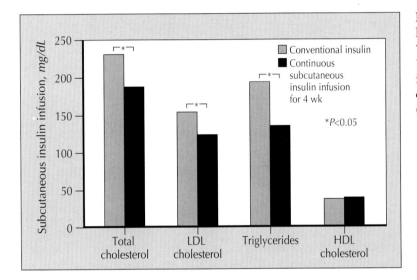

FIGURE 11-27. Intensive insulin therapy can actually reduce levels of triglyceride and LDL cholesterol to better than "normal" levels. In this study by Dunn *et al.* [26], treatment of 10 patients with subcutaneous insulin infusion resulted in an improved plasma lipid profile in a group of IDDM patients compared with levels present during conventional therapy. (*Adapted from* Dunn *et al.* [26].)

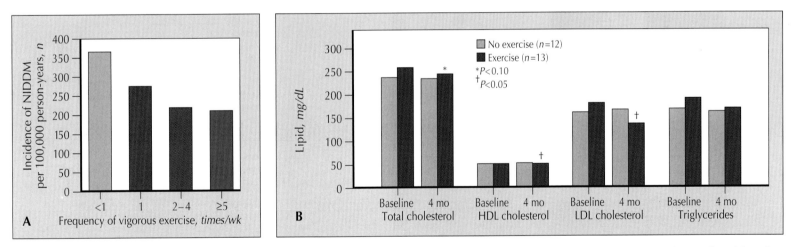

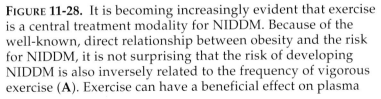

FIGURE 11-28. It is becoming increasingly evident that exercise is a central treatment modality for NIDDM. Because of the well-known, direct relationship between obesity and the risk for NIDDM, it is not surprising that the risk of developing NIDDM is also inversely related to the frequency of vigorous exercise (**A**). Exercise can have a beneficial effect on plasma glucose control and a significant impact on plasma lipid levels in NIDDM. In this randomized study (**B**), 4 months of exercise were associated with improved lipid levels compared with a nonexercising control group. HDL cholesterol also rose significantly in the exercising group. (*Adapted from* Manson *et al.* [27].)

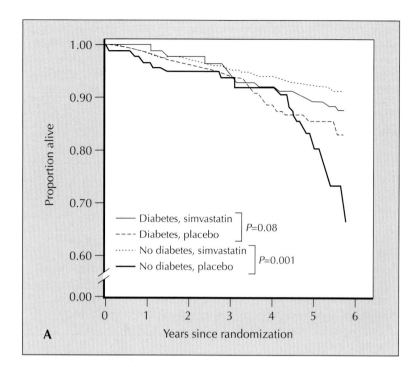

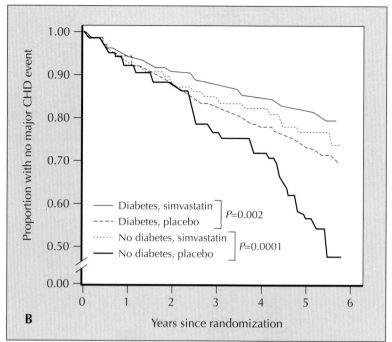

FIGURE 11-29. **A** and **B**, Effects of cholesterol-lowering therapy on survival of diabetics with known coronary heart disease (CHD) from the Scandinavian Simvastatin Survival Study (4S) [28]. The effects of simvastatin-induced reduction of cholesterol on recurrent cardiovascular events and overall survival was assessed in a subgroup of 202 diabetic subjects who were included in 4S. Not unexpectedly, the diabetic group also benefited from cholesterol reduction in this hypercholesterolemic cohort; average baseline cholesterol was 260 mg/dL. The diabetics with reduced choles-

terol while taking simvastatin had an incidence of recurrent events and survival that was slightly less than that of the untreated nondiabetic patients. When compared with the untreated diabetic groups, the data suggest that reducing cholesterol eliminates more than 70% of the increased risk of death and recurrent events in diabetics. These data are similar to those comparing Japanese and American diabetics and suggest that much of the macrovascular morbidity of diabetes is eliminated if patients have low cholesterol. (*Adapted from* Pyörälä *et al.* [28].)

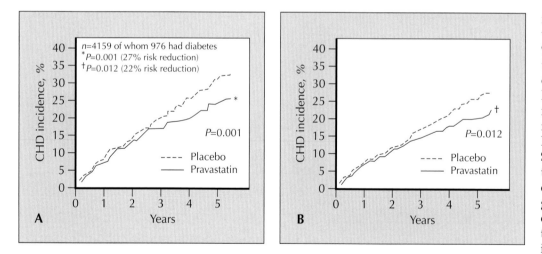

FIGURE 11-30. Effects of therapy on coronary heart disease (CHD) in diabetic in CARE. In this 5-year study, patients with more "average" plasma cholesterol levels (approximately 210 mg/dL) who had had coronary events were randomized to control or pravastatin therapy. A significant

reduction of recurrent major cardiac events was found in the treated group. More than 900 patients in this study had diabetes, and the effect of therapy in the diabetics was comparable to that in the nondiabetic population. As in the nondiabetics, patients receiving pravastatin had a significant reduction in repeat cardiovascular events. Moreover, as in the Scandinavian Simvastatin Survival Study (4S) [28], the treated diabetic group had a slightly better outcome than the untreated nondiabetic group. It should be noted that the incidence of events was less in this population that in the 4S subjects. Perhaps for this reason the improvement in treatment was not as dramatic as that seen with simvastatin. In addition, the cholesterol lowering was not as great. (*Adapted from* Goldberg *et al.* [29].)

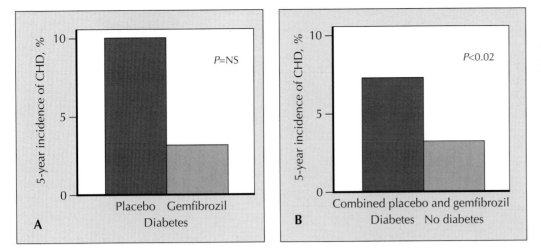

FIGURE 11-31. Effects of gemfibrozil therapy in diabetics in the Helsinki Trial. The Helsinki Trial, performed in the 1980s, studied the effects of gemfibrozil on development of cardiovascular disease. As opposed to CARE and the Scandinavian Simvastatin Survival Study (4S), this was a primary prevention trial. Gemfibrozil lowered LDL in these patients, but its primary effect was an approximately 40% reduction in triglyceride. HDL also increased on drug therapy. Of the more than 4081 subjects in this trial, 135 had type 2 diabetes.

A, Although the gemfibrozil-treated diabetic group had a reduction in the number of cardiovascular events, this did not reach statistical significance because of the relatively small number of subjects.

B, The overall increase in cardiac events in the diabetic group was significant; the diabetics had a 7.4% incidence of myocardial infarction and coronary heart disease mortality compared with 3.3% for the nondiabetic group. These data suggest that fibric acid therapy is beneficial in diabetic patients.

As shown in Figure 11-10*B*, the occurrence of cardiovascular events in middle-aged type 2 diabetics is equal to that found in patients with known coronary disease. For this reason, it is argued that all diabetics should be treated as if they have preexisting disease and their LDL cholesterol should be reduced to less than 100 mg/dL. CHD—coronary heart disease. (*Adapted from* Koskinen *et al.* [30].)

OTHER POSSIBLE CAUSES OF INCREASED CORONARY ARTERY DISEASE IN DIABETES

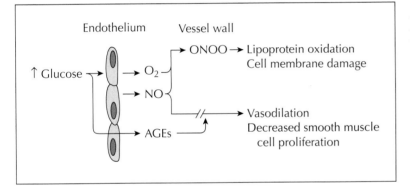

FIGURE 11-32. Hyperglycemia has complex effects on the vasculature. Glucose reacts nonenzymatically with the lysine residue of proteins to form a Schiff base. This base rearranges to form fructoselysine, the Amadori product. Hemoglobin A_{1c}, the standard

clinical measure of long-term glycemic control, is the Amadori product of hemoglobin. A protein carrying the Amadori product can react with other proteins in a complex series of reactions yielding advanced glycosylation end products (AGEs). Two important AGEs are carboxymethyllysine (CML) and pentosidine. AGEs may promote vascular disease by cross-linking proteins in the vessel wall, interacting with receptors that promote oxidant stress [31], or interfering with anti-atherogenic processes. Hyperglycemia increases superoxide (O_2^-) and nitric oxide (NO) production by the endothelium. These products react with each other to form peroxynitrite (ONOO⁻), an oxidant that can modify lipoproteins and disrupt cell membranes leading to vascular dysfunction. NO alone promotes vasodilation and may protect the vasculature by inhibiting platelet aggregation and smooth muscle cell proliferation. However, AGEs scavenge NO and prevent its beneficial effects. (*Adapted from* Semenkovich and Heinecke [32].)

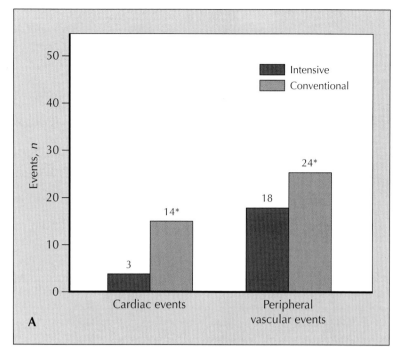

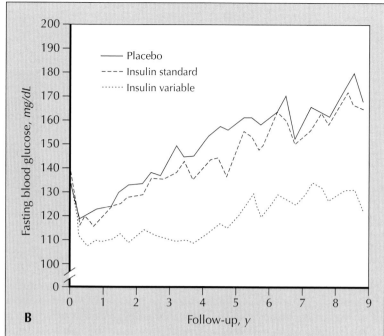

FIGURE 11-33. Effects of treatment of hyperglycemia. Although it is logical to assume that the macrovascular complications of diabetes should be reduced with better glycemic control, clinical data supporting this assumption are limited. In the Diabetes Control and Complications Trials (DCCTs), better control of blood sugar reduced microvascular disease (*ie*, retinopathy and nephropathy) in type 1 diabetic patients (**A**). Other smaller trials have also shown that better blood glucose control prevents retinopathy. Since the presence of microvascular disease often predicts the development of disease of large arteries, a similar beneficial effect of better glycemic therapy would be expected. As illustrated in this figure showing macrovascular events in the DCCT, there were relatively few events, and the difference in events between treatment groups was not significant. Moreover, the events were tabulated and in some cases represent multiple events in the same patient. Therefore, the difference in development of disease between patients in the two different treatment protocols was even less than suggested by these data.

B and **C,** The University Group Diabetes Program (UGDP) began in 1961 and was designed to test the glucose hypothesis (better glycemic control decreases cardiovascular events) in patients with type 2 diabetes. About 200 subjects were enrolled in each of five study arms: 1) placebo plus diet; 2) tolbutamide (a sulfonylurea); 3) phenformin (a drug similar to metformin); 4) insulin standard (a fixed amount of insulin regardless of control); and 5) insulin variable (insulin administered with a goal of normalizing glucose levels). The tolbutamide arm was discontinued in 1969 because of an unexpected increase in mortality, mostly due to cardiovascular events [33]. This move was widely criticized because of potential randomization flaws, protocol violations, and striking differences in event rates between study

centers. In 1998, the US FDA required that package inserts for sulfonylurea drugs contain information about possible cardiovascular side effects based on the UGDP. The placebo and insulin arms of the UGDP were continued through 1975 [34]. Fasting blood glucose levels were lower in the insulin variable compared to the insulin standard and placebo groups (*B*). There were no differences in all-cause mortality between these three groups (*C*). At the end of the study, there were 54 deaths in the placebo group (*n*=205), 48 deaths in the insulin standard group (*n*=210), and 49 deaths in the insulin variable group (*n*=204). There were 29 cardiovascular deaths in the placebo group, 27 in the insulin standard group, and 29 in the insulin variable group. In retrospect, the UGDP probably did not achieve a sufficient difference in glucose levels to test the glucose hypothesis. However, the study supports the notion that insulin treatment of type 2 diabetes does not promote cardiovascular disease. Rapid improvement in metabolic control decreases myocardial infarction mortality in patients with diabetes (**D**). The DIGAMI (Diabetes mellitus Insulin-Glucose infusion in Acute Myocardial Infarction) study was designed to test the hypothesis that decreasing glucose levels in the postinfarction period decreases the high initial mortality rate in diabetics. A total of 83% of the subjects had type 2 diabetes. At the time of presentation with a myocardial infarction, subjects were randomly assigned to usual care (control group; *n* = 304) or insulin-glucose infusion to achieve a blood glucose between 126 and 196 mg/dL (infusion group; *n* = 306). After the first 24 hours, subjects in the infusion group received multiple daily injections of insulin for at least 3 months. After 1 year of follow-up, total mortality was 29% lower for the infusion group. (*Part D adapted from* Malmberg *et al.* [35].)

(continued)

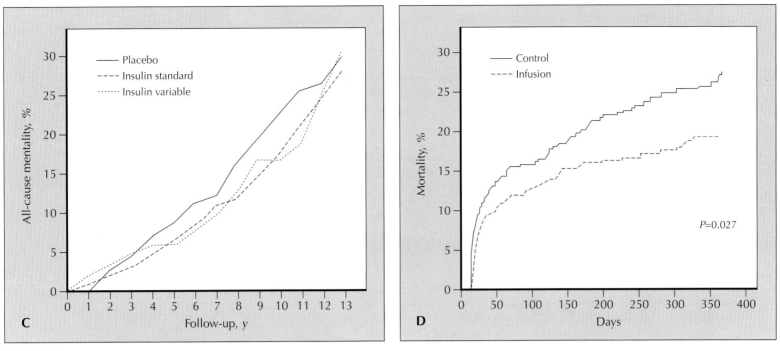

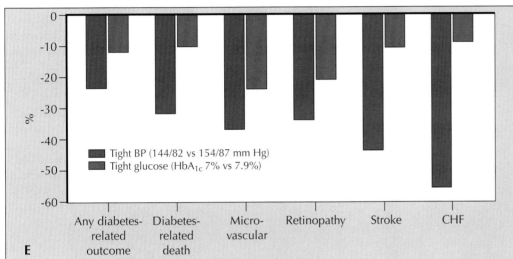

3867 patients with type 2 diabetes were randomly assigned to diet or more intensive therapy with sulfonylurea or insulin [36]. Glycosylated hemoglobin averaged 7.0% in the intensive treatment groups and 7.9% in the conventional group. The lower blood sugar was associated with lower incidence of microvascular disease. Although the overall reduction in macrovascular events did not reach statistical significance, there was no difference between the insulin and sulfonylurea groups; sulfonylureas did not increase cardiovascular disease. A subgroup of patients were treated with metformin, and this group had the lowest cardiovascular event rate.

In UKPDS, microvascular complications were markedly reduced. Moreover, treatment of hypertension markedly reduced both micro- and macrovascular disease (**E**).

FIGURE 11-33. (*continued*) The concern that sulfonylurea treatment may increase cardiovascular events in patients with diabetes has existed since the UGDP study. Recently the UKPDS (UK Prospective Diabetes Study) has reduced this concern. In this study,

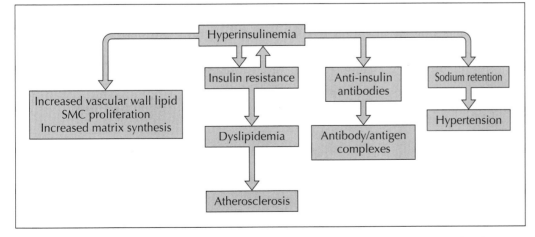

lates sodium reabsorption in the kidney. Alternatively, it may be because both hyperinsulinemia and hypertension are more prevalent in obese, nonexercising individuals. Therapeutic insulin is not provided via an intraperitoneal route; rather, it bypasses the liver. Providing enough insulin action to control blood sugar by blocking hepatic gluconeogenesis requires the peripheral tissues to be exposed to greater-than-normal concentrations of insulin. This may promote insulin resistance. In addition, despite the more widespread use of human insulin, the crystallization of the insulin protein to provide an injectable and slowly diffuseable source of hormone may lead to structural changes that provoke immune reactions. It has been postulated that antibody-antigen reactions involving insulin may occur along the artery wall and lead to endothelial damage.

FIGURE 11-34. Postulated atherogenic actions of insulin. Although insulin reduces blood glucose, it has a number of other physiologic and potentially pathophysiologic actions. Insulin is growth factors for a number of cells. In part, this is because higher levels of insulin will stimulate cell growth via interaction with the insulin-like growth factor (IGF) receptors. Hyperinsulinemia is associated with hypertension. This may occur because insulin acts on blood vessels or stimu-

PROSPECTIVE STUDIES OF INSULIN IN RELATION TO CARDIOVASCULAR DISEASE

STUDY	YEAR	MEN	WOMEN
Pyörälä et al. [37]	1985	S	—
Welborn and Wearne [38]	1979	S	NS
Eschwêge et al. [39]	1985	S	—
Welin et al. [40]	1992	NS	—
Orchard et al. [41]	1994	NS	—
Ferrara et al. [42]	1994	NS	NS
Després et al. [43]	1996	S	—

FIGURE 11-35. Studies of insulin and cardiovascular disease. Hyperinsulinemia is thought to be a risk factor for macrovascular disease. This compilation of studies by Haffner and Miettinen [45] shows that some, but not all, investigators found a relationship between disease and hyperinsulinemia. As noted previously, even if all the studies were in agreement because hyperinsulinemia occurs with obesity and inactivity, a cause-and-effect relationship would not be proven. (*Adapted from* Haffner and Miettinen [44].)

POTENTIAL IMPACT OF INSULIN RESISTANCE AND DIABETES ON THROMBOSIS AND FIBRINOLYSIS

Factors predisposing to thrombosis
  Platelet hyperaggregability
    ↓ Platelet cAMP and cGMP
    ↑ Thromboxane synthesis
  Elevated concentrations of procoagulants
    ↑ Fibrinogen
    ↑ von Willebrand factor and procoagulant activity
    ↑ Thrombin activity
  Decreased concentration and activity of antithrombotic factors
    ↓ Antithrombin III activity
    ↓ Sulfation of endogenous heparin
Factors attenuating fibrinolysis
  Decreased t-PA activity
  Increased PAI-1 synthesis and activity (directly increased by insulin and IGF-1)
  Decreased concentrations of α_2-antiplasmin

FIGURE 11-36. Coagulation abnormalities in diabetes. Diabetes has been shown to affect factors altering both coagulation and fibrinolysis. These are listed here. Evidence exists that both platelet and clotting factors mediated coagulation are accelerated in diabetes; perhaps this leads to an increase in thrombosis. In addition, degradation of the fibrin clot is impaired. A number of elements of the fibrinolytic system have been studied. Hyperinsulinemia, hypertriglyceridemia, and hyperglycemia all increase PAI-1; this may prevent normal fibrinolysis. cAMP—cyclic adenosine monophosphate; cGMP—cyclic guanosine monophosphate; t-PA—tissue plasminogen activator. (*Adapted from* Schneider et al. [45].)

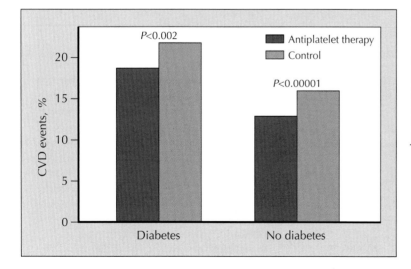

FIGURE 11-37. Antiplatelet agents prevent cardiovascular disease (CVD) events in patients with diabetes. In a meta-analysis of 145 trials of antiplatelet agents, there were 4502 diabetic subjects. Most of these trials used aspirin. When this subgroup was analyzed, the incidence of cardiovascular events (*ie*, cardiovascular death, myocardial infarction, and stroke) was reduced from 22.3% to 18.5% by the antiplatelet agents (significant $P<0.002$). Antiplatelet therapy also provided benefit to the nondiabetic subjects. (*Adapted from* Antiplatelet Trialists' Collaboration [46].)

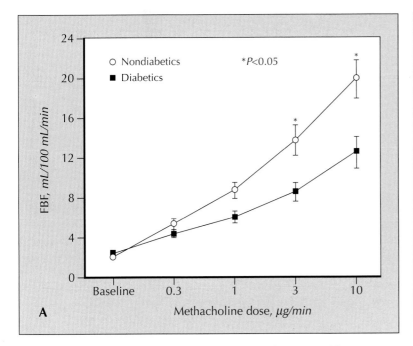

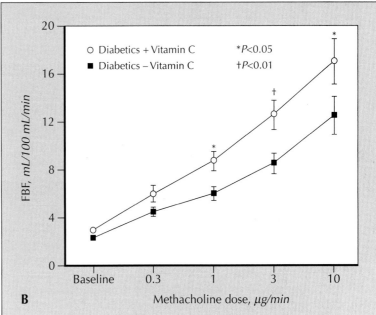

FIGURE 11-38. Impaired endothelium-dependent vasodilation is improved by vitamin C in patients with type 2 diabetes. Endothelium-dependent vasodilation is decreased in patients with diabetes [47], and diabetics have lower tissue levels of vitamin C [48]. **A,** Forearm blood flow (FBF) responses to increasing concentrations of methacholine (which causes endothelium-dependent vasodilation) were greater in nondiabetics (*open circles*) than patients with type 2 diabetes (*closed circles*). **B,** Intravenous administration of 1000 mg of vitamin C to the diabetics (*open circles*) improved FBF compared with responses in the same subjects before vitamin C administration (*closed circles*). (*Adapted from* Ting *et al* [49].)

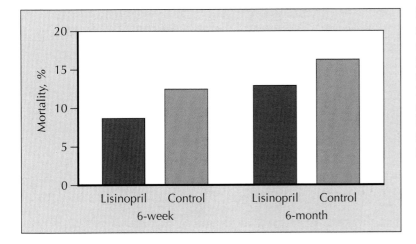

FIGURE 11-39. Angiotensin-converting enzyme (ACE) inhibitors reduce cardiovascular mortality in diabetes. GISSI 3 was a controlled multicenter trial comparing treatment with lisinopril plus nitrates with only nitrates beginning within 24 hours immediately after an acute myocardial infarction. There were more than 19,000 patients and 2790 patients with diabetes. The data shown are the 6-week and 6-month mortality rates in the two groups. Lisinopril reduced mortality by 30% at 6 weeks. This effect was statistically significant and was still evident after 6 months. (*Adapted from* Zuanetti *et al.* [50].)

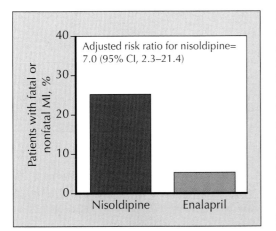

FIGURE 11-40. Angiotensin-converting enzyme (ACE) inhibitors are preferred over dihydropyridine calcium channel blockers for the treatment of hypertension in diabetes. The ABCD (Appropriate Blood pressure Control in Diabetes) trial [51] was designed to test the primary hypothesis that intensive control of hypertension will decrease complications in patients with type 2 diabetes. The secondary hypothesis was that the long-acting dihydropyridine calcium channel blocker nisoldipine would have the same beneficial effect as the ACE inhibitor enalapril. After 5 years of follow-up, nisoldipine treatment was stopped because it was associated with a higher incidence of fatal and nonfatal myocardial infarctions (MIs). After adjustment for numerous variables, including blood pressure, smoking, age, gender, duration of diabetes, glucose control, serum lipids, and medications, the risk ratio for fatal and nonfatal MI was 7.0 (95% CI, 2.3 to 21.4) with nisoldipine. There were 25 events in the nisoldipine group (*n*=235) and five in the enalapril group (*n*=235). This study does not prove that calcium channel blockers increase cardiovascular event rates in type 2 diabetes; rates in the nisoldipine group may simply reflect a lack of benefit from taking an ACE inhibitor. However, taken together with other data suggesting that calcium channel blockers may increase cardiovascular event rates in nondiabetics, this study provides compelling evidence that the treatment of hypertension in people with type 2 diabetes should include an ACE inhibitor.

BLOOD PRESSURE, mm Hg	EVENTS, n	EVENTS/1000 PATIENT YEARS	P FOR TREND	COMPARISON	RELATIVE RISK (95% CI)
≤90 (n=501)	45	24.4		90 vs 85	1.32 (0.84–2.06)
≤85 (n=501)	34	18.6		85 vs 80	1.56 (0.91–2.67)
≤80 (n=499)	22	11.9	0.005	90 vs 80	2.06 (1.24–3.44)

MAJOR CARDIOVASCULAR EVENTS IN PATIENTS WITH DIABETES MELLITUS IN RELATION TO TARGET BLOOD PRESSURE GROUPS

FIGURE 11-41. Major cardiovascular events in patients with diabetes mellitus in relation to target blood pressure groups. A recent study compared the effects of different levels of hypertension treatment on the development of cardiovascular events. This study, the HOT (Hypertension Optimal Treatment) study, included 18,790 patients from 26 counties [52]. Blood pressure was reduced with felodipine and additional agents to achieve three different target levels of diastolic blood pressure. The study included 1501 patients with diabetes. A remarkable reduction in major cardiovascular events was found in the group having the lowest blood pressure, less than 80 mm Hg; the number of events was approximately half of that found in the group having blood pressure of more than 90 mm Hg. (*Adapted from* Hansson *et al* [52].)

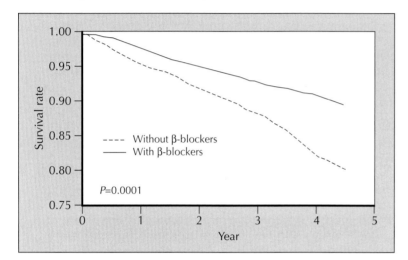

FIGURE 11-42. β-Blockers improve survival of diabetic patients with coronary artery disease (CAD). Despite concerns about the effects of β-blockers on hypoglycemia awareness and myocardial contractility, data have established that these drugs are beneficial. Shown are data from the BIP (Bezafibrate Infarction Prevention) study. The analysis is of 2723 patients with type 2 diabetes and established CAD; 33% of the patients (n=911) received the β-blocker propranolol. Over 5 years, the β-blocker–treated patients had a 44% lower mortality, most of which was due to a decrease in cardiovascular deaths. (*Adapted from* Jonas *et al.* [53].)

OVERALL APPROACH

CRITERIA FOR DIAGNOSIS OF DIABETES MELLITUS

Diabetes symptoms (polyuria, polydipsia, unexplained weight loss) + casual plasma glucose ≥ 200 mg/dL, *OR*

Fasting plasma glucose ≥ 126 mg/dL (no caloric intake for ≥ 8 h), *OR*

2-h plasma glucose ≥ 200 mg/dL during OGTT

Confirmation of diagnosis on subsequent day by any one of three methods

FIGURE 11-43. Criteria for the diagnosis of diabetes mellitus. These criteria have been redefined by the American Diabetes Association. A fasting glucose greater than 126 mg/dL is now defined as diabetes. An additional category of glucose between 109 and 125 is termed "impaired glucose tolerance." Inclusion in this latter category is one criteria for the metabolic syndrome. OGTT—oral glucose tolerance test.

DIABETES AND CHD: EQUIVALENT IN RISK

10-year risk for CHD is about 20%
High mortality with established CHD
High mortality with acute MI
High mortality after acute MI

FIGURE 11-44. The NCEP-ATPIII considers diabetes mellitus as a risk equivalent for coronary heart disease (CHD). This conclusion is based on data showing that patients with diabetes mellitus and no overt CHD have the same rate of cardiovascular events as those with an established diagnosis of CHD (see Fig. 11-10). For this reason, the guidelines for treatment of these patients are now the same as for those with established CHD. MI—myocardial infarction.

EARLY DETECTION OF ATHEROSCLEROSIS IN PATIENTS WITH DIABETES

EKG
Microalbuminuria
? Exercise testing
? Ultrafast CT scanning
? Carotid Doppler studies
Alternative: Treat as if atherosclerosis is present

FIGURE 11-45. Early detection of atherosclerosis in patients with diabetes. The approach to establishing the presence of asymptomatic cardiovascular disease is still evolving. The early diagnosis and institution of prevention and treatment is most important in patients with diabetes. Standard evaluation includes an electrocardiogram (EKG) even in younger type 1 patients. Since microalbuminuria is a marker for atherosclerotic disease, it should be analyzed. The role of additional screening measures, including exercise tolerance testing, ultrafast computed tomography (CT) scanning, and carotid Doppler studies, is unclear. Because diabetics have a greater incidence of silent ischemia, exercise testing is favored by some cardiologists. On the other hand, some argue that all diabetic patients should be treated as if they have coronary artery disease, and they should receive intensive risk factor intervention.

SPECIFIC DYSLIPIDEMIAS

Diabetic dyslipidemia
Lipoprotein pattern: atherogenic dyslipidemia (high TG, low HDL, small LDL particles)
LDL cholesterol goal: < 100 mg/dL
Baseline LDL cholesterol ≥ 130 mg/dL (most patients require LDL-lowering drugs)
Baseline LDL cholesterol, 100–129 mg/dL
    Consider therapeutic options
Baseline triglycerides, ≥ 200 mg/dL
    Non-HDL cholesterol: secondary target of therapy
Elevated triglycerides (non-HDL cholesterol: secondary target)
Non-HDL cholesterol = VLDL + LDL cholesterol = (total cholesterol - HDL cholesterol)
VLDL cholesterol: denotes atherogenic remnant lipoproteins
Non-HDL cholesterol: secondary target of therapy when serum triglycerides are ≥ 200 mg/dL (especially 200–499 mg/dL)
Non-HDL cholesterol goal: LDL cholesterol goal + 30 mg/dL

FIGURE 11-46. The NCEP-ATPIII guidelines for primary prevention of CHD in patients with diabetes mellitus are now identical to those for CHD patients. The primary target is to reduce LDL below 100. A secondary target is the reduction of non-HDL cholesterol to less than 130. This means that patients with elevated triglyceride levels should received triglyceride-lowering therapies [l].

The greater emphasis on non-HDL cholesterol as a target of therapy has major implications for the treatment of patients with type 2 diabetes. These patients are often hypertriglyceridemic. A sometimes effective first approach is the use of therapeutic liftestyles through weight loss, exercise, and diet. A second approach is the improvement of diabetes control. Many patients will, however, still require additional medications and two lipid-lowering drugs are often required.

BENEFIT BEYOND LDL LOWERING: THE METABOLIC SYNDROME AS A SECONDARY TARGET OF THERAPY

General features of the metabolic syndrome
Abdominal obesity
Atherogenic dyslipidemia
    Elevated triglycerides
    Small LDL particles
    Low HDL cholesterol
Raised blood pressure
Insulin resistance (± glucose intolerance)
Prothrombotic state

FIGURE 11-47. The metabolic syndrome as a secondary target of therapy.

A. GUIDELINES FOR PREVENTING OR AMELIORATING ATHEROSCLEROSIS IN PATIENTS WITH DIABETES

Glycemic control
Weight reduction
Exercise
Cigarette smoking cessation
Lowering blood pressure
Controlling lipid abnormalities

FIGURE 11-48. Guidelines for prevention or amelioration of atherosclerosis in patients with diabetes (**A** and **B**). The approach must stress intensive management of the usual coronary risk factors using lifestyle and medication approaches. In addition, although it does not have proven benefits for large vessel disease, control of blood sugar is a cornerstone of diabetes therapy and prevents microvascular and neurologic complications. Exercise and weight loss reduce cardiovascular risk and improve glycemic control. Cigarette smoking and hypertension are especially deleterious in patients with diabetes. Finally, reduction of low-density lipoprotein cholesterol makes a large impact, and triglyceride reduction is also likely to be beneficial.

B. ADA RECOMMENDATIONS FOR PHARMACOLOGIC THERAPY IN ADULTS

THERAPY GOALS	TOTAL CHOLESTEROL, mg/dL	HDL CHOLESTEROL, mg/dL	LDL CHOLESTEROL, mg/dL	TRIGLYCERIDES, mg/dL
Macrovascular disease (+)	—	—	≤100	≤150
Macrovascular disease (–)	<200	—	<130	<200

REFERENCES

1. American Diabetes Association: *Managing Diabetes in the 1990s*. Alexandria, VA: American Diabetes Association; 1989.

2. Krolewski AS, Kosinski EJ, Warram JH, *et al*.: Magnitude and determinants of coronary artery disease in juvenile-onset, insulin-dependent diabetes mellitus. *Am J Cardiol* 1987, 59:750–755.

3. Krolewski AS, Warram JH, Valsania P, *et al*.: Evolving natural history of coronary artery disease in diabetes mellitus. *Am J Med* 1991, 90(suppl 2A):56S–61S.

4. Wilson PWF, Kannel WB: Epidemiology of hyperglycemia and atherosclerosis. In *Hyperglycemia, Diabetes, and Vascular Disease*. Edited by Ruderman N, Williamson J, Brownlee M. New York: Oxford; 1992:21–29.

5. Stolar MW: Atherosclerosis in diabetes: the role of hyperinsulinemia. *Metabolism* 1988, 38(suppl 1):1–9.

6. Assmann G, Schulte H: The Prospective Cardiovascular Munster (PROCAM) Study: prevalence of hyperlipidemia in persons with hypertension and/or diabetes mellitus and the relationship to coronary heart disease. *Am Heart J* 1988, 116:1713–1724.

7. Stamler J, Wentworth D, Neaton J, *et al*.: Diabetes and risk of coronary, cardiovascular, and all causes mortality: findings for 356,000 men screened by the Multiple Risk Factor Intervention Trial (MRFIT). *Circulation* 1984, 70(suppl 2):161.

8. American Diabetes Association: Consensus statement. *Diabetes Care* 1989, 12:573–579.

9. Ledet T, Heickendorff L, Rasmussen LM: Cellular mechanisms of diabetic large vessel disease. In *International Textbook of Diabetes Mellitus*. Edited by Alverti KGMM, DeFronzo RA, Keen H, Zimmet P. New York: John Wiley & Sons Ltd; 1992:1435–1446.

10. Detrano RC, Wong ND, French WJ, *et al*.: Prevalence of fluoroscopic coronary calcific deposits in high-risk asymptomatic persons. *Am Heart J* 1994, 127:1526–1532.

11. Lehto S, Niskanen L, Suhonen M *et al*.: Medical artery calcification: a neglected harbinger of cardiovascular complications in non-insulin-dependent diabetes mellitus. *Arterioscl Thromb Vasc Biol* 1996, 16:978–983.

12. Yokoyama I, Momomura S-I, Ohtake T, *et al*.: Reduced myocardial flow reserve in non-insulin dependent diabetes mellitus. *J Am Coll Cardiol* 1997, 30:1472–1477.

13. Abbott RD, Donahue PR, Kannel WB, *et al*.: The impact of diabetes survival following myocardial infarction in men vs women: the Framingham Study. *JAMA* 1988, 260:3456–3460.

14. Sprafka JM, Burke GL, McGovern PG, Hahn LP: Trends in prevalence of diabetes mellitus in patients with myocardial infarction and effect of diabetes on survival. *Diabet Care* 1991, 537–543.

15. Woodfield SL, Lundergan CF, Reiner JS, *et al*.: Angiographic findings and outcomes in diabetic patients treated with thrombolytic therapy for acute myocardial infarction: the GUSTO-I experience. *J Am Coll Cardiol* 1996, 28:1661–1669.

16. Haffner SM, Lehto S, Ronnemaa T, *et al*.: Mortality from coronary heart disease in subjects with type 2 diabetes and in nondiabetic subjects with and without prior myocardial infarction. *New Engl J Med* 1998, 339:229–234.

17. BARI Investigators: Comparison of coronary bypass surgery with angioplasty in patients with multivessel disease. *N Engl J Med* 1996, 335:217–225.

18. Nordestgaard BG, Agerholm-Larsen B, Stender S: Effect of exogenous hyperinsulinemia on atherogenesis in cholesterol-fed rabbits. *Diabetologia* 1997, 40:512–520.

19. Bierman EL: Atherosclerosis in diabetes. *Arterioscler Throm* 1992, 12:647–656.

19a. Duff G, Mar Millan G: The effect of all oxan diabetes on experimental atherosclerosis in the rabbit. *J Exp Med* 1949, 89:611–612.

20. Kunjathoor VV, Wilson DL, LeBoeuf RC: Increased atherosclerosis in streptozotocin-induced diabetic mice. *J Clin Invest* 1996, 97:1767–1773.

21. Matsumoto T, Ohashi Y, Yamada N, Kikuchi M: Coronary heart disease mortality is actually low in diabetic Japanese by direct comparison with the Joslin cohort. *Diabetes Care* 1994, 17:1062–1063.

22. Taskinen M-R, Beltz WF, Harper I, *et al.*: Effects of NIDDM on very-low-density lipoprotein triglyceride and apolipoprotein B metabolism: studies before and after sulfonylurea therapy. *Diabetes* 1986, 35:1268–1277.

23. Garg A, Grundy SM: Management of dyslipidemia in NIDDM. *Diabetes Care* 1990, 13:153–164.

24. DeFronzo RA, Goodman AM: Efficacy of metformin in patients with non-insulin-dependent diabetes mellitus: the Multicenter Metformin Study Group. *N Engl J Med* 1995, 333:541–549.

25. Ghazzi MN, Perez JE, Antonucci TK, *et al.*: Cardiac and glycemic benefits of troglitazone treatment in NIDDM: the Troglitazone Study Group. *Diabetes* 1997, 46:433–439.

26. Dunn FL, Pietri A, Raskin P, *et al.*: Plasma lipid and lipoprotein levels with continuous subcutaneous insulin infusion in type I diabetes mellitus. *Ann Intern Med* 1981, 95:426–431.

27. Manson JE, Colditz GA, Stampfer MJ, *et al.*: A prospective study of maturity-onset diabetes mellitus and risk of coronary heart disease and stroke in women. *Arch Intern Med* 1991, 151:1141–1147.

28. Pyörälä K, Pedersen JR, Kjekshus J, *et al.*: Cholesterol lowering with simvastatin improves prognosis of diabetic patients with coronary heart disease. *Diabet Care* 1997, 20:614–620.

29. Goldberg R, *et al.*: Hyperlipidemia and cardiovascular factors in patients with type 2 diabetes. *Am J Manag Care* 2000, 56:82–91.

30. Koskinen P, Mannttari M, Manninen V, *et al.*: Coronary heart disease incidence in NIDDM patients in the Helsinki Heart Study. *Diabet Care* 1992, 15:820–825.

31. Yan SD, Schmidt, Anderson GM, *et al.*: Enhanced cellular oxidant stress by the interaction of advanced glycation end products with their receptors/binding proteins. *J Biol Chem* 1994, 269:9889–9897.

32. Semenkovich CF, Heinecke JW: The mystery of diabetes and atherosclerosis: time for a new plot. *Diabetes* 1997, 46:327–334.

33. Meinert CL, Knatterud GL, Prout TE, Klimt CR: A study of the effects of hypoglycemic agents on vascular complications in patients with adult-onset diabetes. II. Mortality results. *Diabetes* 1970, 19(suppl 2):789–830.

34. Knatterud GL, Klimt CR, Levin, *et al.*: Effects of hypoglycemic agents on vascular complications in patients with adult-onset diabetes. VII. Mortality and selected nonfatal events with insulin treatment. *JAMA* 1978, 240:37–42.

35. Malmberg K, Ryden L, Efendic S, *et al.*: Randomized trial of insulin-glucose infusion followed by subcutaneous insulin treatment in diabetic patients with acute myocardial infarction (DIGAMI study): effects on mortality at 1 year. *J Am Coll Cardiol* 1995, 26:57–65.

36. Turner R: Intensive blood-glucose control with sulfonylureas or insulin compared with conventional treatment and risk of complications in patients with type 2 diabetes (UKPDS 33). *Lancet* 1998, 352:837–853.

37. Pyörälä K, Savolainen E, Kaukola S, Haapakoski J: Plasma insulin as coronary heart disease risk factor: relationship to other risk factors and predictive during 9 1/2 year follow-up of the Helsinki Policeman Study population. *Acta Med Scand* 1985, 701(suppl):38–52.

38. Welborn TA, Wearne K: Coronary heart disease incidence and cardiovascular mortality in Busselton with reference to glucose and insulin concentration. *Diabet Care* 1979, 2:154–160.

39. Eschwêge E, Richard JL, Thibult N, *et al.*: Coronary heart disease mortality in relation with diabetes, blood glucose and plasma insulin levels: the Paris Prospective Study 10 years later. *Hormone Metab Res* 1985, 15(suppl):41–46.

40. Welin L, Eriksson H, Larsson B, *et al.*: Hyperinsulinemia is not a major coronary risk factor in elderly men: the study of men born in 1913. *Diabetologia* 1992, 35:766–770.

41. Orchard TJ, Eichner J, Kuller LH, *et al.*: Insulin as a predictor of coronary heart disease: interaction with apolipoprotein E phenotype: a report from the Multiple Risk Factor Intervention Trial. *Ann Epidemiol* 1994, 4:40–45.

42. Ferrara A, Barrett-Connor EL, Edelstein SL: Hyperinsulinemia does not increase the risk of fatal cardiovascular disease in elderly men or women without diabetes: the Rancho Bernardo Study, 1984–1991. *Am J Epidemiol* 1994, 140:857–869.

43. Després JP, Lamarche B, Mauriege P, *et al.*: Hyperinsulinemia as an independent risk factor for ischemic heart disease. *N Engl J Med* 1996, 334:952–957.

44. Haffner SM, Miettinen H: Insulin resistance implications for type II diabetes mellitus and coronary heart disease. *Am J Med* 1997, 103:152–162.

45. Schneider DJ, *et al.*: *Coronary Artery Dis* 1992, 3:26–32.

46. Antiplatelet Trialists' Collaboration: Collaborative overview of randomized trials of antiplatelet therapy. I: Prevention of death, myocardial infarction, and stroke by prolonged antiplatelet therapy in various categories of patients. *Br Med J* 1994, 308:81–106.

47. McVeigh GE, Brennan GM, Johnston BJ, *et al.*: Impaired endothelium-dependent and independent vasodilation in patients with type 2 (non-insulin-dependent) diabetes mellitus. *Diabetologia* 1992, 35:771–776.

48. Cunningham JJ, Ellis SL, McVeigh GE, *et al.*: Reduced mononuclear leukocyte ascorbic acid content in adults with insulin-dependent diabetes mellitus consuming adequate dietary vitamin C. *Metabolism* 1991, 40:146–149.

49. Ting HH, Timimi FK, Boles KS, *et al.*: Vitamin C improves endothelium-dependent vasodilation in patients with non-insulin-dependent diabetes mellitus. *J Clin Invest* 1996, 97:22–28.

50. Zuanetti G, Latini R, Maggioni AP, *et al.*: Effect of the ACE inhibitor lisinopril on mortality in diabetic patients with acute myocardial infarction: data from the GISSI-3 study. *Circulation* 1997, 96:4239–4245.

51. Estacio RO, Jeffers BW, Hiatt WR, *et al.*: The effect of nisoldipine as compared with enalapril on cardiovascular outcomes in patients with non-insulin-dependent diabetes and hypertension. *N Engl J Med* 1998, 338:645–652.

52. Hansson L, Zanchett A, Carruthers SG, *et al.*: Effects of intensive blood-pressure lowering and low-dose aspirin in patients with hypertension: principal results of the Hypertension Optimal Treatment (HOT) randomized trial. *Lancet* 1998, 351:1755–1762.

53. Jonas M, Reicher-Reiss H, Boyko V, *et al.*: Usefulness of beta-blocker therapy in patients with non-insulin-dependent diabetes mellitus and coronary artery disease: Bezafibrate Infarction Prevention (BIP) Study Group. *Am J Cardiol* 1996, 77:1273–1277.

GENDER DIFFERENCES IN CORONARY RISK FACTORS AND RISK INTERVENTIONS

CHAPTER 12

Nanette K. Wenger

As was noted in the Framingham Heart Study [1,2], women develop any initial manifestations of coronary heart disease (CHD) approximately 10 years later than men and incur myocardial infarction (MI) on average as much as 20 years later. With progressive aging of the US population and more women surviving to an older age when CHD becomes clinically manifest, several gender differences have been highlighted. The more adverse outcome has been prominent, with increased case fatality rates and greater morbidity of women after both MI [2–4] and myocardial revascularization procedures [5]. Since 1984, more women than men die of cardiovascular disease in the United States. This underscores the need to undertake preventive interventions across the lifespan [4].

Because of the virtual exclusion until recent years of elderly individuals of both genders from clinical trials of CHD prevention, and the limited participation of women of all ages in these studies, there are sparse data regarding the coronary risk characteristics of women and responses to risk reduction. Recently reported studies show substantial benefit of selected interventions designed to reduce coronary risk in women. During the past few decades the decrease in cardiovascular and coronary mortality has been less pronounced for women than for men [1]; concomitantly, the reduction in coronary risk factors has been less prominent among women [6]. A 1998 Centers for Disease Control National Ambulatory Medical Care Survey showed that, in office practice, fewer women than men were counseled about exercise, nutrition, and weight reduction [7].

This chapter addresses the epidemiologic and interventional data for which gender-specific analyses are about coronary risk attributes. In general, risk factors for CHD are similar in both genders, and correlation is comparable between the major risk factors and rates of CHD for women and for men: both coronary risk attributes and coronary risk interventions in women differ qualitatively and quantitatively from those for men. Finally, coronary risk attributes unique to women such as estrogen and menopausal status and the gonadal hormones administered for oral contraception and postmenopausal hormone replacement are discussed.

The American Heart Association has provided a guide to preventive cardiology for women [8] outlining the goals, screening measures, and recommendations for lifestyle factors, risk factors, and pharmacologic therapies.

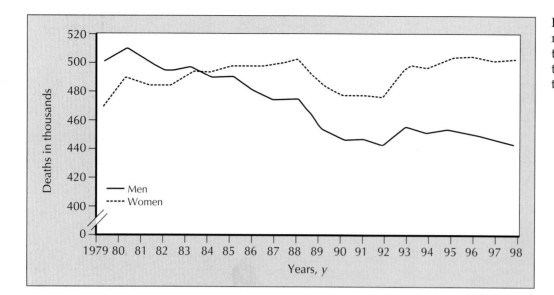

FIGURE 12-1. Cardiovascular disease mortality trends for males and females in the United States, 1979 to 1998, according to the National Center for Health Statistics and the American Heart Association.

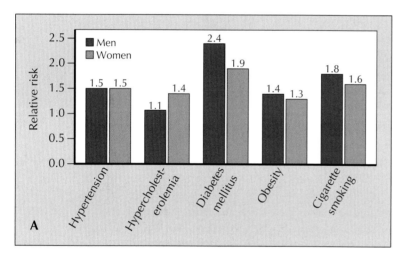

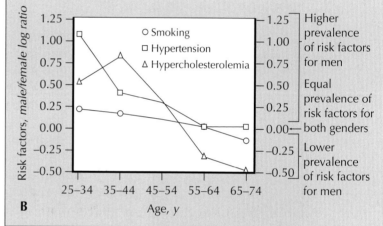

FIGURE 12-2. A, Based on follow-up data from the National Health and Nutrition Examination Survey (NHANES) I [9], the relative risk of coronary heart disease by gender for women and men (compared with 1.0), respectively, for hypertension is 1.5:1.5; for hypercholesterolemia, 1.1:1.4; for diabetes mellitus, 2.4:1.9; for obesity, 1.4:1.3; and for cigarette smoking, 1.8:1.6.

The gender prevalence of risk attributes also varies with age [10]. B, In the Stanford Five-City Project, there was a female-male crossover effect in coronary risk factors with aging such that although hypertension, hypercholesterolemia, and smoking were more prevalent among younger men than younger women, the opposite was true at an older age; older women thus had a more adverse coronary risk profile, with the change being most prominent for hypercholesterolemia [10]. After age 45 years, more women than men develop diabetes (not illustrated). (*Adapted from* Williams *et al.* [10].)

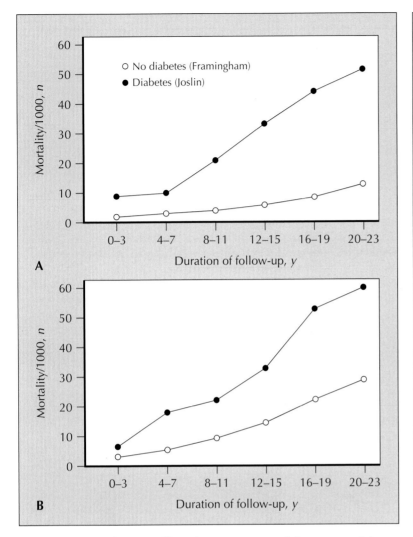

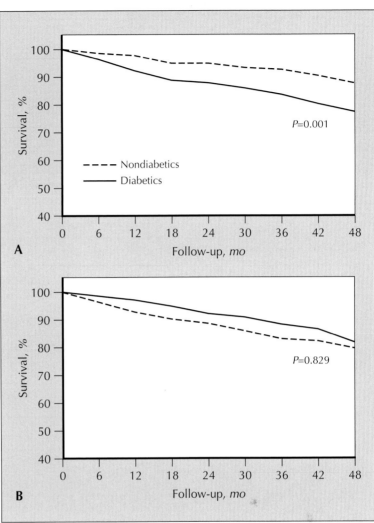

FIGURE 12-3. Diabetes mellitus is a more powerful coronary risk factor for women (**A**) than for men (**B**), virtually negating the protective effect of female gender on coronary risk [11,12], even among premenopausal women. Twenty-four–year follow-up data of diabetic patients 35 to 64 years of age at the Joslin Clinic were compared with data for nondiabetic participants of similar ages in the Framingham Study with regard to coronary mortality. Differences for diabetic versus nondiabetic individuals [13] were far more pronounced for women than for men.

In the Nurses' Health Study [14], a three- to sevenfold excess of cardiovascular events occurred among women with maturity-–onset diabetes mellitus, but was more likely with than without associated coronary risk factors. (*Adapted from* Krolewski *et al.* [13].)

FIGURE 12-4. Diabetes mellitus also confers a substantially higher risk of mortality in women (**A**) than in men (**B**) with angiographically documented coronary heart disease [15]. The 48-month survival rate is examined by gender and diabetic status in this figure. The greater adverse effect of diabetes mellitus on mortality in women was apparent for both cardiac and noncardiovascular disease. (*Adapted from* Liao *et al.* [15].)

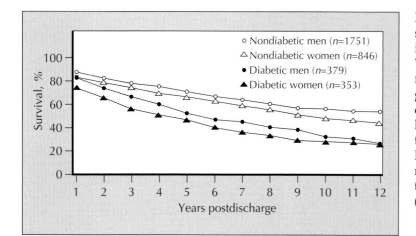

FIGURE 12-5. In the Worcester Heart Study, diabetics had lower survival rates than nondiabetics of either gender after myocardial infarction for both the short-term (1 year) and long-term (12 years). Women experienced lower survival rates than men at the end of the first year, but thereafter the mortality rates were equivalent for both genders. Among nondiabetic subjects, men had a 17% excess risk of death compared with women; there was no gender difference in long-term mortality among diabetic persons (*ie*, the "female advantage" was eliminated in diabetic patients). In the Framingham Heart Study, women with diabetes had twice the rate of recurrent myocardial infarction [3], and the rate of heart failure was four times greater for diabetic women compared with nondiabetics. (*Adapted from* Donahue *et al.* [16].)

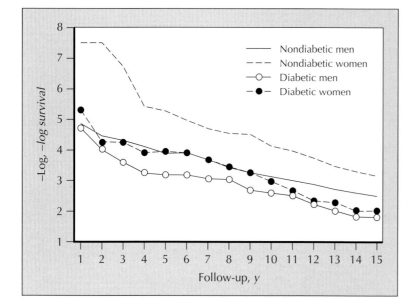

FIGURE 12-6. Although diabetes mellitus exerted a more adverse effect on the risk of fatal coronary heart disease (CHD) in women than in men in the Rancho Bernardo Study, the mechanisms require elucidation. The curves displayed were estimated by a Cox model blocked on both gender and diabetes status and adjusted for age [8]; shown here are age-adjusted ischemic heart disease - log (-log survival) by gender and diabetes status. The gender difference in the independent contribution of diabetes to fatal CHD appeared largely explained by the persistently more favorable survival rate of women than that of men without diabetes. Diabetic women are described to have more favorable lipid profiles than diabetic men, although they have more hypertension. Others have suggested the importance of lipid abnormalities [17]. The relationship with insulin resistance and hyperinsulinemia and upper body obesity remains controversial, in that some workers describe hyperinsulinemia as a coronary risk factor for men only [18]. (*Adapted from* Barrett-Connor *et al.* [11].)

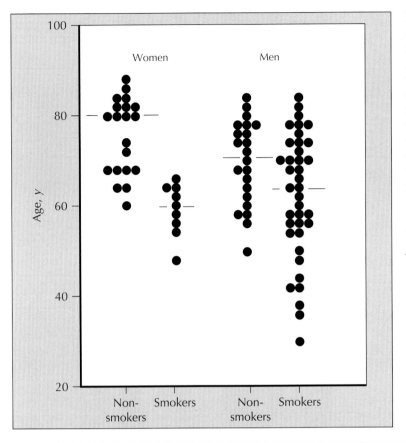

FIGURE 12-7. Cigarette smoking lowers the age of initial myocardial infarction (MI) more for women than for men; whether this relates to the younger age of menopause among women smokers remains to be determined [19,20]. This figure shows the age at the time of initial acute MI by gender and smoking status among 89 consecutively admitted patients whose smoking status was recorded [19]. Cigarette smoking imparts a threefold greater risk of MI in women, including premenopausal women, than in men; the risk of an initial MI attributable to cigarette smoking is significantly greater for women than men. In the Nurses' Health Study, the number of cigarettes smoked daily correlated with the risk of fatal coronary heart disease [17]. Even after initial MI, smoking substantially decreases survival among women [21]. As with men, smoking predominates in less-educated women of lower socioeconomic status [1]. *Horizontal bars* indicate median values. (*Adapted from* Hansen *et al.* [19].)

RISK OF MYOCARDIAL INFARCTION OR DEATH BY SMOKING STATUS AFTER CABG SURGERY

	DEATH, n			MI OR DEATH, n		
AGE GROUP, y	SUBJECTS SMOKING 1 y BEFORE ENROLLMENT, n	TOTAL, n	RELATIVE RISK (95% CL)	SUBJECTS SMOKING 1 y BEFORE ENROLLMENT, n	TOTAL, n	RELATIVE RISK (95% CL)
55–59	265	974	1.5(1.1, 2.0)	318	955	1.5(1.2, 1.9)
Quitters	80	368		99	360	
Continuers	185	606		219	595	
60–64	204	561	2.0(1.5, 2.6)	236	545	1.4(1.1, 1.9)
Quitters	66	254		92	244	
Continuers	138	307		144	301	
65–69	94	203	1.4(0.9, 2.0)	95	189	1.5(1.0, 2.3)
Quitters	48	107		48	100	
Continuers	46	96		47	89	
70+	38	60	3.3(1.5, 7.1)	41	59	2.9(1.4, 5.9)
Quitters	16	30		17	29	
Continuers	22	30		24	30	

FIGURE 12-8. Risk of myocardial infarction (MI) or death by smoking status after coronary artery bypass graft (CABG) surgery. Smoking cessation after CABG in the Coronary Artery Surgery Study (CASS) registry improved survival in both genders, with the benefit persisting into older age [22]. The combined endpoint of MI or death was also improved. Relative risks were determined by the Cox regression model after adjustment for covariates. Continuers were subjects who smoked at enrollment and at all follow-up visits; quitters were subjects who stopped smoking during the year before enrollment and reported being nonsmokers at all follow-up visits. Men comprised 79% of quitters and 77% of continuers. All studies of smoking cessation are descriptive rather than randomized trial reports. Smoking cessation is more likely to occur at older age (65–75 y) and in men; white race, higher socioeconomic status, and being married are other favorable predictors of smoking cessation [23]. Because women former smokers have rates of MI and fatal coronary heart disease comparable to those of nonsmoking women [24], the coronary risks of smoking likely involve relatively acute mechanisms such as platelet aggregation and coagulation factors; cardiovascular risk is also accentuated in women smokers who use oral contraceptives. CL—confidence limits. (*Adapted from* Hermanson *et al.* [22].)

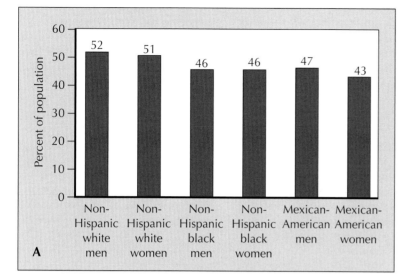
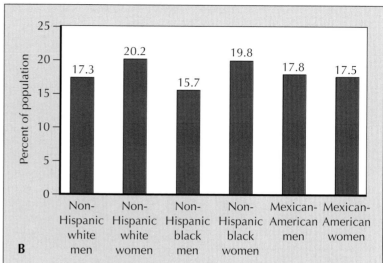

FIGURE 12-9. Although there has been a continuing and substantial decline in cholesterol levels in both women and men in the United States [25], more than one third of US women between 50 and 59 years of age and more than 40% of those older than 60 years of age in the 1988 to 1991 NHANES III survey had serum cholesterol levels above 240 mg/dL. Based on unpublished data from

NHANES III, 1988 to 1994, almost 50% of all Americans had cholesterol levels above 200 mg/dL, and more women than men had cholesterol levels above 240 mg/dL. Shown are the estimated percentages of Americans ages 20 to 74 years with blood cholesterol levels of 200 mg/dL or more (**A**) and 240 mg/dL or more (**B**).

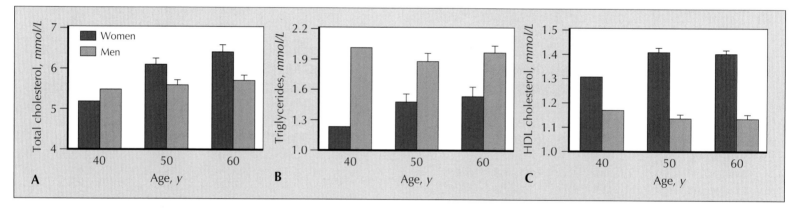

FIGURE 12-10. Based on Framingham data [21,26], high serum cholesterol levels are more prevalent in young men than young women, and total cholesterol levels in older women exceed those in their male counterparts (**A**). At all ages, triglyceride levels are higher in men (**B**), and high-density lipoprotein (HDL) cholesterol levels are higher in women (**C**). Nevertheless, triglyceride levels in

women rise following menopause (*panel B*), which appears to be associated with adverse lipid and lipoprotein changes in women [27]. In the Women's Healthy Lifestyle Project Clinical Trial [28], diet and physical activity reduced the perimenopause to postmenopause rise in LDL cholesterol and prevented weight gain both in hormone users and nonusers. (*Adapted from* Razay *et al.* [27].)

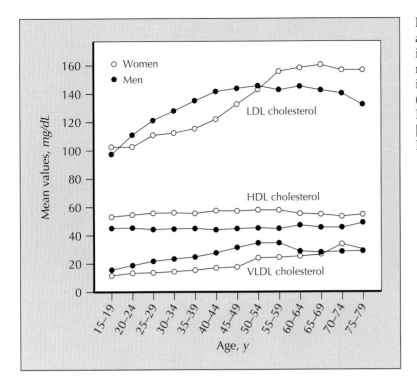

FIGURE 12-11. Data from the Framingham Study define that, although higher high-density lipoprotein (HDL) cholesterol levels in women than men are present from adolescence through menopause and into older age, total cholesterol levels in women increase with aging, at least to age 70 [29]. Low-density lipoprotein (LDL) cholesterol levels in women also rise with aging, such that LDL levels in postmenopausal women exceed those in men [27,29]. VLDL—very low-density lipoprotein (*Adapted from* Kannel [29].)

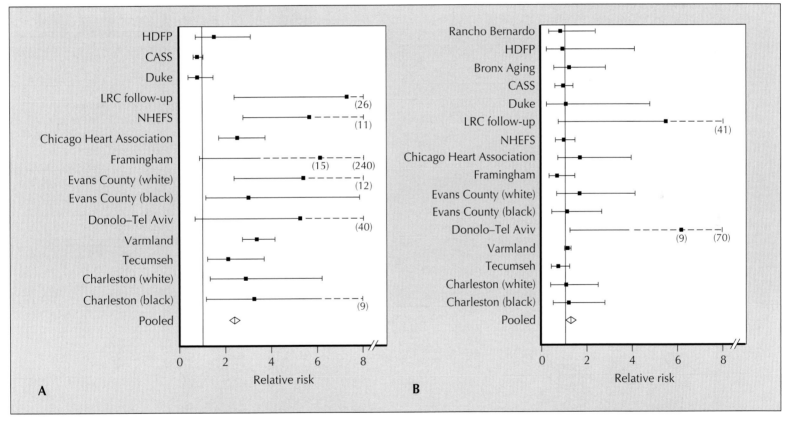

FIGURE 12-12. Data from a large number of population studies demonstrate that cholesterol levels continue to predict coronary heart disease (CHD) risk in middle-aged (younger than 65 years) and, to a lesser extent, older (65 years or older) women [30]. The relative risk and 95% confidence intervals of fatal CHD associated with cholesterol levels of 6.20 mmol/L (240 mg/dL) or higher are compared with cholesterol levels of less than 5.17 mmol/L (200 mg/dL) in middle-aged (**A**) and older (**B**) women. Where studied, the cholesterol–CHD relationship appeared less prominent among black than white women. CASS—Coronary Artery Surgery Study; HDFP—Hypertension Detection and Follow-up Program; LRC—Lipid Research Clinics; NHEFS—NHANES I Epidemiologic Follow-up Study. (*Adapted from* Manolio *et al.* [30].)

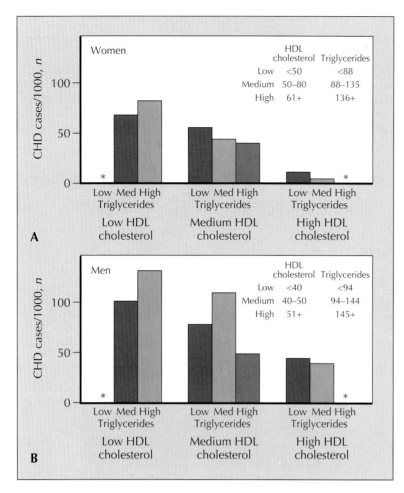

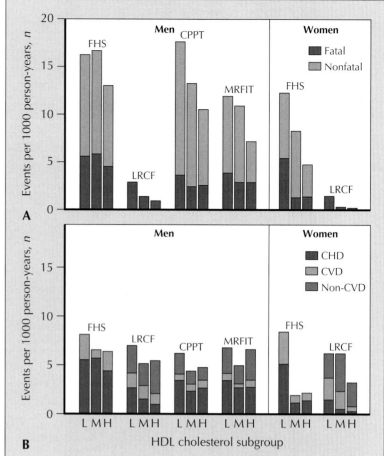

FIGURE 12-13. Based on Framingham data, elevated triglyceride levels [31] appear as more powerful coronary risk factors for women (**A**) than for men (**B**) [32] in determining the incidence of coronary heart disease (CHD). The incidence of CHD by gender and levels of high-density lipoprotein (HDL) cholesterol and triglycerides is shown [27]. Increased CHD risk occurs with elevated triglycerides when the HDL cholesterol concentration is low (<40 mg/dL). However, recent data from the Lipid Research Clinics Follow-up Study [33] failed to demonstrate an independent effect of triglycerides on coronary mortality among women after adjustment for covariates. Also, hypertriglyceridemia did not impart independent risk in the Prospective Cardiovascular Munster (PROCAM) Study [34]. *Asterisks* indicate fewer than 86 persons at risk. (*Adapted from* Castelli [31].)

FIGURE 12-14. Lower levels of high-density lipoprotein (HDL) cholesterol are more powerful coronary risk factors for women than for men in determining both incidence of and mortality from coronary heart disease (CHD). CHD incidence rates (**A**) and cause-specific mortality rates (**B**) in low (L), middle (M), and high (H) HDL cholesterol subgroups are shown. Respective numbers of subjects in the low, medium, and high subgroups of each study were Framingham Heart Study (FHS) (men): 235, 216, 253; Lipid Research Clinics Prevalence Mortality Follow-up Study (LRCF) (men): 1576, 1216, 1145; Lipid Research Clinics Coronary Primary Prevention Trial (CPPT) (men): 597, 713, 498; Multiple Risk Factor Intervention Trial (MRFIT) (men): 2861, 1807, 1124; FHS (women): 60, 170, 484; LRCF (women): 302, 520, 1476. CVD—cardiovascular disease. (*Adapted from* Gordon *et al.* [35].)

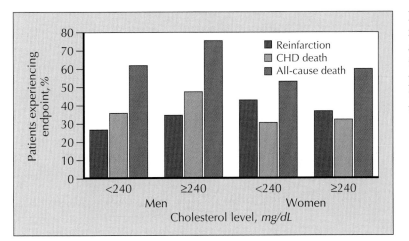

FIGURE 12-15. Framingham data show an increased risk of recurrent myocardial infarction (MI), coronary heart disease (CHD), and all-cause mortality with an elevated total cholesterol concentration; this association is particularly prominent in the elderly [36]. In this population from the Framingham Study with a previous MI, the total cholesterol CHD risk association was stronger for men than for women. (*Adapted from* Wong *et al.* [36].)

EFFECT OF CHOLESTEROL LOWERING ON DEATH AND MAJOR CORONARY EVENTS

	PATIENTS, *N* (%)		
	PLACEBO	SIMVASTATIN	RELATIVE RISK (95% CI)
Death			
Women	25(6.0)	27(6.6)	1.12(0.65–1.93)
Men	231(12.8)	155(8.5)	0.66(0.53–0.80)
Age <60 y	89(8.1)	55(5.2)	0.63(0.45–0.88)
Age ≥60 y	167(14.8)	127(11.0)	0.73(0.58–0.92)
Major coronary event			
Women	91(21.7)	59(14.5)	0.65(0.47–0.91)
Men	531(29.4)	372(20.5)	0.66(0.58–0.76)
Age <60 y	303(27.6)	188(17.6)	0.61(0.51–0.73)
Age ≥60 y	319(28.3)	243(21.0)	0.71(0.60–0.86)

FIGURE 12-16. Effect of cholesterol lowering on death and major coronary events. In the Scandinavian Simvastatin Survival Study [37], which examined the effect of cholesterol lowering in patients with angina pectoris or myocardial infarction, benefit at a median 5.4 years of follow-up showed a decrease in relative risk of a major coronary event in both genders; relative risk was calculated by Cox regression analysis. The benefit persisted in persons older than 60 years of age. This is the first trial to document that cholesterol lowering decreases major coronary events in women. Because only 19% of the study population were women and only 52 deaths occurred, demonstration of improved survival in this subgroup was unlikely. Survival was improved in older patients, not subdivided by gender. (*Adapted from* the Scandinavian Simvastatin Survival Study Group [37].)

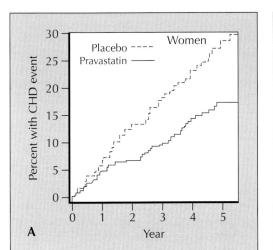
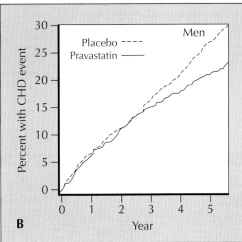

FIGURE 12-17. The CARE (Cholesterol and Recurrent Events) study was a secondary prevention trial in patients with average cholesterol levels. The decrease in death and reinfarction was more prominent for women (**A**) than for men (**B**) [38]. Pravastatin also decreased stroke risk and the performance of myocardial revascularization procedures. The overall risk reduction was 46% for women and 20% for men; *P*=0.001 for both. CHD—coronary heart disease.

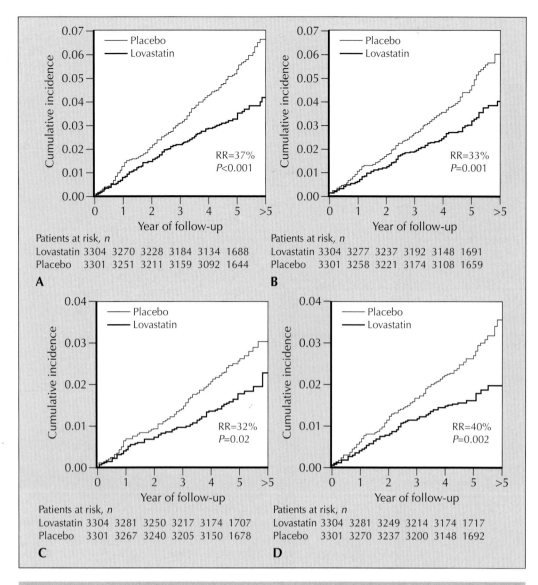

FIGURE 12-18. In the AFCAPS/TexCAPS (Air Force/Texas Coronary Atherosclerosis Prevention Study) primary prevention trial of lipid lowering with lovastatin, treatment reduced the risk of fatal or nonfatal myocardial infarction (MI), unstable angina, or sudden cardiac death. Benefit was more marked in women than in men; relative risk was 46% for women and 37% for men [39]. **A,** Composite primary endpoint: fatal or nonfatal MI, sudden death, or unstable angina. **B,** Secondary endpoint: revascularizations. **C,** Secondary endpoint: unstable angina. **D,** Secondary endpoint: fatal and nonfatal MI.

MAJOR CORONARY HEART DISEASE LIPID TRIALS

STUDY	PATIENTS, N	WOMEN, N (%)	PREVENTION CATEGORY	RISK REDUCTION OF MAJOR CHD EVENTS IN WOMEN, %
4S	4444	827 (19)	Secondary	35
CARE	4159	576 (14)	Secondary	46
LIPID	9014	1516 (17)	Secondary	11
WOSCOPS	6595	0	Primary	—
AFCAPS/TexCAPS	6605	997 (15)	Primary	46

FIGURE 12-19. Major coronary heart disease (CHD) prevention lipid trials. Risk reduction for women was demonstrated in both primary and secondary prevention statin trials [40]. In the recently reported Heart Protection Study [41], risk reduction was comparable for statin-treated women and men. In this study, antioxidant vitamins C and E and β-carotene failed to provide benefit for women or men.

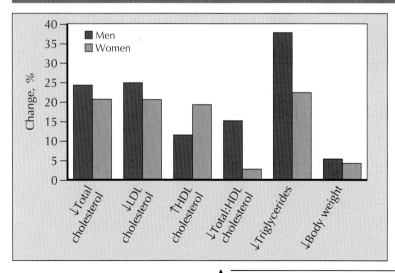

FIGURE 12-20. Examination of the effects of short-term lifestyle modification demonstrates that dietary fat and cholesterol restriction appears less effective in lowering circulating lipoprotein and triglyceride levels in postmenopausal women than in comparably aged men. These data were derived from 4587 adults who attended a 21-day residential lifestyle modification program of diet and exercise [42]. All values after intervention were significantly different (P<0.01) from values before intervention, except for the total:HDL cholesterol ratio for women. (*Adapted from* Barnard [42].) HDL—high-density lipoprotein; LDL—low-density lipoprotein.

CARDIOVASCULAR EVENTS ACCORDING TO HYPERTENSIVE STATUS, GENDER, AND AGE

VARIABLE	WOMEN, n			MEN, n		
Age, y	45–54	55–64	65–74	45–54	55–64	65–74
Hypertensive status						
Normal (<140/90 mm Hg)	27,327	63,556	69,720	82,956	143,926	106,533
Hypertensive (>160/95 mm Hg)	98,174	246,930	288,609	227,646	405,021	317,730
Events attributable to hypertension ($I_H - I_N$), n	70,847	183,374	218,889	144,690	261,095	211,197

FIGURE 12-21. Cardiovascular events according to hypertensive status, gender, and age. Whereas systolic blood pressure in men peaks at middle age, it increases in women at least to the age of 80 years. The numbers of all cardiovascular events comparing normotensive status with hypertensive status by gender and age, based on Framingham data extrapolated to the white US population between the ages of 45 and 74 years, is shown. Cardiovascular events in women attributable to hypertension increased with increasing age in the Framingham cohort [43]. The absolute number of cardiovascular complications attributable to hypertension may be greater for women than men by 65 to 74 years of age. Cardiovascular disease death rates in women in the Lipid Research Clinics Follow-up Study also increased progressively with quartiles of both systolic and diastolic blood pressures [32].

Forty-five percent of US women in the 45- to 64-year age group have hypertension, with the percentage rising to 71% after age 65 years. The black-to-white ratio discrepancy in the increased prevalence of hypertension is more pronounced for women than for men [1,44]. (*Adapted from* Anastos *et al.* [43].)

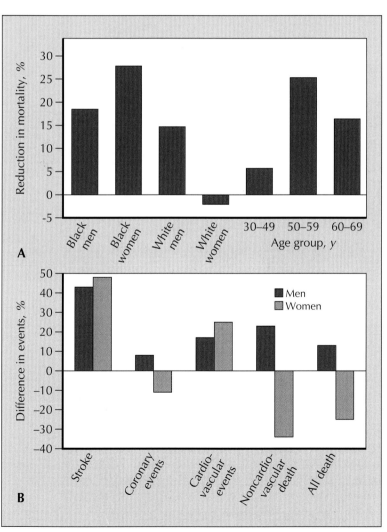

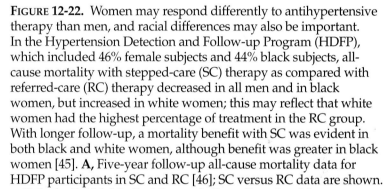

FIGURE 12-22. Women may respond differently to antihypertensive therapy than men, and racial differences may also be important. In the Hypertension Detection and Follow-up Program (HDFP), which included 46% female subjects and 44% black subjects, all-cause mortality with stepped-care (SC) therapy as compared with referred-care (RC) therapy decreased in all men and in black women, but increased in white women; this may reflect that white women had the highest percentage of treatment in the RC group. With longer follow-up, a mortality benefit with SC was evident in both black and white women, although benefit was greater in black women [45]. **A,** Five-year follow-up all-cause mortality data for HDFP participants in SC and RC [46]; SC versus RC data are shown.

B, In the British Medical Research Council study of the treatment of mild hypertension, which encompassed 48% female subjects but had virtually all white participants, all-cause mortality decreased by 15% in treated men but increased by 26% in treated women [47]. In the Systolic Hypertension in the Elderly Program (SHEP) [48], which enrolled 57% women, treatment of isolated systolic hypertension with chlorthalidone and atenolol added as needed provided comparable gender benefit. (Part A *adapted from* the Hypertension Detection and Follow-up Program Cooperative Group [46]; part B *adapted from* the Medical Research Council Working Party [47].)

OBESITY AND BODY FAT DISTRIBUTION

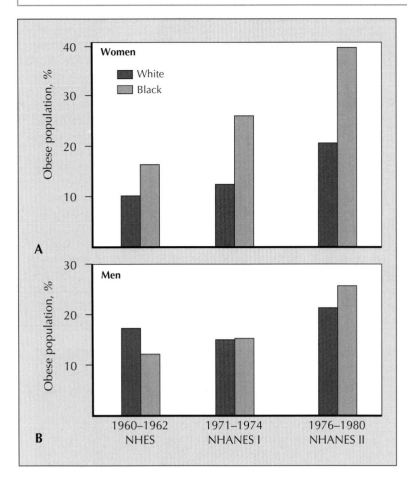

A

B

FIGURE 12-23. Although the prevalence of obesity in the United States has increased for both women (**A**) and men (**B**) in recent years [49,50], it is greater among black, Hispanic, and native American women [44]. The percentage of population classified as obese in three surveys of representative samples of the US population is shown by gender, race, and years of study. NHES—National Health Examination Survey; NHANES—National Health and Nutrition Examination Survey [50]. (*Adapted from* Spelsberg *et al.* [50].)

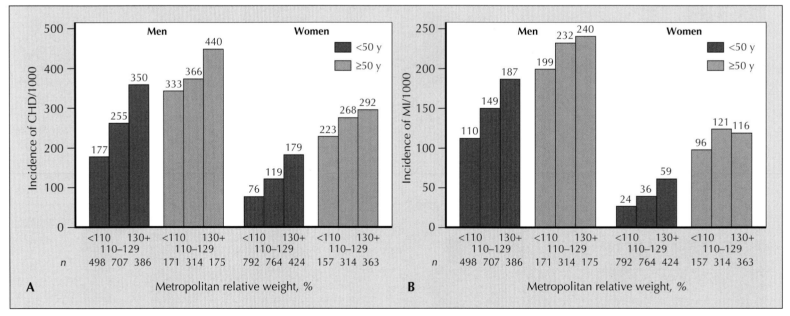

A Metropolitan relative weight, %

B Metropolitan relative weight, %

FIGURE 12-24. The 26 years of follow-up data from the Framingham Heart Study document that obesity significantly and independently predicted cardiovascular disease: coronary heart disease (CHD) incidence, myocardial infarction (MI), stroke, congestive heart failure, and coronary and cardiovascular death, particularly among women [51]. Recently published 14-year follow-up data from the Nurses' Health Study [52] confirmed a direct relationship between increased body weight and all-cause mortality, without excess mortality in lean women when smokers were excluded.

A, The 26-year incidence of CHD. **B,** The 26-year incidence of MI by Metropolitan Relative Weight (Metropolitan Life

Insurance Company's desirable weights, derived from the mortality experiences of subscribers) at entry among Framingham men and women younger and older than 50 years of age. In the Lipid Research Clinics Follow-up Study, cardiovascular disease mortality rates in women increased by the quartile of body mass [32]. Weight loss in women is described as less effective in lowering low-density lipoprotein cholesterol levels and raising high-density lipoprotein cholesterol levels than for men [53]. *Numbers above the bars* give the actual incidence rates per 1000 [51]. *n*—number at risk for an event. (*Adapted from* Hubert *et al.* [51].)

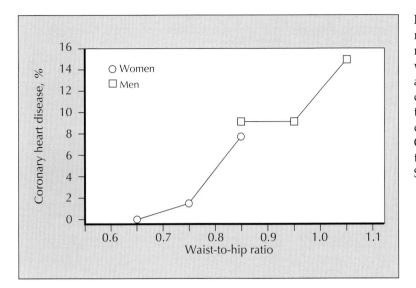

FIGURE 12-25. Waist-to-hip ratio and coronary heart disease (CHD) risk. Although being overweight imparts greater risk for elderly men than for elderly women, the pattern of body fat distribution warrants attention such that an increased waist-to-hip ratio was associated with an atherogenic lipid profile in women, independent of body mass index [54]. Waist-to-hip ratio, or a factor related to this parameter, was considered to explain much of the gender difference in the incidence of myocardial infarction in the Goteborg Study. Twelve-year incidence of CHD related to waist-to-hip ratio and gender are presented in the study in Goteborg, Sweden [55]. (*Adapted from* Larsson *et al.* [55].)

EXERCISE AND PHYSICAL FITNESS

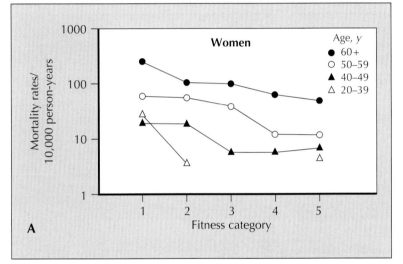

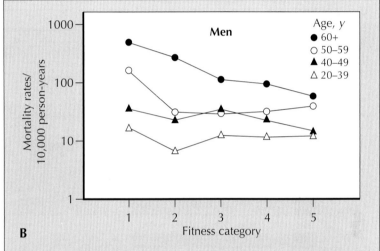

FIGURE 12-26. Physical activity and coronary heart disease (CHD) risk. Although there was no evidence in the Framingham Heart Study that physical activity was significantly related to CHD death in women [56], this and other questionnaire assessments of physical inactivity in women were likely due to inadequate questionnaire measures that failed to focus on physical activities characteristic for women. Physical fitness, as measured by treadmill exercise testing, showed a strong, graded, and consistent relation-ship to decreased total mortality rates in both genders; this study involved 3120 healthy women (**A**) and 10,224 healthy men (**B**), categorized by physical fitness quintiles as determined by maximal treadmill exercise tests [57]. Regular moderate intensity leisure time exercise, even in older age, is associated with favorably altered lipoprotein levels in both genders [58]. (*Adapted from* Blair *et al.* [57].)

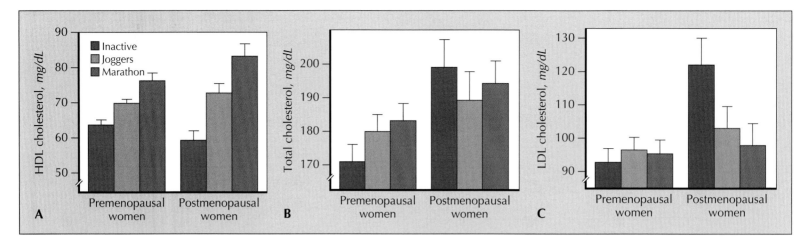

FIGURE 12-27. A–C, Meta-analysis of exercise training studies in women [59] showed that exercise-related lowering of low-density lipoprotein (LDL) cholesterol and increase in high-density lipoprotein (HDL) cholesterol was not significant, despite lowering of both total cholesterol and triglyceride levels. Weight loss with exercise resulted in larger decreases in cholesterol and triglyceride concentra-

tions in women than did exercise per se. All exercise-related changes were less marked for women than for men. One study [60] described a more favorable effect on lipids and lipoproteins related to exercise in postmenopausal than in premenopausal women, suggesting that exercise may counteract the unfavorable effects of menopause and aging on lipids and coronary risk. (*Adapted from* Hartung *et al.* [60].)

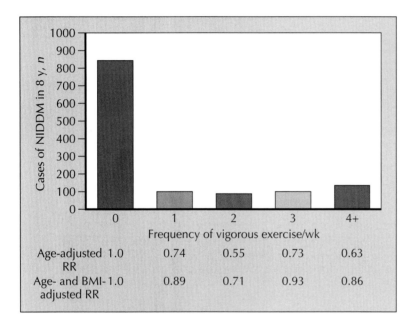

FIGURE 12-28. In the Nurses' Health Study [61], during 8 years of follow-up, there was a decreased incidence of non–insulin-dependent diabetes mellitus (NIDDM) among both obese and nonobese women who exercised regularly. Differences in numbers of person-years and cases are due to exclusion of women with missing information on frequency of exercise. BMI—body mass index; RR—relative risk. (*Adapted from* Manson *et al.* [61].)

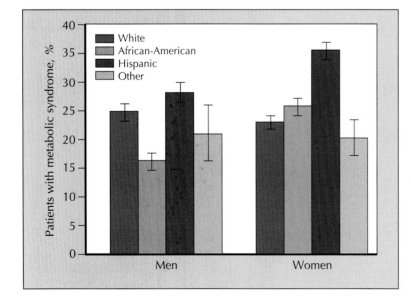

FIGURE 12-29. Prevalence of metabolic syndrome by sex and race, National Health and Nutrition Examination Survey III. The metabolic syndrome is characterized by at least three of the following abnormalities: increased waist circumference, increased serum triglycerides, low high-density lipoprotein cholesterol, increased blood pressure, and increased serum glucose level. In the 1998 to 1994 Third National Health and Nutrition Examination Survey, the age-adjusted prevalence was similar for men and women (about 24%). However, black women had a 57% higher prevalence than men, and Mexican-American women a 26% higher prevalence than men [62]. (*Adapted from* Ford *et al.* [62].)

ESTROGEN STATUS AND EXOGENOUS GONADAL HORMONE THERAPY

ORAL CONTRACEPTIVES

ORAL CONTRACEPTIVE USE AND RISK OF CHD EVENTS

STUDY	DESIGN	CHD EVENTS, n	AGE AT EVENT, y	RISK ESTIMATE (95% CI)
Mann and Inman [63]	Case-referent	153	<50	0.6(NS)
Mann et al. [64]	Case-control	63	<45	0.9(NS)
Mann et al. [65]	Case-referent	106	40–44	1.1(NS)
Shapiro et al. [66]	Case-control	234	25–49	1.2(0.8–1.7)
Petitti et al. [67]	Cohort	26	?	0.8(0.4–1.7)
Rosenberg et al. [68]	Cohort	156	<50	1.0(0.7–1.6)
Slone et al. [69]	Case-control	536	25–49	1.2(0.9–1.4)
Royal College of General Practitioners' Oral Contraception Study [70]	Cohort	17	?	2.0(0.2–17.6)
Stampfer et al. [71]	Cohort	485	?	0.8(0.6–1.0)

FIGURE 12-30. Oral contraceptive use and risk of coronary heart disease (CHD) events. Estrogen-progestin dosage in current oral contraceptives is considerably lower than in prior years, resulting in less adverse effects on lipoproteins, glucose tolerance, and insulin resistance. Despite these changes in laboratory values, there is little evidence that past oral contraceptive use imparts coronary risk before menopausal years [71]. Risk appears confined to older users who smoke cigarettes or have other coronary risk factors. Meta-analysis of both case-control and prospective studies of past use of oral contraceptives and CHD found an overall 1.01 risk for CHD and 1.05 risk for myocardial infarction among past oral contraceptive users compared with nonusers [72], with risk estimates of individual studies varying from 0.6 to 2.0 [73]. NS—not significant. (*Adapted from* Barrett-Connor and Bush [73].)

POSTMENOPAUSAL HORMONE THERAPY

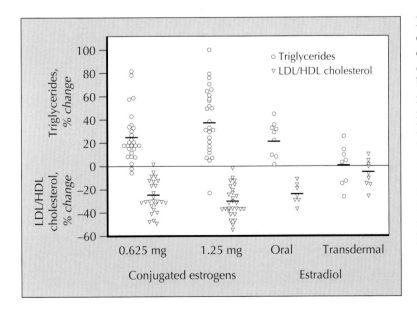

FIGURE 12-31. The increased risk in postmenopausal women of coronary heart disease has been partly attributed to unfavorable changes in circulating lipoprotein levels in part mediated by decreased estrogen status, changes in body weight, and changes in body fat distribution, among others. Early menopause increased the risk of myocardial infarction [74], suggesting that the increase in risk relates to early cessation of ovulatory function. Postmenopausal estrogen therapy decreases low-density lipoprotein (LDL) cholesterol levels and increases high-density lipoprotein (HDL) cholesterol levels, but increases plasma triglyceride levels [75,76]. The effects of estrogen treatments on the LDL/HDL cholesterol ratio and on triglyceride levels are shown [76]. Each point represents the individual percentage change with estrogen compared with placebo. *Horizontal bars* denote the mean of the percentage changes. (*Adapted from* Walsh et al. [76].)

EFFECTS OF HORMONE REPLACEMENT THERAPY ON GLUCOSE AND INSULIN LEVELS

CHARACTERISTICS	NO ESTROGEN (n=275)	UNOPPOSED PREMARIN (n=81)	PREMARIN + PROVERA (n=45)
Age, y	70.8±7.8	65.8±5.9*	64.8±5.6*
BMI, kg/m^2	24.3±3.6	23.9±3.9	23.8–3.2
Fasting glucose, $mmol/L$ (adjusted for age, BMI)	5.34	5.17[†]	5.21
2-h glucose, $mmol/L$ (adjusted for age, BMI)	6.97	7.55[†]	7.14
Fasting insulin, $pmol/L$ (adjusted for age, BMI, fasting glucose, alcohol use, physical exercise)	97.7	76.3[†]	81.3
2-h insulin, $pmol/L$ (adjusted for age, BMI, 2-h glucose, alcohol use, physical activity)	714.8	620.4	633.5

*$P<0.05$,
[†]$P<0.001$: Premarin, or Premarin + Provera versus no estrogen.

FIGURE 12-32. Effects of hormone replacement therapy on glucose and insulin levels. Improved glucose and insulin levels are also described with postmenopausal estrogen replacement. This figure from the Rancho-Bernardo Study shows the effects of control status versus unopposed Premarin (Wyeth-Ayerst Laboratories, Philadelphia, PA) versus Premarin and Provera (Upjohn Company, Kalamazoo, MI) [77]. Estrogen use was not associated with impaired glucose tolerance. It was associated with lower levels of insulin, with differences not explained by characteristics such as age, obesity, or glucose intolerance. Glucose and insulin levels were comparable with Premarin alone and Premarin and Provera. BMI—body mass index. (*Adapted from* Barrett-Connor and Laakso [77].)

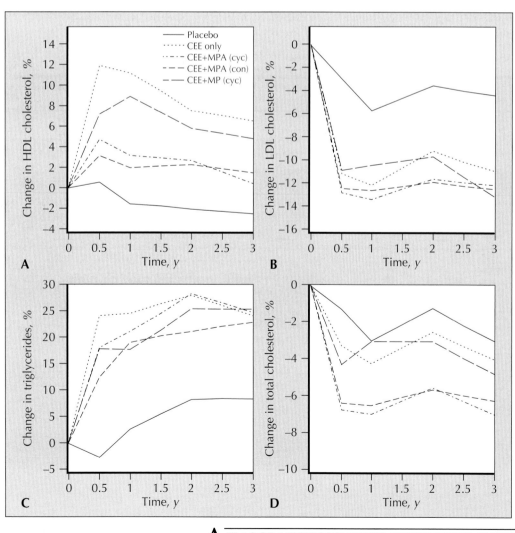

A, **B**, **C**, **D**

FIGURE 12-33. In the Postmenopausal Estrogen/Progestin Interventions (PEPI) study [78], estrogen alone or in combination with a progestin improved lipoprotein levels, without adverse effects on insulin or blood pressure. The mean percent changes from baseline for high-density lipoprotein (HDL) cholesterol (**A**), low-density lipoprotein (LDL) cholesterol (**B**), triglycerides (**C**), and total cholesterol (**D**) are shown for all treatment groups. Unopposed conjugated equine estrogen (CEE) effected the greatest increase in HDL cholesterol but should be restricted to use in women without a uterus, owing to the high rate of endometrial hyperplasia. CEE with micronized progesterone had the second most favorable effect on HDL cholesterol. All hormone regimens decreased LDL cholesterol and increased triglyceride levels compared with placebo. Con—consecutive; cyc—cyclic; MP—micronized progesterone; MPA—medroxyprogesterone acetate. However, all hormone regimens increased the levels of high sensitivity C-reactive protein (CRP), an independent predictor of coronary risk [79]. (*Adapted from* The Writing Group for the PEPI Trial [78].)

RISK OF A CORONARY EVENT ASSOCIATED WITH POSTMENOPAUSAL ESTROGEN USE

STUDY	STUDY DESIGN	STUDY SIZE	ENDPOINT	RISK ESTIMATE
Lafferty and Helmuth [80]	Cohort 1100 PY	124 women	MI	0.16*
Stampfer et al. [81]	Cohort 129,000 PY	32,317 women	All CVD	0.30*
Nachtigall et al. [82]	Clinical trial 1680 PY	168 women	MI	0.33
Hammond et al. [83]	Cohort 3000 PY	610 women	All CVD	0.33*
Bush et al. [84]	Cohort 19,300 PY	2270 women	CVD death	0.34*
Talbott et al. [85]	Case-control Controls = 64	Cases = 64	Sudden death	0.34
Rosenberg et al. [86]	Case-control Controls = 6730	Cases = 336	Nonfatal MI	0.47
Henderson et al. [87]	Cohort 39,600 PY	8807 women	MI	0.54*
Beard et al. [88]	Case-control Controls = 150	Cases = 86	MI and sudden death	0.55
Petitti et al. [89]	Cohort PY?	3437 women	All CVD	0.60
Avila et al. [90]	Cohort 128,500 PY	24,900 women	Nonfatal MI	0.70
Adam et al. [91]	Case-control Controls = 151	Cases = 76	Nonfatal MI	0.79
Szklo et al. [92]	Case-control Controls = 39	Cases = 36	Nonfatal MI	0.83
Rosenberg et al. [93]	Case-control Controls = 303	Cases = 105	Nonfatal MI	1.05
Thompson et al. [94]	Case-control Controls = 1206	Cases = 603	MI and stroke	1.36*
La Vecchia et al. [95]	Case-control Controls = 160	Cases = 116	Nonfatal MI	1.62
Wilson et al. [96]	Cohort PY?	1234 women	All CVD	1.76*
Jick et al. [97]	Case-control Controls = 34	Cases = 17	Nonfatal MI	7.50*

*$P<0.05$.

FIGURE 12-34. Risk of a coronary event associated with post-menopausal estrogen use. Most case-control and prospective epidemiologic data show an approximately 50% reduction in the risk of a coronary event associated with postmenopausal estrogen use. There is also a favorable effect on cardiovascular and all-cause mortality rates [75]. This was also evident in the Lipid Research Clinics Program Follow-up Study [84] and in the Nurses' Health Study [98]. Despite their consistency, these data are limited by lack of randomized controlled trials such that selection bias by treating physicians or self-selection by the women may have influenced the results. The specific fatal and nonfatal cardiovascular disease (CVD) endpoints and risk estimates are shown for a number of studies of estrogen use [73]. MI—myocardial infarction. PY—person-years. (Adapted from Barrett-Connor and Bush [73].)

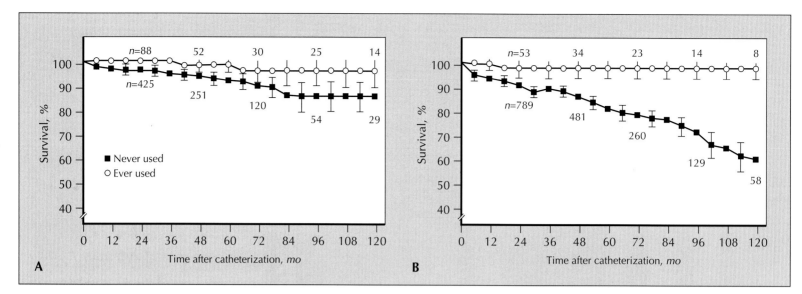

FIGURE 12-35. In postmenopausal women with angiographically defined coronary heart disease (CHD), 10-year survival was improved among "ever used" compared with "never used" estrogen (**A**; coronary stenosis detectable up to 69%). The benefit is more pronounced with more severe CHD (**B**; left main coronary stenosis of 50% or greater or other stenosis of 70% or greater) [99]. The study was a retrospective review of women who underwent coronary angiography and is limited by small numbers, especially in the "ever used" group at 10-year follow-up. *T-bars* represent standard error of mean. By contrast, an angiographic randomized controlled trial of estrogen and estrogen/progestin versus placebo in women with documented coronary heart disease, the Estrogen Replacement and Atherosclerosis (ERA) trial showed no difference in regression or progression of coronary atherosclerotic lesions [100]. (*Adapted from* Sullivan *et al.* [99].)

EFFECT OF CURRENT AND PRIOR ESTROGEN USE ON ALL-CAUSE MORTALITY

	FOLLOW-UP PATIENT-YEARS	DEATHS, *n*	FREQUENCY/1000	AGE-ADJUSTED RR	95% CI
Estrogen use					
No	23,938	809	28.7	1.0	—
Yes	32,082	638	22.5	0.8*	0.70–0.87
Dosage, *mg/d*					
<0.625	9474	157	20.4	0.73†	0.61–0.87
≥1.25	11,126	185	23.3	0.79‡	0.67–0.93
Duration, *y*					
≤3	9573	221	24.2	0.83§	0.71–0.96
4–14	11,676	204	21.0	0.76	0.65–0.89
≥15	10,005	172	19.5	0.69¶	0.58–0.82
Years since last use					
≥15	9847	268	23.8	0.80‡	0.70–0.92
2–14	12,476	217	22.0	0.79‡	0.68–0.92
0–1	9091	116	18.2	0.64¶	0.52–0.78

*P<0.0001.
†P<0.001.
‡P<0.01.
§P<0.05.
¶P<0.001, test for trend.

FIGURE 12-36. Effect of current and prior estrogen use on all-cause mortality. In a prospective observational study of 8881 postmenopausal women, all-cause mortality decreased with increasing duration of estrogen use and was lower for current users than for women who used estrogen only in the distant past [101]. The age-adjusted all-cause mortality data and relative risk are presented by history of estrogen use. Follow-up patient-years and number of deaths do not always total 56,020 and 1447, respectively, because of women with missing values on some variables. CI—confidence interval; RR—relative risk. (*Adapted from* Henderson *et al.* [101].)

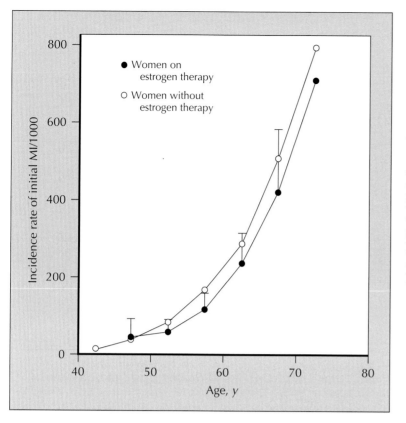

FIGURE 12-37. Estrogen therapy and incidence of initial myocardial infarction (MI). Unopposed estrogen therapy is not recommended for women with an intact uterus because of the estrogen-mediated endometrial hyperplasia and sixfold increased risk of uterine cancer. Few data are available regarding estrogen/progestin combination therapy and the current recommended regimens. In a population-based, prospective cohort Swedish study [102], estrogen alone and combined estrogen/progestin was associated with decreased coronary risk and decreased risk of initial MI. Age-specific rates for initial MI compared women receiving all types of estrogens with women in the general population. Women prescribed estrogen demonstrated a significant 30% reduction of relative risk of initial MI; this was also seen in women taking combined estrogen/progestin. Incidence rates of initial MI resemble the background population at 45 to 49 years but were lower in older age groups, especially 55 to 59 years (increased duration of hormone use). *T-bars* indicate 95% error. (*Adapted from* Falkeborn *et al.* [102].)

ADVERSE EFFECTS OF POSTMENOPAUSAL HORMONE THERAPY IN WOMEN WITHOUT HYSTERECTOMY (PEPI)

			TREATMENT GROUP				
EVENT	PLACEBO	CEE ONLY	CEE+MPA (cyc)	CEE+MPA (con)	CEE+MP (cyc)	TOTAL	*P* VALUE
Cancer							
Endometrial	1	1	0	0	0	2	0.60
Breast	1	1	2	0	4	8	0.29
Other*	2	0	4	1	1	8	0.20
Cardiovascular disease	0	1	1	0	3	5	0.29
Thromboembolic disease	0	4	2	2	2	10	0.42
Endometrial hyperplasia (adenomatous or atypical)	*2*	*41*	*2*	*0*	*1*	*46*	*<0.001[†]*
Gall bladder disease	2	2	4	5	4	17	0.73
Hysterectomy	2	7	3	0	2	14	0.04[†]
Total, *n*[‡]	10(8)	57(47)	18(18)	8(8)	17(16)	110(97)	

*Excluding nonmelanomatous skin cancer.

[†]For women with a uterus at baseline.

[‡]Total number of specific events; numbers in parentheses are the numbers of patients who suffered the events. Some patients suffered more than one event.

FIGURE 12-38. Adverse effects of postmenopausal hormone therapy in women without hysterectomy. In the Postmenopausal Estrogen/Progestin Inteventions (PEPI) study [78], unopposed estrogen therapy in women with an intact uterus was also associated with significantly more adenomatous and atypical endometrial hyperplasia and an increased likelihood of hysterectomy during the course of the study. No other adverse events were significantly different between groups. There were 174 to 178 women in each group. CEE—conjugated equine estrogen; con—consecutive; cyc—cyclic; MP—micronized progesterone; MPA—medroxyprogesterone acetate. (*Adapted from* The Writing Group for the PEPI Trial [78].)

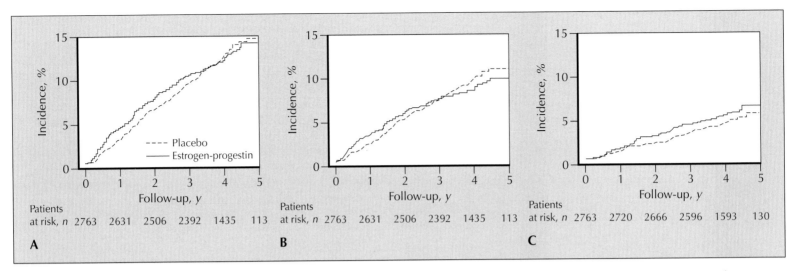

A **B** **C**

FIGURE 12-39. Estrogen plus progestin for the treatment of coronary heart disease (CHD). Estrogen plus progestin, in the first randomized controlled trial of such therapy in postmenopausal women with defined coronary disease, the Heart and Estrogen/progestin Replacement Study (HERS) [103], did not reduce the overall rate of CHD events. More CHD events occurred in the hormone group than in the placebo group in year 1 and fewer in years 4 and 5. Therefore, starting this treatment is not recommended for women with secondary CHD prevention; however, given its favorable effect after several years of treatment, it may be appropriate for women already receiving this therapy to continue with it. As in previous studies, hormone use increased the rates of venous thromboembolic events [104] and gallbladder disease. Shown are Kaplan-Meier estimates of the cumulative incidence of primary CHD (**A**), nonfatal myocardial infarction (**B**), and CHD death (**C**). (*Adapted from* Hulley *et al.* [103].)

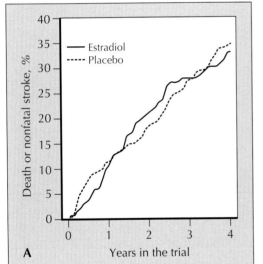

A

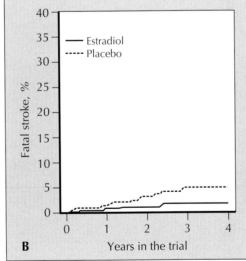

B

FIGURE 12-40. Occurrence of death, nonfatal stroke, and fatal stroke. Comparable lack of benefit was shown for stroke in this trial. 17 β-estradiol in women with a recent transient ischemic attack or ischemic stroke did not increase the risk of death or nonfatal stroke; the risk of fatal stroke increased and neurologic and functional deficits were greater in women with nonfatal stroke. (*Adapted from* Viscoli *et al.* [105].)

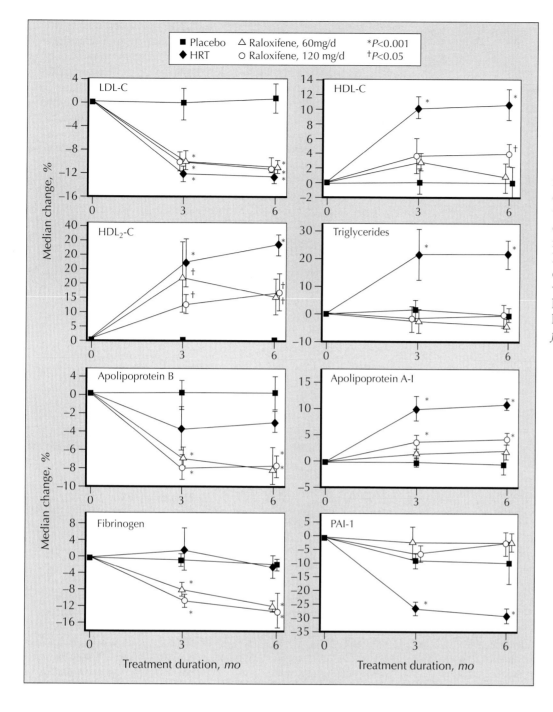

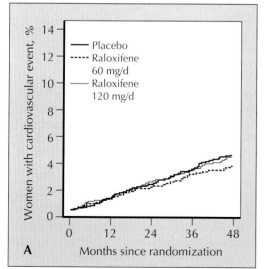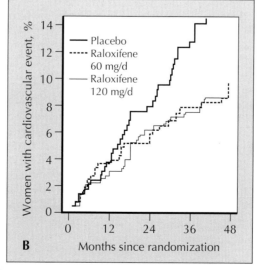

FIGURE 12-41. Selective estrogen receptor modulators in reducing markers of cardiovascular risk. These modulators, which have estrogen-agonist effects on bone and coronary risk factors and estrogen-antagonist effect on the breast and uterus, favorably alter markers of cardiovascular risk [106]. Raloxifene decreased low-density lipoprotein cholesterol (LDL-C), fibrinogen, and lipoprotein(a) and increased high-density lipoprotein–2 cholesterol (HDL$_2$-C) without increasing triglyceride levels. There was no effect on HDL-C and plasminogen activator inhibitor 1(PAI-1). An ongoing clinical trial, Raloxifene Use for The Heart (RUTH), is designed to assess clinical outcomes in women with coronary heart disease or at high risk for its occurrence [107]. HRT—hormone replacement therapy. (*Adapted from* Walsh *et al.* [106].)

FIGURE 12-42. Incidence of cardiovascular events. This retrospective examination of the cardiovascular effect of raloxifene, a selective estrogen receptor modulator in a randomized, controlled trial in women at risk of osteoporosis [108] showed no increase in early cardiovascular events. In women at increased cardiovascular risk based on RUTH criteria, raloxifene use was associated with significantly fewer cardiovascular events. (*Adapted from* Barrett-Connor *et al.* [108].)

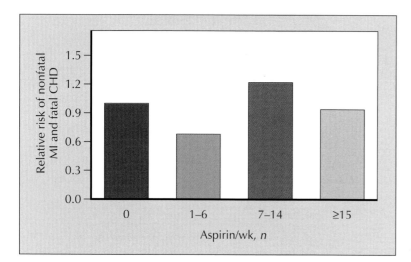

FIGURE 12-43. The Nurses' Health Study [109] provided data that suggest that regular aspirin use (1–6/week) may protect against the initial myocardial infarction (MI) in women, including the subset of women with diabetes mellitus; risk reduction was most prominent for women who were smokers or who had hypercholesterolemia or hypertension. Higher doses did not appear to offer significant protection. Relative risks of nonfatal MI, fatal coronary heart disease (CHD), and the combined endpoint are presented according to aspirin use.

Compared with women who did not take any aspirin, women who consumed between one and six aspirins per week had a 32% reduction in the age-adjusted risk of MI (*ie*, nonfatal MI and fatal CHD). Results were nearly identical to the consumption of one to three and four to six aspirins per week. Results were similar when nonfatal and fatal coronary events were examined separately. No reduction in MI risk occurred in women taking 7 to 14 or 15 or more aspirins per week. The American Diabetes Association recommends consideration of aspirin use for diabetic patients 30 years of age and older or with cardiovascular risk factors [110]. The US Preventive Services Task Force suggests that the net effect of aspirin improves with increasing risk for coronary heart disease [111,112]. (*Adapted from* Manson *et al.* [109].)

REFERENCES

1. American Heart Association: *2001 Heart and Stroke Statistical Update*. Dallas: American Heart Association; 2000.

2. Kannel WB, Abbott RD: Incidence and prognosis of myocardial infarction in women: the Framingham Study. In *Coronary Heart Disease in Women*. Edited by Eaker ED, Packard B, Wenger NK, *et al.* New York: Haymarket Doyma Inc.; 1987:208–214.

3. Abbott RD, Donahue RP, Kannel WB, *et al.*: The impact of diabetes on survival following myocardial infarction in men vs women. The Framingham Study. *JAMA* 1988, 260:3456–3460.

4. Wenger NK: Clinical characteristics of coronary heart disease in women: emphasis on gender differences. *Cardiovasc Res* 2002, 53:558–567.

5. Edwards FH, Carey JS, Grover FL, *et al.*: Impact of gender on coronary bypass operative mortality. *Ann Thorac Surg* 1998, 66:125–131.

6. Eaker ED, Chesebro JH, Sacks FM, *et al.*: Cardiovascular disease in women. *Circulation* 1993, 88:1999–2009.

7. Centers for Disease Control and Prevention: Missed opportunities in preventive counseling for cardiovascular disease: United States 1995. *MMWR Morb Mortal Wkly Rep* 1998, 47:91–95.

8. Mosca L, Grundy SM, Judelson D, *et al.*: Guide to preventive cardiology for women. *Circulation* 1999, 99:2480–2484.

9. Centers for Disease Control: Coronary heart disease incidence by sex—United States, 1971–1987. *MMWR Morb Mortal Wkly Rep* 992, 41:526–529.

10. Williams EL, Winkleby MA, Fortmann SP: Changes in coronary heart disease risk factors in the 1980s: evidence of a male-female crossover effect with age. *Am J Epidemiol* 1993, 137:1056–1067.

11. Barrett-Connor EL, Cohn BA, Wingard DL, *et al.*: Why is diabetes mellitus a stronger risk factor for fatal ischemic heart disease in women than in men? The Rancho Bernardo Study. *JAMA* 1991, 265:627–631.

12. Kannel WB, McGee DL: Diabetes and glucose tolerance as risk factors for cardiovascular disease: the Framingham Study. *Diabetes Care* 1979, 2:120–126.

13. Krolewski AS, Warram JH, Valsania P, *et al.*: Evolving natural history of coronary artery disease in diabetes mellitus. *Am J Med* 1991, 90(suppl 2A):56s–61s.

14. Manson JE, Colditz GA, Stampfer MJ, *et al.*: A prospective study on maturity-onset diabetes mellitus and risk of coronary heart disease and stroke in women. *Arch Intern Med* 1991, 151:1141–1147.

15. Liao Y, Cooper RS, Ghali JK, *et al.*: Sex differences in the impact of coexistent diabetes on survival in patients with coronary heart disease. *Diabetes Care* 1993, 16:708–713.

16. Donahue RP, Goldberg RJ, Chen Z, *et al.*: The influence of sex and diabetes mellitus on survival following acute myocardial infarction: a community-wide perspective. *J Clin Epidemiol* 1993, 46:245–252.

17. Goldschmid MG, Barrett-Connor E, Edelstein SL, *et al.*: Dyslipidemia and ischemic heart disease mortality among men and women with diabetes. *Circulation* 1994, 89:991–997.

18. Modan M, Or J, Karasik A, *et al.*: Hyperinsulinemia, sex, and risk of atherosclerotic cardiovascular disease. *Circulation* 1991, 84:1165–1175.

19. Hansen EF, Andersen LT, Von Eyben FE: Cigarette smoking and age at first acute myocardial infarction, and influence of gender and extent of smoking. *Am J Cardiol* 1993, 71:1439–1442.

20. Willett WC, Green A, Stampfer MJ, *et al.*: Relative and absolute excess risks of coronary heart disease among women who smoke cigarettes. *N Engl J Med* 1987, 317:1303–1309.

21. Perkins J, Dick TBS: Smoking and myocardial infarction: secondary prevention. *Postgrad Med J* 1985, 61:295–300.

22. Hermanson B, Omenn GS, Kronmal RA, *et al.*, and Participants in the Coronary Artery Surgery Study: Beneficial six-year outcome of smoking cessation in older men and women with coronary artery disease. Results from the CASS Registry. *N Engl J Med* 1988, 319:1365–1369.

23. Coambs RB, Li S, Kozlowski LT: Age interacts with heaviness of smoking in predicting success in cessation of smoking. *Am J Epidemiol* 1992, 135:240–246.

24. Rosenberg L, Kaufman DW, Helmrich SP, *et al.*: Myocardial infarction and cigarette smoking in women younger than 50 years of age. *JAMA* 1985, 253:2965–2969.

25. Johnson CL, Rifkind BM, Sempos CT, *et al.*: Declining serum total cholesterol levels among US adults. The National Health and Nutrition Examination Surveys. *JAMA* 1993, 269:3002–3008.

26. Campos H, McNamara JR, Wilson PWF, *et al.*: Differences in low density lipoprotein subfractions and apolipoproteins in premenopausal and postmenopausal women. *J Clin Endocrinol Metab* 1988, 67:30–35.

27. Razay G, Heaton KW, Bolton CH: Coronary heart disease risk factors in relation to the menopause. *Q J Med* 1992, 85:889–896.

28. Kuller LH, Simkin-Silverman LR, Wing RR, *et al.*: Women's healthy lifestyle project: a randomized clinical trial: results at 54 months. *Circulation* 2001, 103:32–37.

29. Kannel WB: Nutrition and the occurrence and prevention of cardiovascular disease in the elderly. *Nutr Rev* 1988, 46:68–78.

30. Manolio TA, Pearson TA, Wenger NK, *et al.*: Cholesterol and heart disease in older persons and women. Review of an NHLBI workshop. *Ann Epidemiol* 1992, 2:161–176.

31. Castelli WP: The triglycerides issue: a view from Framingham. *Am Heart J* 1986, 112:432–437.

32. Bush TL, Criqui MH, Cowan LD, *et al.*: Cardiovascular disease mortality in women: results from the Lipid Research Clinics Follow-up Study. In *Coronary Heart Disease in Women*. Edited by Eaker ED, Packard B, Wenger NK, *et al.* New York: Haymarket Doyma Inc.; 1987:106–111.

33. Criqui MH, Heiss G, Cohn R, *et al.*: Plasma triglyceride level and mortality from coronary heart disease. *N Engl J Med* 1993, 328:1220–1225.

34. Assmann G, Schulte H: The importance of triglycerides: results from the Prospective Cardiovascular Munster (PROCAM) Study. *Eur J Epidemiol* 1992, 8(suppl 1):99–103.

35. Gordon DJ, Probstfield JL, Garrison RJ, *et al.*: High-density lipoprotein cholesterol and cardiovascular disease: four prospective American studies. *Circulation* 1989, 79:8–15.

36. Wong ND, Wilson PWF, Kannel WB: Serum cholesterol as a prognostic factor after myocardial infarction: the Framingham Study. *Ann Intern Med* 1991, 115:687–693.

37. Scandinavian Simvastatin Survival Study Group: Randomised trial of cholesterol lowering in 4444 patients with coronary heart disease: the Scandinavian Simvastatin Survival Study (4S). *Lancet* 1994, 344:1383–1389.

38. Lewis SJ, Sacks FM, Mitchell JS, *et al.*, for the CARE Investigators: Effect of pravastatin on cardiovascular events in women after myocardial infarction: the Cholesterol and Recurrent Events (CARE) Trial. *J Am Coll Cardiol* 1998, 32:140–146.

39. Downs JR, Clearfield M, Weis S, *et al.*, for the AFCAPS/TexCAPS Research Group: Primary prevention of acute coronary events with lovastatin in men and women with average cholesterol levels: results of AFCAPS/TexCAPS. *JAMA* 1998, 279:1615–1622.

40. Long-term Intervention with Pravastatin in Ischemic Disease (LIPID) Study Group: Prevention of cardiovascular events and death with pravastatin in patients with coronary heart disease and a broad range of initial cholesterol levels. The Long-term Intervention with Pravastatin in Ischemic Disease (LIPID) Study Group. *N Engl J Med* 1998, 339:1349–1357.

41. Clinical Trial Service Unit: HPS MRC/BHF Heart Protection Study. Accessible at http://www.hpsinfo.org

42. Barnard RJ: Effects of life-style modification on serum lipids. *Arch Intern Med* 1991, 151:1389–1394.

43. Anastos K, Charney P, Charon RA, *et al.*: Hypertension in women: what is really known? The Women's Caucus, Working Group on Women's Health of the Society of General Internal Medicine. *Ann Intern Med* 1991, 115:287–293.

44. National Center for Health Statistics: *Health: United States, 1990*. Hyattsville, MD: U.S. Public Health Service, Centers for Disease Control; 1991.

45. Hypertension Detection and Follow-up Program Cooperative Group: Persistence of reduction in blood pressure and mortality of participants in the Hypertension Detection and Follow-up Program. *JAMA* 1988, 259:2113–2122.

46. Hypertension Detection and Follow-up Program Cooperative Group: Five-year findings of the Hypertension Detection and Follow-up Program. II: mortality by race-sex and age. *JAMA* 1979, 242:2572–2577.

47. Medical Research Council Working Party: MRC trial of treatment of mild hypertension: principal results. *BMJ* 1985, 291:97–104.

48. SHEP Cooperative Research Group: Prevention of stroke by antihypertensive drug treatment in older persons with isolated hypertension. Final results of the Systolic Hypertension in the Elderly Program (SHEP). *JAMA* 1991, 265:3255–3264.

49. Barrett-Connor EL: Obesity, atherosclerosis and coronary artery disease. *Ann Intern Med* 1985, 103:1010–1019.

50. Spelsberg A, Ridker PM, Manson JE: Carbohydrate metabolism, obesity, and diabetes. In *Cardiovascular Health and Disease in Women*. Edited by Douglas PS. Philadelphia: WB Saunders Co.; 1993:191–216.

51. Hubert HB, Feinleib M, McNamara PM, *et al.*: Obesity as an independent risk factor for cardiovascular disease: a 26-year follow-up of participants in the Framingham Heart Study. *Circulation* 1983, 67:968–977.

52. Willett WC, Manson JE, Stampfer MJ, *et al.*: Weight, weight change, and coronary heart disease in women: risk within the 'normal' weight range. *JAMA* 1995, 273:461–465.

53. Brownell KD, Stunkard AJ: Differential changes in plasma high-density lipoprotein-cholesterol levels in obese men and women during weight reduction. *Arch Intern Med* 1981, 141:1142–1146.

54. Soler JT, Folsom AR, Kushi LH, *et al.*: Association of body fat distribution with plasma lipids, lipoprotein, apolipoproteins AI and B in postmenopausal women. *J Clin Epidemiol* 1988, 41:1075–1081.

55. Larsson B, Bengtsson C, Bjorntorp P, *et al.*: Is abdominal body fat distribution a major explanation for the sex difference in the incidence of myocardial infarction? The Study of Men Born in 1913 and the Study of Women, Goteborg, Sweden. *Am J Epidemiol* 1992, 135:266–273.

56. Kannel WB, Sorlie P: Some health benefits of physical activity. The Framingham Study. *Arch Intern Med* 1979, 139:857–861.

57. Blair SN, Kohl HW III, Paffenbarger RS Jr, *et al.*: Physical fitness and all-cause mortality. A prospective study of healthy men and women. *JAMA* 1989, 262:2395–2401.

58. Reaven PD, McPhillips JB, Barrett-Connor EL, *et al.*: Leisure time exercise and lipid and lipoprotein levels in an older population. *J Am Geriatr Soc* 1990, 38:847–854.

59. Lokey EZ, Tran ZV: Effects of exercise training on serum lipid and lipoprotein concentrations in women: a meta-analysis. *Int J Sports Med* 1989, 10:424–429.

60. Hartung GH, Moore CE, Mitchell R, *et al.*: Relationship of menopausal status and exercise level to HDL cholesterol in women. *Exp Aging Res* 1984, 10:13–18.

61. Manson JE, Rimm EB, Stampfer MJ, *et al.*: Physical activity and incidence of non-insulin dependent diabetes mellitus in women. *Lancet* 1991, 338:774–778.

62. Ford ES, Giles WH, Dietz WH: Prevalence of the metabolic syndrome among US adults: findings from the Third National Health and Nutrition Examination Survey. *JAMA* 2002, 287:356–359.

63. Mann JI, Inman WHW: Oral contraceptives and death from myocardial infarction. *BMJ* 1975, 2:245–248.

64. Mann JI, Vessey MP, Thorogood M, *et al.*: Myocardial infarction in young women with special reference to oral contraceptive practice. *BMJ* 1975, 2:241–245.

65. Mann JI, Inman WHW, Thorogood M: Oral contraceptive use in older women and fatal myocardial infarction. *BMJ* 1976, 2:445–447.

66. Shapiro S, Slone D, Rosenberg L, *et al.*: Oral-contraceptive use in relation to myocardial infarction. *Lancet* 1979, 1:743–747.

67. Petitti DB, Wingerd J, Pellegrin F, *et al.*: Risk of vascular disease in women: smoking, oral contraceptives, noncontraceptive estrogens, and other factors. *JAMA* 1979, 242:1150–1154.

68. Rosenberg L, Hennekens CH, Rosner B, *et al.*: Oral contraceptive use in relation to nonfatal myocardial infarction. *Am J Epidemiol* 1980, 111:59–66.

69. Slone D, Shapiro S, Kaufman DW, *et al.*: Risk of myocardial infarction in relation to current and discontinued use of oral contraceptives. *N Engl J Med* 1981, 305:420–424.

70. Royal College of General Practitioners' Oral Contraception Study: Further analyses of mortality in oral contraceptive users. *Lancet* 1981, 1:541–546.

71. Stampfer MJ, Willett WC, Colditz GA, *et al.*: A prospective study of past use of oral contraceptive agents and risk of cardiovascular disease. *N Engl J Med* 1988, 319:1313–1317.

G ENDER DIFFERENCES IN CORONARY RISK FACTORS AND RISK INTERVENTIONS

72. Stampfer MJ, Willett WC, Colditz GA, *et al.*: Past use of oral contraceptives and cardiovascular disease: a meta-analysis in the context of the Nurses' Health Study. *Am J Obstet Gynecol* 1990, 163:285–291.

73. Barrett-Connor E, Bush TL: Estrogen and coronary heart disease in women. *JAMA* 1991, 265:1861–1867.

74. Palmer JR, Rosenberg L, Shapiro S: Reproductive factors and risk of myocardial infarction. *Am J Epidemiol* 1992, 136:408–416.

75. Knopp RH: The effects of postmenopausal estrogen therapy on the incidence of arteriosclerotic vascular disease. *Obstet Gynecol* 1988, 72(suppl 5):23s–30s.

76. Walsh BW, Schiff I, Rosner B, *et al.*: Effects of postmenopausal estrogen replacement on the concentration and metabolism of plasma lipoproteins. *N Engl J Med* 1991, 325:1196–1204.

77. Barrett-Connor E, Laakso M: Ischemic heart disease risk in post-menopausal women. Effects of estrogen use on glucose and insulin levels. *Arteriosclerosis* 1990, 10:531–534.

78. The Writing Group for the PEPI Trial: Effects of estrogen or estrogen/progestin regimens on heart disease risk factors in post-menopausal women. The Postmenopausal Estrogen/Progestin Interventions (PEPI) Trial. *JAMA* 1995, 273:199–208.

79. Cushman M, Legault C, Barrett-Connor E, *et al.*: Effect of post-menopausal hormones on inflammation-sensitive proteins: the Postmenopausal Estrogen Progestin Interventions (PEPI) Study. *Circulation* 1999, 100:717–722.

80. Lafferty FW, Helmuth DO: Post-menopausal estrogen replacement: the prevention of osteoporsis and systemic effects. *Maturitas* 1985, 7: 47–59.

81. Stampfer MJ, Willet WC, Colditz GA, *et al.*: A prospective study of postmenopausal estrogen therapy and coronary heart disease. *N Engl J Med* 1985, 313:1044–1049.

82. Nachtigall LE, Nachtigall RH, Nachtigall RD, *et al.*: Estrogen replacement therapy, II: a prospective study in the relationship to carcinoma and cardiovascular and metabolic problems. *Obstet Gynecol* 1979, 54:74–79.

83. Hammond CB, Jelovsek FR, Lee KL, *et al.*: Effects of long-term estrogen replacement therapy. I: metabolic effects. *Am J Obstet Gynecol* 1979, 133:525–536.

84. Bush TL, Barrett-Connor E, Cowan LD, *et al.*: Cardiovascular mortality and noncontraceptive use of estrogen in women: results from the Lipid Research Clinics Program Follow-up Study. *Circulation* 1987, 75:1102–1109.

85. Talbott E, Kuller LH, Detre K, *et al.*: Biologic and psychosocial risk factors of sudden death from coronary disease in white women. *Am J Cardiol* 1977, 39:858–864.

86. Rosenberg L, Armstrong B, Jick H, *et al.*: Myocardial infarction and estrogen therapy in postmenopausal women. *N Engl J Med* 1976, 294:1256–1259.

87. Henderson BE, Paganini-Hill A, Ross RK: Estrogen replacement therapy and protection from acute myocardial infarction. *Am J Obstet Gynecol* 1988, 159:312–317.

88. Beard CM, Kottke TE, Annegers JF, *et al.*: The Rochester Coronary Heart Disease Project: effect of cigarette smoking, hypertension, diabetes, and steroidal estrogen use on coronary heart disease among 40- to 59-year old women, 1969 through 1982. *Mayo Clin Proc* 1989, 64:1471–1480.

89. Petitti DB, Perlman JA, Sidney S: Noncontraceptive estrogens and mortality: long-term followup of women in the Walnut Creek study. *Obstet Gynecol* 1987, 70:289–293.

90. Avila MH, Walker AM, Jick H: Use of replacement estrogens and the risk of myocardial infarction. *Epidemiology* 1990, 1:128–135.

91. Adam S, Williams V, Vessey MP: Cardiovascular disease and hormone replacement treatment: a pilot case-control study. *BMJ* 1981, 282:1277–1278.

92. Szklo M, Tonascia J, Gordis L, *et al.*: Estrogen use and myocardial infarction risk: a case-control study. *Prev Med* 1984, 13:510–516.

93. Rosenberg L, Slone D, Shapiro S, *et al.*: Noncontraceptive estrogens and myocardial infarction in young women. *JAMA* 1980, 244:339–342.

94. Thompson SG, Meade TW, Greenberg G: The use of hormonal replacement therapy and the risk of stroke and myocardial infarction in women. *J Epidemiol Commun Health* 1989, 43:173–178.

95. LaVecchia C, Franceschi S, Decarli AS, *et al.*: Risk factors for myocardial infarction in young women. *Am J Epidemiol* 1987, 125:832–843.

96. Wilson PWF, Garrison RJ, Castelli WP: Postmenopausal estrogen use and heart disease. *N Engl J Med* 1986, 315:135.

97. Jick H, Dinan B, Rothman KJ: Noncontraceptive estrogens and nonfatal myocardial infarction. *JAMA* 1978, 239:1407–1409.

98. Stampfer MJ, Colditz GA, Willett WC, *et al.*: Postmenopausal estrogen therapy and cardiovascular disease. Ten-year follow-up from the Nurses' Health Study. *N Engl J Med* 1991, 325:756–762.

99. Sullivan JM, Vander Zwaag R, Hughes JP, *et al.*: Estrogen replacement and coronary artery disease. Effect on survival in post-menopausal women. *Arch Intern Med* 1990, 150:2557–2562.

100. Herrington DM, Reboussin DM, Brosnihan KB, *et al.*: Effects of estrogen replacement on the progression of coronary-artery atherosclerosis. *N Engl J Med* 2000, 343:522–529.

101. Henderson BE, Paganini-Hill A, Ross RK: Decreased mortality in users of estrogen replacement therapy. *Arch Intern Med* 1991, 151:75–78.

102. Falkeborn M, Persson I, Adami H-O, *et al.*: The risk of acute myocardial infarction after oestrogen and oestrogen-progestogen replacement. *Br J Obstet Gynecol* 1992, 99:821–828.

103. Hulley S, Grady D, Bush T, *et al.*, for the Heart and Estrogen/progestin Replacement Study (HERS) Research Group: Randomized trial of estrogen plus progestin for secondary prevention of coronary heart disease in postmenopausal women. *JAMA* 1998, 280:605–613.

104. Grady D, Wenger NK, Herrington D, *et al.*, for the Heart and Estrogen/progestin Replacement Study Research Group: Postmenopausal hormone therapy increases risk for venous thromboembolic disease. The Heart and Estrogen/progestin Replacement Study. *Ann Intern Med* 2000, 132:689–696.

105. Viscoli CM, Brass LM, Kernan WN, *et al.*: A clinical trial of estrogen-replacement therapy after ischemic stroke. *N Engl J Med* 2001, 345:1243–1249.

106. Walsh BW, Kuller LH, Wild RA, *et al.*: Effects of raloxifene on serum lipids and coagulation factors in healthy postmenopausal women. *JAMA* 1998, 279:1445–1451.

107. Barrett-Connor E, Wenger NK, Grady D, *et al.*: Hormone and nonhormone therapy for the maintenance of postmenopausal health: the need for randomized controlled trials of estrogen and raloxifene. *J Women's Health* 1998, 7:839–847.

108. Barrett-Connor E, Grady D, Sashegyi A, *et al.*: Raloxifene and cardiovascular events in osteoporotic postmenopausal women: four-year results from the MORE (Multiple Outcomes of Raloxifene Evaluation) randomized trial. *JAMA* 2002, 287:847–857.

109. Manson JE, Stampfer MJ, Colditz GA, *et al.*: A prospective study of aspirin use and primary prevention of cardiovascular disease in women. *JAMA* 1991, 266:521–527.

110. American Diabetes Association: Aspirin therapy in diabetes. *Diabetes Care* 2001, 24 (suppl 10):S62–S63.

111. US Preventive Services Task Force: Aspirin for the primary prevention of cardiovascular events: recommendation and rationale. *Ann Intern Med* 2002, 136:157–160.

112. Hayden M, Pignone M, Phillips C, *et al.*: Aspirin for the primary prevention of cardiovascular events: a summary of the evidence for the US Preventive Services Task Force. *Ann Intern Med* 2002, 136:161–172.

COST-EFFECTIVENESS OF RISK FACTORS

13

CHAPTER

Paul A. Heidenreich and Harlan M. Krumholz

The identification of risk factors for cardiovascular disease prompts questions about the organization and implementation of risk factor modification programs. Are resources better spent on treating cardiovascular disease or preventing it? Should programs be adopted that screen all persons for risk factors or should the efforts be targeted to certain patient groups? Should all risk factors receive equal attention or are resources better directed toward certain risk factors? How can these different strategies be compared? These questions are difficult to answer and, in many cases, cannot be resolved easily. One method of addressing these questions is to compare the costs and benefits of alternative uses of health care resources.

Cost-effectiveness analysis has evolved as a method to facilitate the comparison of various uses of resources. These analyses compare alternative programs by explicitly estimating their costs and benefits. Because escalating health care costs have focused attention on the efficient allocation of health care resources, the use of these analyses may increase dramatically. Although these analyses cannot dictate which programs should be implemented, they do demonstrate the relative attractiveness of programs in producing a health benefit.

The growing literature to address the cost-effectiveness of various strategies to prevent cardiovascular disease has included analyses of blood pressure, cholesterol, and smoking. The results of these analyses suggest that selected programs for the treatment of hypertension, hypercholesterolemia, and smoking have favorable cost-effectiveness ratios. There is a continuing need, however, to refine estimates of the costs and benefits of these programs so that informed policy choices can be made.

OVERVIEW

HEALTH CARE COSTS

Health care costs in the United States are high and increasing

Health spending is expected to increase as a share of gross domestic product from 13.0% in 1999 to 15.9% by 2010

National health care spending is projected to increase from $1.2 trillion in 1996 to $2.6 trillion by 2010

FIGURE 13-1. The costs for health care in the United States are high and rising. Economists have estimated that health spending will increase over the next decade [1]. The high costs will place increasing pressure on decisions about the allocation of resources.

POSSIBLE PRINCIPLES FOR ALLOCATING SCARCE RESOURCES

Maximize health outcomes
Minimize total costs to society
Maximize outcomes with available resources

FIGURE 13-3. Possible principles for allocating scarce resources. Policy-makers may choose a variety of ways to allocate scarce resources. They may choose to maximize health outcomes at any cost, minimize costs despite their health implications, or maximize outcomes with available resources. It is not possible to maximize outcomes while simultaneously minimizing costs. The cost-effectiveness analysis is most useful when policy-makers seek to maximize outcomes with available resources. The analysis provides information about the relative costs and benefits of programs competing for resources.

COSTS VERSUS CHARGES

Costs
  The price paid for the resources consumed in providing a service
Charges
  The price requested for reimbursement for providing a service

OBJECTIVE OF COST-EFFECTIVENESS ANALYSIS

The comparison of alternative strategies in terms of their costs and consequences

FIGURE 13-2. Objective of cost-effectiveness analysis. Resources are finite. Limited resources ultimately force choices among various alternatives. In the health care system, cost-effectiveness analysis is a method to examine explicitly the costs and benefits of a medical technology or program in order to facilitate decisions about the allocation of scarce resources. Each cost-effectiveness ratio specifies the incremental cost that is required to produce an incremental benefit when one strategy is compared with another.

DEFINITION OF THE COST-EFFECTIVENESS RATIO

$$\text{Cost per unit of benefit} = \frac{\text{Cost of strategy A - Cost of strategy B}}{\text{Benefit with A - Benefit with B}}$$

FIGURE 13-4. Definition of the cost-effectiveness ratio. The cost-effectiveness ratio is calculated by dividing the net increase in health costs associated with one program compared with another by the net effectiveness of one program over another. The lower the value of the ratio, the more favorable the program. Low-ratio programs are more efficient than high-ratio programs for producing a health benefit.

FIGURE 13-5. Costs versus charges. The costs of a program are not equivalent to what is charged for the program or intervention. *Costs* represent the monetary value of the resources consumed in providing the service. *Charges* are what a business is asking for that service. In a health care environment where a third party is commonly responsible for payment, the charge often is not closely related to the worth of the service.

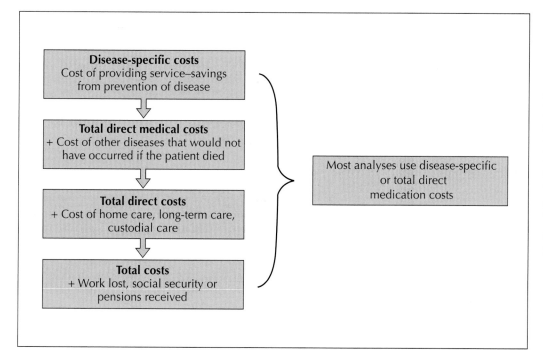

FIGURE 13-6. The layers of cost. The total costs are much more than merely the *disease-specific costs* involved in providing the service. The disease-specific costs plus the costs relating to adverse events and costs relating to the illness that would not have occurred if the patient had died represent the *total direct medical costs*. The total direct medical costs plus the cost of home care, long-term care, and custodial care equal the *total direct costs*. Finally, the total direct costs plus indirect costs such as lost work days comprise the *total costs*. Therefore, the total costs are almost always greater than the cost of providing the service.

BENEFIT OF THE INTERVENTION

The effectiveness must be a measure of the benefit of the intervention. Without a benefit, it is not possible (or necessary) to calculate cost-effectiveness.

FIGURE 13-7. Benefit of the intervention. In the comparison of two strategies, the cost-effectiveness methodology is appropriate only if the more costly approach is also more effective. If it is not more effective, then the other strategy is preferred. Each cost-effectiveness ratio must specify explicitly the benefit of the program or technology being studied.

MEASURES OF HEALTH BENEFIT

Improvements in physiologic endpoints
Years of life gained
Healthy years of life gained
Quality-adjusted life-years gained

FIGURE 13-8. Measures of health benefit. Although the costs of a program are always expressed in monetary terms, health benefits can be measured in several ways. The many ways of measuring health benefits have led to different types of cost-effectiveness ratios. For example, the benefit may be expressed as a physiologic endpoint such as cost per mm Hg decrease in blood pressure. It may also be expressed as years of life gained, healthy years of life gained, or quality-adjusted years of life gained. The existence of many types of ratios can sometimes make it difficult to compare different analyses with each other.

Is the benefit worth the cost?

Dialysis has been used as a benchmark for the amount that the public is willing to pay for 1 year of life.

FIGURE 13-9. Is the benefit worth the cost? Cost-effective analyses cannot indicate which programs ought to be adopted. The decision about what cost-effectiveness ratio is acceptable to society is arbitrary. These analyses can show only the value of one program relative to another. The approximately $35,000 per year cost (in 1990 dollars, $44,000 in 2001 dollars) of renal dialysis has been used as a benchmark for the amount that the public has been willing to pay to prolong life by 1 year [2].

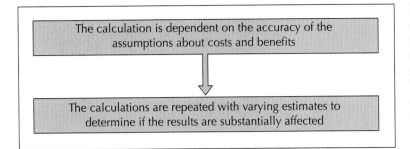

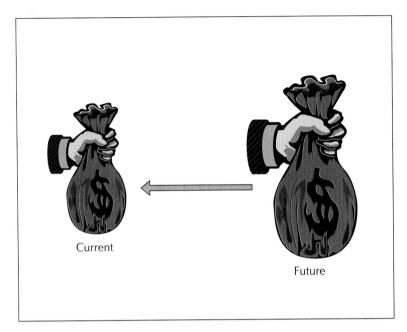

FIGURE 13-10. Varying the assumptions. Most cost-effectiveness analyses are dependent on many assumptions, many of which represent "best estimates" because there are no large studies of the subject. Because these assumptions may not be accurate, it is important for the analysis to be repeated with varying estimates. The investigators determine whether the results of the analysis change substantially if the assumptions are changed to a reasonable extent. The repeated analyses with varying assumptions is termed "the sensitivity analysis" and is a critical component to every economic evaluation.

FIGURE 13-11. Discounting future costs and benefits. Discounting is another important concept in the calculation of cost-effectiveness ratios. Current dollars (and benefits) are more highly valued than the promise of future dollars and benefits. Therefore, if costs and benefits accrue during different periods, then the future events must be "discounted" so that their value may be compared with the current costs and benefits. Future costs and benefits are commonly discounted by approximately 3% per year [3].

DISCOUNTING AND PREVENTION

In risk factor modification, the costs begin immediately and the benefits are in the future

FIGURE 13-12. Discounting and prevention. As with costs, future benefits are also discounted. The discounting tends to make cost-effectiveness ratios for preventive programs less favorable because costs begin immediately, but benefits are in the future.

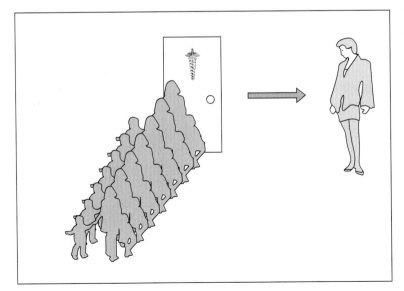

FIGURE 13-13. An important determinant of the cost is the number of people who must be treated to produce a benefit. In risk factor modification, unlike therapeutic interventions such as dialysis, most people would not have died without the intervention. Commonly, many people must be treated to produce a benefit, *eg*, to save a single life. The importance of the risk factor and the effectiveness of its modification will determine how many people must be treated to produce a benefit. If more people must be treated to produce a benefit, it is less likely that the intervention will be cost-effective.

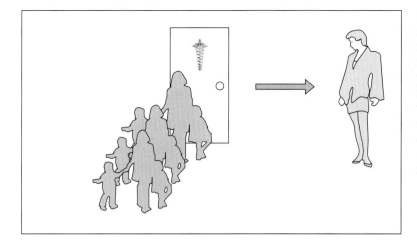

FIGURE 13-14. Impact of risk factor clustering. Risk factor modification in patients with multiple risk factors tends to be more efficient than similar programs for individuals with a single risk factor. When cardiovascular risk factors present together, the patient's risk of disease increases. Because the incidence of disease is higher in this group, fewer people would have to be treated with risk factor modification to produce a benefit, *eg*, to save a single life (assuming that the relative reduction in risk does not change). Therefore, interventions in this group are more efficient (cost-effective) relative to interventions in groups with any single risk factor.

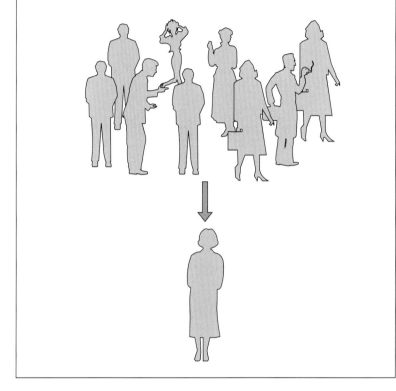

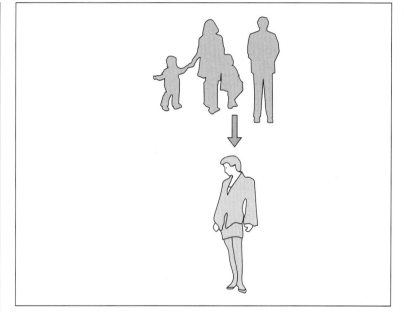

FIGURE 13-15. Risk factor modification for primary prevention. Primary prevention targets individuals who do not have any manifestations of the disease. Risk factor modification as a primary prevention strategy can be costly because many people may have to be screened in order to identify one person with the risk factor and many people with the risk factor may have to be treated for one person to benefit. The prevalence of the disease in the population and their susceptibility to the outcome influence the cost-effectiveness of the program.

FIGURE 13-16. Risk factor modification and secondary prevention. Secondary prevention often produces more favorable cost-effectiveness ratios than primary prevention, *ie*, fewer people must be screened and treated to benefit one person with the risk factor. First, the secondary prevention population has manifest cardiovascular disease and has a high prevalence of individuals with modifiable risk factors. Screening in this population is more efficient. Second, this group has a high likelihood of recurrent events and may have more to gain by reducing their risk.

CHOLESTEROL REDUCTION

THE EPIDEMIOLOGY OF CHOLESTEROL

Elevated cholesterol is highly prevalent

Elevated cholesterol is associated with an increased risk of heart disease

The treatment of hypercholesterolemia reduces the risk of heart disease

Potential pharmacologic costs of treating hypercholesterolemia in the US has been estimated to be from $3–$17 billion/y

FIGURE 13-17. The epidemiology of cholesterol and the rationale for cost-effectiveness analysis of the treatment of hypercholesterolemia. The estimated cost of treating hypercholesterolemia ($3 to $17 billion/y) is based on past National Cholesterol Education Program guidelines [4] and the distribution of risk factors in the Framingham Offspring study [5].

COST OF SCREENING TESTS

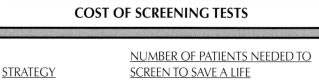

STRATEGY	NUMBER OF PATIENTS NEEDED TO SCREEN TO SAVE A LIFE
Screening + pravastatin	418 (95% CI 235 to 79,720)
Screening + resin	846 (95% CI 325 to -799)
Screening + diet	590 (95% CI 292 to -610)

FIGURE 13-18. Cost of screening tests. Most of the published estimates of the cost-effectiveness of cholesterol-lowering therapy have neglected the cost of screening tests. Rembold [6] has provided an estimate, based on the clinical trials, of the number needed to be screened for hyperlipidemia over 5 years to prevent one death [6,7].

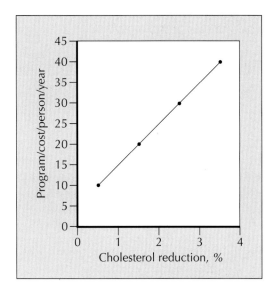

FIGURE 13-19. Cost-effectiveness of population approaches to cholesterol reduction. Investigators used the Coronary Heart Disease Policy Model, a state-transition, computer-based model, to estimate the cost-effectiveness of population approaches to reducing serum cholesterol levels in the US adult population [8]. They calculated that a national program with the costs ($4.95 per year) and cholesterol-lowering benefits (2%) of the Stanford Five-City Project [9] would have a cost-effectiveness ratio of $3200 per year of life saved. They found that the cost-effectiveness of a program would be less than $50,000 per year of life saved if it 1) cost less than $10 per person and produced a 1% reduction in cholesterol; 2) cost less than $20 per person and produced a 2% reduction in cholesterol; 3) cost less than $30 per person and produced a 3% reduction in cholesterol; or 4) cost less than $40 per person and produced a 4% reduction in cholesterol.

CHOLESTEROL REDUCTION AND MORTALITY

Primary prevention
  West of Scotland Coronary Prevention Study
Secondary prevention
  Scandinavian Simvastatin Survival Study
  Long-term Intervention with Pravastatin in Ischemic Disease (LIPID) study

FIGURE 13-20. Cholesterol reduction and mortality. Cost-effectiveness analyses are commonly expressed as dollars per year of life saved. Only two secondary prevention trials [10] and one primary prevention trial [11] have shown a reduction in all-cause mortality with cholesterol-lowering therapy. Both of these studies used statins to achieve cholesterol reduction. Other studies have demonstrated substantial reductions in cardiovascular events. Many earlier studies demonstrated reductions in cardiovascular mortality that were offset by death from other causes.

BENEFIT OF LOWERING CHOLESTEROL

For every 10 percentage points of cholesterol lowered → CHD mortality risk is reduced by 15% and total mortality risk is reduced by 11%

FIGURE 13-21. Benefit of lowering cholesterol. Gould *et al.* [12] conducted a meta-analysis of cholesterol reduction trials, including eight trials of statins. They found that the only significant factor that affected coronary heart disease (CHD) mortality risk is net cholesterol reduction. In addition, the statins did not appear to have any specific effects on CHD mortality risk. When considering all of the trials, they concluded that for every 10 percentage points of cholesterol reduction, CHD mortality was reduced by 15% and the total mortality risk was reduced by 11%.

WEST OF SCOTLAND CORONARY PREVENTION STUDY: ECONOMIC ANALYSIS

For every 10,000 asymptomatic men with hypercholesterolemia treated with pravastatin for 5 years

318 avoid the transition to cardiovascular disease

2017 hospital days are avoided

2460 years of life are saved

Cost-effectiveness ratio <$50,000/year of life saved

FIGURE 13-22. West of Scotland Coronary Prevention Study: economic analysis. This study showed that using pravastatin in men who have hypercholesterolemia but no symptoms prevents 318 individuals from making the transition to cardiovascular disease for every 10,000 treated (31 individuals need to be treated over 5 years to prevent one transition) [13]. They undertook an economic analysis and estimated that for every 10,000 individuals treated, there would be a savings of 2017 hospital days and a savings of 2460 years of life. They estimate that the use of pravastatin for these individuals has a cost-effectiveness ratio of less than $50,000 per year of life saved.

REDUCTION IN HEALTH CARE UTILIZATION IN THE 4S TRIAL

Simvastatin therapy compared with placebo:

Reduced hospitalization for acute coronary disease by 26%

Reduced the average length of stay by 10%

Reduced overall total hospital days by 34%

Estimated reduction in costs associated with hospitalizations for total cardiovascular disease over 5.4-year median follow-up period is $4350 per randomized patient

FIGURE 13-23. Reduction in health care utilization in the Scandinavian Simvastatin Survival Study (4S). The investigators from the 4S trial sought to determine the impact of simvastatin on the use of health care resources for cardiovascular disease hospitalizations and revascularization procedures. They found that simvastatin was associated with a reduction in hospitalizations and length of stay. As a result, over the 5.4-year median follow-up of the trial, $4350 in hospitalization costs were saved per patient randomized to simvastatin. These reductions, however, did not completely offset the cost of the drug [14]. (Cost expressed in 2002 dollars.)

COST-EFFECTIVENESS OF SIMVASTATIN FOR SECONDARY PREVENTION

TOTAL CHOLESTEROL BEFORE TREATMENT	COST-EFFECTIVENESS, *DOLLAR/YOLS*					
	MEN (35 YEARS)	WOMEN (35 YEARS)	MEN (55 YEARS)	WOMEN (55 YEARS)	MEN (70 YEARS)	WOMEN (70 YEARS)
213	12,768	30,688	7840	18,368	6944	14,896
261	9856	21,056	6160	11,536	5264	9520
309	7504	14,784	4704	7952	4256	6944

FIGURE 13-24. Cost-effectiveness of simvastatin for secondary prevention. Investigators from the Scandinavian Simvastatin Survival Study (4S) used a Markov model to estimate the cost-effectiveness of simvastatin for lowering cholesterol levels in patients with coronary heart disease, using data from their trial. In the analysis of direct costs, the investigators calculated that the cost per year of life saved ranged from $4256 for 70-year-old men with a cholesterol of 309 mg/dL to $30,688 for 35-year-old women with a 213 mg/dL cholesterol level. For all assumptions, the cost per year was less than $56,000 per year of life saved [15]. (Cost expressed in 2001 dollars.) YOL—years of life saved.

FIGURE 13-25. Reduction in healthcare utilization: the Long-term Intervention with Provastatin in Ischemic Disease (LIPID) trial. The investigators from the LIPID study reported that pravastatin reduced the risk of acute myocardial infarction (AMI) by 29% and coronary revascularization by 20%. These reductions would be expected to reduce short-term medical costs. In addition, the treatment was associated with a 24% reduction in death from coronary heart disease and a 29% reduction in all-cause mortality. (*Data from* the LIPID study group [16].)

FIGURE 13-26. Reduction in health care utilization in the Cholesterol and Recurrent Events (CARE) trial. The West of Scotland Study and the Scandinavian Simvastatin Survival Study (4S) trial focused on patients with hypercholesterolemia. The CARE trial enrolled patients with an average cholesterol level after myocardial infarction (MI) [17]. Their primary endpoint was a fatal coronary event or nonfatal MI, which was reduced by 24% in the pravastatin group. They did not have a significant reduction in overall mortality. The use of pravastatin was associated with substantial reductions in events and procedures associated with higher resource consumption, such as cardiovascular procedures. In a model based on the CARE trial, the cost-effectiveness of pravastatin treatment for patients with low-density lipoprotein (LDL) cholesterol of 211 mg/dL ranged from $13,200 to $26,400 per year of life gained for nondiabetic patients, and $4400 to $11,000 per year of life gained for diabetic patients [18]. CABG—coronary artery bypass graft; PTCA—percutaneous transluminal coronary angioplasty. (Cost expressed in 2002 dollars.)

FIGURE 13-27. Reduction in health care utilization in the Air Force/Texas Coronary Atherosclerosis Prevention Study (AFCAPS/TexCAPS) trial. The West of Scotland Study and the Scandinavian Simvastatin Survival Study (4S) focused on patients with hypercholesterolemia. The AFCAPS/TexCAPS trial enrolled patients with an average cholesterol level and no clinically evident atherosclerotic cardiovascular disease (CVD) [19]. Their primary endpoint was first major acute coronary event, which was reduced by 37% in the lovastatin group. They did not have a significant reduction in overall mortality. The use of lovastatin was associated with substantial reductions in events and procedures associated with higher resource consumption, such as cardiovascular procedures. The reduction in these events would be expected to offset, at least partially, the costs of the cholesterol-lowering agent. HDL—high-density lipoprotein; LDL—low-density lipoprotein; MI—myocardial infarction.

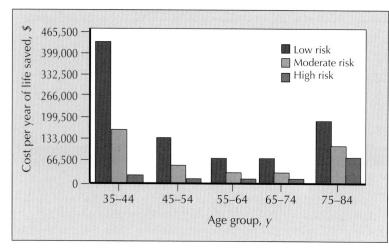
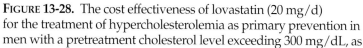

FIGURE 13-28. The cost effectiveness of lovastatin (20 mg/d) for the treatment of hypercholesterolemia as primary prevention in men with a pretreatment cholesterol level exceeding 300 mg/dL, as

reported by Goldman *et al.* [20]. The ratios were derived from a computer simulation using the Coronary Heart Disease (CHD) Policy Model [21]. Estimates of CHD incidence and all-cause mortality were based on data from the Framingham Heart Study 30-year follow-up. The analysis showed that the results were sensitive to the patient's age and risk factors. Middle-age and high-risk individuals had the most favorable ratios. High-risk patients were defined as having a diastolic blood pressure above 105 mm Hg, being a smoker, and weighing more than 130% of ideal body weight. Moderate-risk patients were defined as having a diastolic blood pressure between 95 and 104 mm Hg, being a nonsmoker, and weighing 110% to 129% of ideal body weight. Low-risk patients were defined as having a diastolic blood pressure below 95 mm Hg, being a nonsmoker, and weighing less than 110% of ideal body weight. The authors estimated that 20 mg/d of lovastatin reduced the serum cholesterol level by 19%. The high-risk group had a cost-effectiveness ratio of less than $40,000 per year of life saved until age 75 years. The moderate-risk group had a cost-effectiveness ratio of approximately $40,000 per year of life saved from age 55 years to 74 years. Costs are expressed in 2002 dollars.

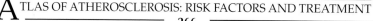

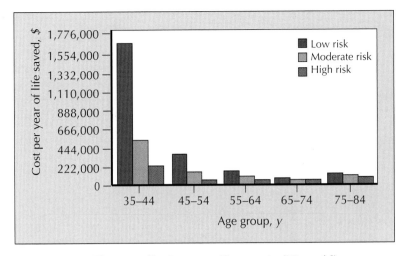

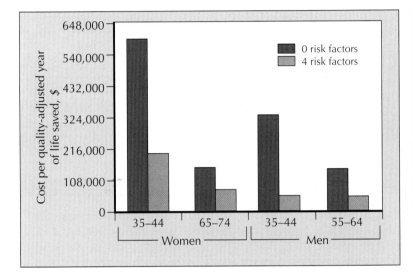

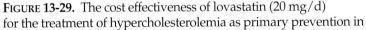

FIGURE 13-29. The cost effectiveness of lovastatin (20 mg/d) for the treatment of hypercholesterolemia as primary prevention in

women with a pretreatment cholesterol level exceeding 300 mg/dL. The cost-effectiveness ratios are derived from a computer simulation using the Coronary Heart Disease Policy Model [21]. Women were stratified by age and risk group. High-risk patients were defined as having a diastolic blood pressure above 105 mm Hg, being a smoker, and weighing more than 130% of ideal body weight. Moderate-risk patients were defined as having a diastolic blood pressure between 95 and 104 mm Hg, being a nonsmoker, and weighing 110% to 129% of ideal body weight. Low-risk patients were defined as having a diastolic blood pressure below 95 mm Hg, being a nonsmoker, and weighing less than 110% of ideal body weight. For each age group, the cost-effectiveness ratio is most favorable for the high-risk group (ie, lowest ratio of cost per life saved). In comparison with men (see Fig. 13-27), the ratios for women are less favorable at every age and for every risk level. Nevertheless, women at high risk who were between 55 and 74 years of age and those at moderate risk who were between 65 and 74 years of age had a cost-effectiveness ratio of less than $56,000 per year of life saved. Costs are expressed in 2002 dollars.

FIGURE 13-30. The cost-effectiveness ratios for the use of statin therapy for primary prevention in men and women with a low-density lipoprotein (LDL) cholesterol of greater than 190 mg/dL and zero to four risk factors for coronary disease. Using the Coronary Heart Disease Policy Model, Prosser [22] demonstrated that for patients with four other risk factors, the treatment with statins costs less than $81,000 per quality-adjusted life year saved. Primary prevention for young women is expensive regardless of the number of risk factors. Costs are expressed in 2002 dollars.

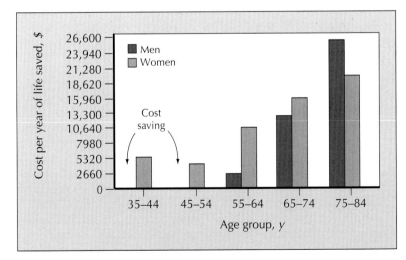

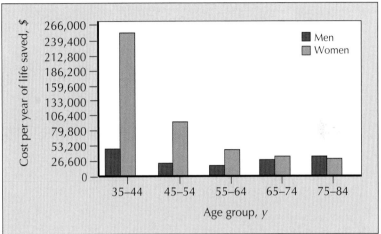

FIGURE 13-31. The cost-effectiveness ratios for the use of lovastatin (20 mg/d) as cholesterol-lowering therapy for secondary prevention in subjects with a pretreatment cholesterol level of less than 250 mg/dL. These estimates were derived from the Coronary Heart Disease Policy Model [21]. The therapy is more cost-effective for men than women and for older subjects compared with younger subjects. Cost are expressed in 2002 dollars.

FIGURE 13-32. The cost-effectiveness ratios for the use of lovastatin (20 mg/d) as cholesterol-lowering therapy for secondary prevention in subjects with a pretreatment cholesterol level of 250 mg/dL or more. These estimates were derived from the Coronary Heart Disease Policy Model [21]. In these subjects, the therapy is very cost-effective for men and women at all ages. For men between 35 and 54 years of age, the therapy saves both lives and money. The cost-effectiveness ratio does not exceed $40,000 per year of life saved for any group.

The interpretation of all of the analyses in this section must take into account the constantly changing costs of medications. After the publication of these analyses, competition has reduced the cost of medications by as much as 50%. Sensitivity analyses performed with various assumptions about the cost of medications may be more relevant today than the original estimates used in the analysis. Costs are expressed in 2002 dollars.

HYPERTENSION TREATMENT

THE EPIDEMIOLOGY OF HYPERTENSION

Hypertension is highly prevalent

Hypertension is associated with an increased risk of heart disease, stroke, renal failure, and death

The treatment of moderate and severe hypertension reduces the risk of hypertensive complications

The treatment of mild hypertension decreases the incidence of strokes and probably reduces the incidence of CHD

The treatment of hypertension is widespread, and approximately $10 billion/y is spent on therapy

FIGURE 13-33. The epidemiology and rationale for cost-effectiveness analysis of the treatment of hypertension. CHD—coronary heart disease.

NUMBER OF PATIENTS NEEDED TO SCREEN FOR HYPERTENSION PRIMARY PREVENTION

STRATEGY	NUMBER NEEDED TO SCREEN TO SAVE A LIFE
Screening + treatment with diuretics (with diastolic blood pressure decrease of 10 mm Hg)	274 (95% CI 165 to 1546)
Screening + treatment with diuretics (with diastolic blood pressure decrease of 6 mm Hg)	1307 (95% CI 834 to 3386)

FIGURE 13-34. Number of patients needed to screen for hypertension: primary prevention. Rembold [6] has provided an estimate, based on the clinical trials, of the number of patients needed to be screened for hypertension over 5 years to prevent one death [6]. Although this estimate is not economic, it does provide a perspective on the resources required to prevent an adverse event. He used the Atherosclerosis Risk in Communities Study for an estimate of the prevalence of hypertension [23].

COST-EFFECTIVENESS OF SCREENING FOR HYPERTENSION

AGE GROUP, y	MEN, $/QALY	WOMEN, $/QALY
20	37,492	56,847
40	20,838	29,716
60	10,719	15,877

FIGURE 13-35. Cost-effectiveness of screening for hypertension. The identification of hypertensive individuals requires screening. Littenberg et al. [24] estimated the costs and effects of life expectancy of screening with sphygmomanometry for diastolic blood pressures in the range of 90 to 105 mm Hg. They assumed that adults who were screened would be treated if they have persistent hypertension. The estimates of the benefit of therapy were based on a published meta-analysis. Costs for treatment were estimated to be approximately $384 per year and included the cost of the medication as well as follow-up visits and laboratory tests. Costs and benefits were discounted by 5% per year. The results suggest that screening is cost-effective in men and women of all ages. Men and older adults have more favorable ratios because they are more likely to have high blood pressure. In the sensitivity analysis, the ratio became less favorable as the benefit of the therapy decreased and as the cost of the medication increased. Costs are expressed in 2002 dollars per quality-adjusted life year (QALY).

COST OF THERAPY FOR MILD TO MODERATE HYPERTENSION: US POPULATION, 1990–2010

MEDICATION	COST OF TREATMENT, $	CHD SAVINGS, $	NET COST, $
Propranolol	121.8	56.4	65.5
HCTZ	91.2	27.5	63.8
Nifedipine	234.3	56.2	178.1
Prazosin	397.6	61.3	336.3
Captopril	334.8	37.5	297.4

FIGURE 13-36. Cost of therapy for mild to moderate hypertension: US population, 1990–2010. Using the Coronary Heart Disease (CHD) Policy Model, which is a computer simulation model, Edelson et al. [25] estimated the total costs associated with the use of various antihypertensive treatments from 1990 through 2010. The net costs were calculated by subtracting the savings induced by lowering the incidence of CHD and of death related to hypertension and the diseases it causes from the cost of medications (including physician visits and laboratory tests). Costs were calculated in 2002 dollars (in billions) with a 5% per year discount rate. This analysis suggested that treatment with propranolol or hydrochlorothiazide (HCTZ) is much less expensive than treatment with nifedipine, prazosin, or captopril. (Cost expressed in 2002 dollars.)

BENEFIT OF THERAPY OF MILD TO MODERATE HYPERTENSION: US POPULATION, 1990–2010	
MEDICATION	YEARS OF LIFE SAVED (IN MILLIONS)
Propranolol	4.21
HCTZ	2.74
Nifedipine	3.96
Prazosin	3.82
Captopril	2.90

FIGURE 13-37. Benefit of therapy of mild to moderate hypertension: US population, 1990–2010. The Coronary Heart Disease (CHD) Policy Model was used to estimate the benefit of antihypertensive therapy from 1990 to 2010. The antihypertensive and cholesterol effects of each of the medications were derived from a meta-analysis of trials that evaluated the efficacy of these agents. The effects of these changes in blood pressure and cholesterol on the incidence of CHD were calculated by the CHD Policy Model, based on estimates derived from the Framingham Heart Study [26]. HCTZ—hydrochlorothiazide.

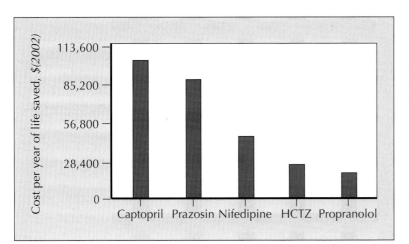

FIGURE 13-38. Comparison of the cost-effectiveness ratios for various initial monotherapies for mild to moderate hypertension. These estimates were derived from a 20-year simulation of the Coronary Heart Disease Policy Model. Costs were based on 2002 dollars, and both costs and years of life saved were discounted by 5% per year. The analysis suggests that the cost-effectiveness of this intervention is very sensitive to the cost of the medication. Of the therapies considered, propranolol is the most cost-effective for the treatment of mild to moderate hypertension, and captopril is the least cost-effective. The analysis also suggests that the treatment of mild to moderate hypertension can have a cost-effectiveness ratio well below $42,600 per year of life saved. HCTZ—hydrochlorothiazide.

SMOKING CESSATION

THE EPIDEMIOLOGY OF SMOKING
Smoking is highly prevalent
Smoking is associated with an increased risk of heart disease, stroke, cancer, and death
Smoking cessation reduces the risk of these smoking-related complications

FIGURE 13-39. The epidemiology and rationale for cost-effectiveness analysis of the treatment of smoking.

CONSEQUENCES OF SMOKING
Health care costs are as much as 40% higher in smokers than in nonsmokers
Life expectancy is shorter
69.7 years for male smokers and 75.6 years for female smokers
77.0 years for male nonsmokers and 81.6 years for female nonsmokers

FIGURE 13-40. Consequences of smoking. Barendregt *et al.* [26] modeled the consequences of smoking based on epidemiologic data. Costs were estimated based on a study of the Dutch population in 1988. They found that annual per capita health care costs for smokers were consistently higher than those for nonsmokers. The difference varied slightly by age group and was highest among men 65 to 74 years of age. They also found that the smokers had a substantially shorter life expectancy.

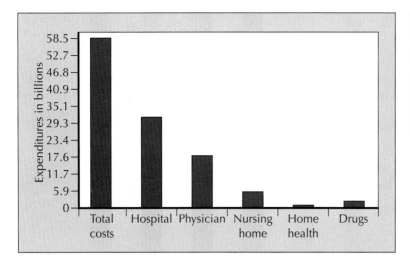

FIGURE 13-41. Medical expenditures associated with smoking. The Centers for Disease Control and Prevention estimated the medical care expenditures attributable to smoking in 1993 [27]. They found that cigarette smoking accounts for a substantial portion of medical care costs in the United States with an overall estimated cost of $59 billion. Public funding paid for 43% of the medical care expenditures attributable to smoking. (Cost expressed in 2002 dollars.)

MEDICAL EXPENDITURES PER PACK OF CIGARETTES

For each of the 24 billion packages of cigarettes sold in 1993:

$2.41 was spent on medical care attributable to smoking

$1.04 was spent through public sources on medical care attributable to smoking

FIGURE 13-42. Medical expenditures per pack of cigarettes. The Centers for Disease Control and Prevention calculated the medical expenditures per pack of cigarettes sold. They demonstrated that the medical expenditures were as much or more than the cost of the cigarettes [27]. (Cost expressed in 2002 dollars.)

IMPACT OF A 1% REDUCTION IN SMOKING PREVALENCE IN THE UNITED STATES

In the first year:

924 fewer hospitalizations for AMI

538 fewer hospitalizations for stroke

$49 million savings

Over 7 years:

63,840 fewer hospitalizations for AMI

34,261 fewer hospitalizations for stroke

$3.6 billion savings

FIGURE 13-43. Impact of a 1% reduction in smoking prevalence in the United States. Lightwood and Glantz [28] performed Monte Carlo simulations to determine the economic benefits of smoking cessation. They calculate that a program that produces a 1% decline in smoking prevalence has substantial economic benefits, even in the first 7 years. They contend that this effect is similar to what was produced by California's large Proposition 99 anti-tobacco education program. (Cost expressed in 2002 dollars.) AMI—acute myocardial infarction.

FIGURE 13-44. Smoking is strongly associated with many causes of mortality, and smoking cessation is effective in improving life expectancy. The estimated gains in life expectancies due to smoking cessation are shown. The values are derived from calculations by Oster *et al.* [29], and are based on life-table data from the American Cancer Society and estimates of the decline in excess mortality after quitting [30].

BENEFITS OF SMOKING CESSATION: GAINS IN DISCOUNTED LIFE EXPECTANCY

AGE GROUP, y	MEN, y	WOMEN, y
35–39	0.99	0.54
40–44	1.07	0.60
45–49	1.10	0.64
50–54	1.07	0.65
55–59	0.97	0.63
60–64	0.83	0.56
65–69	0.66	0.45

COST-EFFECTIVENESS OF NICOTINE REPLACEMENT GUM

AGE GROUP, y	COSTS, $	
	MEN	WOMEN
35–39	6932	13,134
40–44	6282	11,455
45–49	6005	10,493
50–54	6084	10,044
55–59	6567	10,326
60–64	7624	11,449
65–69	9439	13,830

FIGURE 13-45. Oster *et al.* [29] assessed the cost-effectiveness of nicotine gum as an adjunct to a physician's advice to quit smoking. Physician's advice against smoking was estimated to be associated with a success rate of 4.5%. The addition of nicotine replacement was estimated to increase the 1-year rate of smoking cessation by 35% (increasing the quit rate to approximately 6%). Costs are expressed in 2002 dollars.

BENEFIT OF SMOKING CESSATION PROGRAM AFTER ACUTE MYOCARDIAL INFARCTION

STUDY	5-Y MORTALITY AFTER MI, %	
	QUITTERS	SMOKERS
Sparrow *et al.* [31]	12	25
Aberg *et al.* [32]	16	22
Daly *et al.* [33]	20	30
Johansson *et al.* [34]	15	27
Perkins and Dick [35]	21	47
Hedback and Perk [36]	16	31

FIGURE 13-46. Benefit of smoking cessation program after acute myocardial infarction (AMI). Smoking cessation after MI is associated with improved survival. The results of observational studies of the relationship of smoking status with long-term survival after AMI are reported. Values given are 5-year mortality rates after AMI.

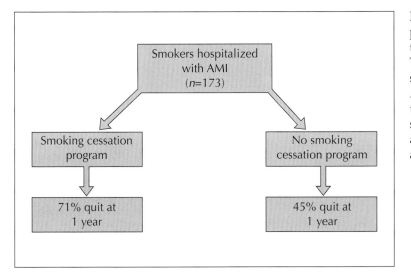

FIGURE 13-47. Benefit of nurse-managed smoking cessation program after acute myocardial infarction (AMI). Smoking cessation programs can be effective in improving quit rates. In 1990, Taylor *et al.* [37] reported the results of a trial of a nurse-managed smoking cessation program for 173 patients hospitalized with an AMI. The program included supportive phone calls as well as the usual hospital counseling, and was effective in increasing the smoking cessation rate at 1 year from 45% to 71%. Smoking status at 1 year was verified by measurement of expired carbon monoxide and serum thiocyanate levels.

COST-EFFECTIVENESS OF A NURSE-MANAGED SMOKING CESSATION PROGRAM

Cost, $: 467
Gain in life expectancy, y: 1.7
Cost-effectiveness, $275/life saved

FIGURE 13-48. Cost-effectiveness of a nurse-managed smoking cessation program that was reported by Taylor *et al.* [37] (*see* Fig. 13-46). Krumholz *et al.* [38] estimated that this program had a cost-effectiveness ratio of $270 per year of life saved. In a sensitivity analysis, they showed that the intervention maintained a favorable cost-effectiveness ratio even if the cost of the program increased substantially or the effectiveness decreased dramatically. For example, the cost-effectiveness of the program remained less than $24,600 per year of life saved even if the program decreased the smoking rate by only three per 1000 smokers (baseline assumption 260/1000 smokers) at its expected cost or if the program costs as much as $10,873 per participant (baseline assumption $100) but had its expected impact. (Cost expressed in 2002 dollars.)

REFERENCES

1. Heffler S, Levit K, Smith S, *et al*.: Health spending growth up in 1999; faster growth expected in the future. *Health Affairs* 2001, 20:193–203.

2. Iglehart J: The end stage renal disease program. *N Engl J Med* 1993, 328:366–4371.

3. Gold M, Siegel J, Russel L, Weinstein M: *Cost Effectiveness in Health and Medicine*. New York: Oxford University Press; 1996.

4. National Cholesterol Education Program: *Second Report of the Expert Panel on Detection, Evaluation, and Treatment of High Blood Cholesterol in Adults*. Washington, DC: US Department of Health and Human Services; 1993. [NIH publication no. 93–3095.]

5. Wilson PWF, Christiansen JC, Anderson KM, *et al*.: Impact of national guidelines for cholesterol risk screening: the Framingham Offspring Study. *JAMA* 1989, 262:41–44.

6. Rembold CM: Number needed to screen: development of a statistic for disease screening. *Br Med J* 1998, 317:302–312.

7. Nieto FG, Alonso J, Chambless LE, *et al*.: Population awareness and control of hypertension and hypercholesterolemia: the atherosclerosis risk in communities study. *Arch Intern Med* 1995, 155:677–84.

8. Tosteson ANA, Weinstein MC, Hunink MGM, *et al*.: Cost-effectiveness of population-wide educational approaches to reduce serum cholesterol levels. *Circulation* 1997, 95:24–30.

9. Farquhar JW, Fortmann SP, Flora JA, *et al*.: Effects of a community-wide education on cardiovascular disease risk factors. *JAMA* 1990, 264:359–365.

10. Scandinavian Simvastatin Survival Study Group: Randomised trial of cholesterol lowering in 444 patients with coronary heart disease: the Scandinavian Simvastatin Survival Study (4S). *Lancet* 1994, 394:1383–1389.

11. Sheperd J, Cabbe SM, Ford I, *et al*.: Prevention of coronary heart disease with pravastatin in men with hypercholesterolemia. *N Engl J Med* 1995, 333:1301–1307.

12. Gould AL, Rossouw JE, Santanello NC, *et al*.: Cholesterol reduction yields clinical benefit. *Circulation* 1998, 97:946–952.

13. Caro J, Klittich A, McGuire A, *et al*.: The West of Scotland coronary prevention study: economic benefit analysis of primary prevention with pravastatin. *Br Med J* 1997, 315:1577–1582.

14. Pedersen TR, Kjekshus J, Berg K, *et al*.: Cholesterol lowering and the use of healthcare resources. *Circulation* 1996, 93:1796–1802.

15. Johannesson M, Jonsson B, Kjekshus J, *et al*.: Cost effectiveness of simvastatin treatment to lower cholesterol levels in patients with coronary heart disease. *N Engl J Med* 1997, 336:332–336.

16. The Long-term Intervention with Pravastatin in Ischemic Disease (LIPID) Study Groups: Prevention of cardiovascular events and death with prevastatin in patients with coronary heart disease and a broad range of initial cholesterol levels. *N Engl J Med* 1998, 339:1349–1357.

17. Sacks FM, Pfeffer MA, Moye LA, *et al*.: The effect of pravastatin on coronary events after myocardial infarction in patients with average cholesterol levels. *N Engl J Med* 1996, 335:1001–1009.

18. Grover SA, Coupal L, Zowall H, Dorais M: Cost-effectiveness of treating hyperlipidemia in the presence of diabetes: who should be treated? *Circulation* 2000, 102:722–777.

19. Downs JR, Clearfield M, Weis S, *et al*.: Primary prevention of acute coronary events with lovastatin in men and women with average cholesterol levels: results of the AFCAPS/TexCAPS. *JAMA* 1998, 279:1615–1622.

20. Goldman L, Weinstein M, Goldman P, *et al*.: Cost-effectiveness of HMG-CoA reductase inhibition for primary and secondary prevention of coronary heart disease. *JAMA* 1991, 265:1145–1151.

21. Weinstein M, Coxson P, Williams L, *et al*.: Forecasting coronary heart disease incidence, mortality, and cost: the coronary heart disease policy model. *Am J Public Health* 1987, 77:1417–1426.

22. Prosser LA, Stinnett AA, Goldman PA, *et al*.: Cost-effectiveness of cholesterol-lowering therapies according to selected patient characteristics. *Ann Intern Med* 2000, 132:769–779.

23. Nieto FG, Alonso J, Chambless LE, *et al*.: Population awareness and control of hypertension and hypercholesterolemia: the atherosclerosis risk in communities study. *Arch Intern Med* 1995, 155:677–84.

24. Littenberg B, Garber A, Sox HJ: Diagnosis and treatment: screening for hypertension. *Ann Intern Med* 1990, 112:192–202.

25. Edelson J, Weinstein M, Tosteson A, *et al*.: Long-term cost-effectiveness of various initial monotherapies for mild to moderate hypertension. *JAMA* 1990, 263:407–413.

26. Barendregt JJ, Bonneux L, van der Maas PJ: The health care costs of smoking. *N Engl J Med* 1997, 337:1052–1057.

27. Bartlett JC, Miller LS, Rice DP, Max WB: Medical-care expenditures attributable to cigarette smoking: United States, 1993. *MMWR Morbid Mortal Wkly Rep* 1994, 43:469–472.

28. Lightwood JM, Glantz SA: Short-term economic and health benefits of smoking cessation. *J Am Coll Cardiol* 1997, 96:1089–1096.

29. Oster G, Huse D, Delea T, *et al*.: Cost-effectiveness of nicotine gum as an adjunct to physician's advice against cigarette smoking. *JAMA* 1986, 256:1315–1318.

30. Doll R, Peto R: Mortality in relation to smoking: twenty years observation on male British doctors. *BMJ* 1976, 2:1525–1536.

31. Sparrow D, Dawber T, Colton T: The influence of cigarette smoking on prognosis after a first myocardial infarction: a report from the Framingham Study. *J Chronic Dis* 1978, 31:425–432.

32. Aberg A, Bergstrand R, Johansson S: Cessation of smoking after myocardial infarction: effects on mortality after 10 years. *Br Heart J* 1983, 49:416–422.

33. Daly L, Mulcahy R, Graham I, *et al*.: Long-term effect on mortality of stopping smoking after unstable angina and myocardial infarction. *BMJ* 1983, 387:324–326.

34. Johansson S, Bergstrand R, Pennert K: Cessation of smoking after myocardial infarction in women: effects on mortality and reinfarctions. *Am J Epidemiol* 1985, 121:823–831.

35. Perkins J, Dick T: Smoking and myocardial infarction: secondary prevention. *Postgrad Med J* 1985, 61:295–300.

36. Hedback B, Perk J: Five-year results of a comprehensive rehabilitation programme after myocardial infarction. *Eur Heart J* 1987, 8:234–242.

37. Taylor A, Houston-Miller N, Killen J, *et al*.: Smoking cessation after acute myocardial infarction: effect of a nurse-managed intervention. *Ann Intern Med* 1990, 113:118–123.

38. Krumholz H, Cohen B, Tsevat J, *et al*.: Cost-effectiveness of a smoking cessation program after myocardial infarction. *J Am Coll Cardiol* 1993, 22:1697–1702.

INDEX

A

ABCA1 transporter, of high-density lipoprotein, 2.65
Abdominal fat deposition, heart disease and, 3.12–3.13
Acetylation, of low-density lipoprotein, 2.50
Acetylcholine, vasomotor tone and, 1.25, 1.29, 1.35–1.36
Adhesion molecules, endothelial dysfunction and, 1.30, 1.42–1.43
    in hyperlipidemia, 2.28
β-Adrenergic blockers, 2.73, 4.38
Adventitia, endothelial, 1.23
    normal aorta, 1.3
    normal coronary artery, 1.2
Advicor, 3.48
Air Force/Texas Coronary Atherosclerosis Prevention Study, 4.52, 4.73
Alcohol consumption, blood pressure and, 3.21
    heart disease risk and, 3.15
    hypertriglyceridemia exacerbated by, 2.24
American Diabetes Association, on aspirin, 4.64
American Heart Association, on women's heart disease, 4.44
Amino acids, in low-density lipoprotein, 2.42
Amphipathic helices, apolipoprotein, 2.1, 2.8–2.9, 2.15, 2.62
Android obesity, 3.12–3.13
Aneurysms, fibrofatty plaques in, 1.17
Angina pectoris, endothelial dysfunction in, 1.26
    hemostatic factors in, 4.4
Angioplasty, in diabetes mellitus, 4.25
Angiotensin-converting enzyme inhibitors, in diabetes mellitus, 4.37
    endothelial function and, 1.36
Antihypertensive therapy, gender differences and, 4.53
Antioxidants, endothelial function and, 1.37
    lipoproteins and, 2.40, 2.50, 3.18–3.19
Aorta, fatty streak in, 1.3, 1.5
    fibrofatty plaques in, 1.9–1.18
    intimal thickening in, 1.7–1.8
    normal histology of, 1.3
Aortic aneurysms, fibrofatty plaques in, 1.17
Apo A-I gene, in familial hyperalphalipoproteinemia, 2.66–2.67
    high-density lipoprotein and, 2.59, 2.68–2.69
Apo B-100 gene, low-density lipoprotein and, 2.40
Apo C-III gene, triglycerides regulated by, 2.35–2.36
Apolipoprotein A-I, 2.61–2.62
Apolipoprotein A-II, 2.61–2.62
Apolipoprotein B-100, in familial combined hyperlipidemia, 2.30
    in low-density lipoprotein, 2.41
Apolipoprotein C-II, in triglyceride metabolism, 2.25–2.26
Apolipoprotein C-III, coronary artery disease risk and, 2.38
    in triglyceride metabolism, 2.20, 2.25–2.27, 2.35–2.36
Apolipoprotein E, in dysbetalipoproteinemia, 2.29
    in low-density lipoprotein, 2.42
    in triglyceride metabolism, 2.20, 2.25, 2.27–2.28, 2.37
Apolipoprotein(a), in atherogenesis, 2.46
Apolipoproteins, classification of, 2.2, 2.5
    coronary artery disease risk and, 2.38, 4.10
    defined, 2.1
    in familial hyperalphalipoproteinemia, 2.67–2.68
    in familial hypoalphalipoproteinemia, 2.69–2.70, 2.72–2.73
    in fibrofatty plaques, 1.16
    functions of, 2.5–2.6
        in triglyceride metabolism, 2.20, 2.25–2.28, 2.35–2.37
    in high-density lipoprotein, 2.61–2.62
    hypertriglyceridemia associated with, 2.24
    lipid bonds with, 2.6–2.8
    in lipoprotein structure, 2.9–2.13, 2.61
Arteries, coronary See Coronary arteries
    extracellular matrix of, 1.46–1.47
    normal histology of, 1.2–1.3
Arteriosclerosis See also Atherosclerosis
    histopathology of, 1.1–1.18 See also Histopathology; specific lesions
    pathogenesis of, 1.1–1.2
Aspirin, heart disease risk and, 4.6–4.8
    in diabetes mellitus, 4.36
    myocardial infarction in, 4.64
Atherogenesis, diet and, 3.3 See also Diet

hypotheses of, intimal thickening in, 1.6–1.7
    response-to-injury, 1.31
    thrombogenic, 1.10, 1.16
lipoproteins in, 2.66
    low-density, 2.39–2.40, 2.45–2.48, 2.51–2.53
    macrophages in, 1.41–1.49
    obesity and, 3.12–3.13
    oxidative stress and, 2.56
    triglycerides in, 2.19–2.22
Atherosclerosis, antioxidants and, 2.40, 2.55–2.56
    as cardiac disease predictor, 1.22–1.23
    in diabetes mellitus, 4.22-4.27, 4.39–4.40
    diet and See also Diet
        trials of, 3.24–3.27
    lesion formation in, 2.55, 2.66
    macrophages and, 1.41–1.49
    oxidized low-density lipoprotein in, 2.51–2.53
    pathogenesis of See Atherogenesis
    risk factors for, elevated triglycerides as, 2.19–2.22
        endothelial dysfunction and, 1.22
        lipoprotein levels as, 2.2
        timeline of, 1.38, 1.45
    treatment of, in diabetes mellitus, 4.39–4.40
        lipid-lowering drugs in, 3.33–3.56
Atherosis, in fibrofatty plaques, 1.9
Atkins diet, 3.30
Atorvastatin, clinical trials of, 3.45
    pharmacologic effects of, 3.41–3.42
    side effects of, 3.46

B

Bacterial infection, in atherogenesis, 1.42, 1.44–1.45
Benefit, in cost-effectiveness analysis, 4.69–4.71
Bile acid sequestrants, 3.38–3.40
    in diabetes mellitus, 4.29
Blood pressure, in diabetes mellitus, 4.38
    diet and, 3.21, 3.23
Bypass Angioplasty Revascularization Investigation, 4.25

C

Calcification of vessels, heart disease risk and, 4.17
    in diabetes mellitus, 4.24
Cardiac death, time of day and, 4.5
Cardiovascular disease, clinical trials in, dietary intervention, 3.26–3.27
        dietary prevention, 3.24–3.25
    dietary changes recommended in, 3.27–3.29
        popular diets and, 3.30–3.31
    endothelial dysfunction in, event-free survival curves and, 1.38
        plaque rupture and, 1.34
    gender-related prevalence of, 4.44
    risk of, alcohol and, 3.15
        antioxidants and, 1.37
        asymptomatic to symptomatic, 1.45
        atherosclerosis as predictor of, 1.22–1.23
        cost-effectiveness and, 4.67–4.79
        diabetes mellitus and, 4.21–4.40, 4.45–4.46
        diet and, 3.1–3.31 See also Diet
        endothelial dysfunction in, 1.26–1.29
        gender differences and, 4.43–4.64
        high-density lipoprotein and, 2.59–2.60, 2.66, 4.10
        low-density lipoprotein and, 2.60, 4.2, 4.8–4.9
        modifiable versus fixed factors in, 3.2
        obesity and, 2.31
        smoking and, 4.47
        tea consumption and, 1.37
        triglycerides and, 2.19–2.22, 2.32–2.34, 2.38
    sudden death in, time of day and, 4.5
    treatment of, endothelial function and, 1.35
        lipid-lowering drugs in, 3.33–3.56
Carotid arteries, treatment of diseased, 4.17–4.18
Central obesity, 3.12–3.13
Cerivastatin, 3.42, 3.46
Charges versus costs of health care, 4.68
Chlamydia, in atherogenesis, 1.42, 1.44–1.45
Cholesterol See also High-density lipoproteins; Low-

density lipoproteins
    atherogenesis and, 2.39
    in diabetes mellitus, 4.27–4.38
    dietary, as cardiovascular risk factor, 3.3–3.11
        fiber and, 3.14
        serum levels and, 3.11, 3.16–3.17
        sources of, 3.11
    in dysbetalipoproteinemia, 2.29
    epidemiology of, 4.72
    gender differences and, 4.48–4.52
    in lipoproteins, 2.2, 2.4–2.5, 2.7, 2.10–2.13, 2.15
    reduction of, cost-effectiveness of, 4.72–4.76
        diets for, 3.24–3.29
        drugs in, 3.33–3.56
        lifestyle therapy in, 3.28
    reverse transport of, 2.64
    screening tests for, 4.72
Cholesterol and Recurrent Events trial, 3.43–3.44, 4.6, 4.51, 4.74
Cholesterol ester transport protein deficiency, 2.59, 2.68
Cholestyramine, 3.38–3.40, 4.29
Chylomicrons See also Triglyceride-rich lipoproteins
    defined, 2.1
    metabolism of, 2.25–2.26, 2.63
        defects in, 2.27–2.28
        in diabetes mellitus, 4.28–4.29
    structure of, 2.5, 2.15
    as triglyceride source, 2.19
Cigarette smoking See Smoking
Clofibrate, 2.32, 3.52, 4.30
Clopidogrel, 4.8
Coagulation, in hypertriglyceridemia, 2.29
Colestipol, 3.38–3.40, 4.29
Collagen, in arterial extracellular matrix, 1.46–1.47
Copenhagen Male Study, 4.9
Corn oil, other dietary fats versus, 3.6
Cornea, in Tangier disease, 2.71–2.72
Coronary arteries, calcification of, 4.17
    fatty streak in, 1.4–1.5
    fibrofatty plaques in, 1.10–1.11, 1.15–1.17
    intimal thickening in, 1.6, 1.9
    normal histology of, 1.2
Coronary artery bypass surgery, smoking and, 4.47
Coronary artery disease See also Cardiovascular disease
    apolipoprotein E and, 2.37
    in diabetes mellitus, 4.24–4.26, 4.33–4.38
    endothelial dysfunction in, 1.26
        fibrofatty plaques and, 1.34
    premyocardial infarction, stenosis and, 1.46
    primary prevention of, 3.35
    risk of, cost-effectiveness and, 4.67–4.79
        dietary factors in, 3.3–3.4, 3.9
        gender differences and, 4.43–4.64
        hematologic factors in, 4.1–4.10
        high-density lipoprotein in, 2.59–2.60, 4.10
        homocysteine in, 4.2, 4.12–4.13
        imaging and, 4.2, 4.15–4.18
        insulin resistance in, 4.2, 4.13–4.15
        low-density lipoprotein in, 4.2, 4.8–4.9
        triglyceride markers of, 2.38
        vitamins in, 4.2, 4.11–4.12
    treatment of, estrogen plus progestin in, 4.62
        lipid-lowering drugs in, 3.33–3.56
Coronary Drug Project, 3.49
Coronary Heart Disease Policy Model, 4.76–4.77
Cost-effectiveness of risk factors, 4.67–4.79
    of cholesterol reduction, 4.72–4.76
    of hypertension treatment, 4.76–4.77
    overview of, 4.68–4.72
    ratio for, 4.68
    of smoking cessation, 4.77–4.79
Costs of health care, 4.68
    analysis of, 4.68–4.71
C-reactive protein, heart disease risk and, 4.1, 4.4, 4.6
Cytokines, in aneurysms, 1.17
    in atherogenesis, 1.42
    endothelial dysfunction and, 1.30, 1.32–1.33
    in fibrofatty plaques, 1.11
Cytomegalovirus, in atherogenesis, 1.42, 1.44–1.45

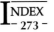

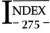

COLOR PLATES

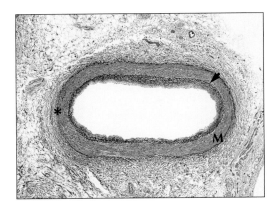

FIGURE 1-1. Page 2

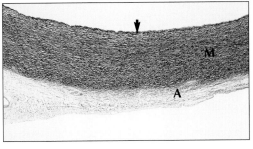

FIGURE 1-2. Page 3

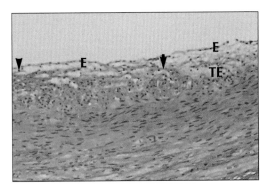

FIGURE 1-3. Page 3

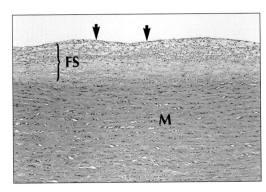

FIGURE 1-4. Page 3

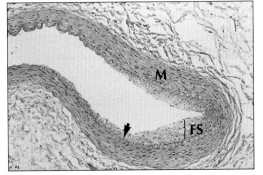

FIGURE 1-5. Page 4

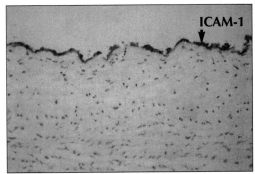

FIGURE 1-7A. Page 4

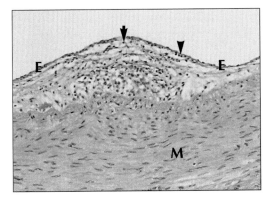

FIGURE 1-10. Page 5

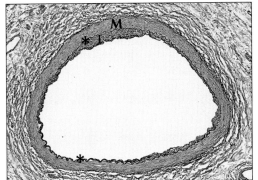

FIGURE 1-11A. Page 6

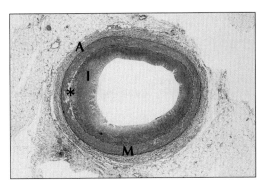

FIGURE 1-11B. Page 6

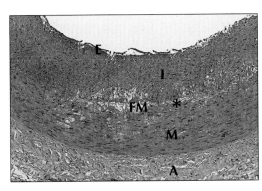

FIGURE 1-11C. Page 6

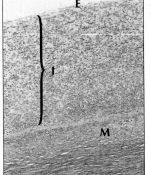

FIGURE 1-12A.
Page 7

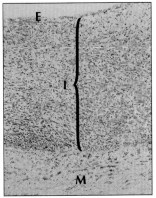

FIGURE 1-12B.
Page 7

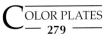

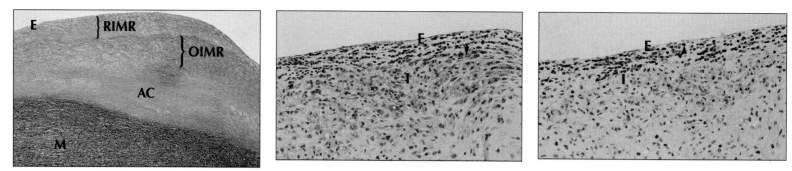

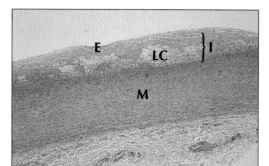 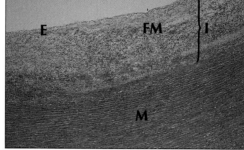 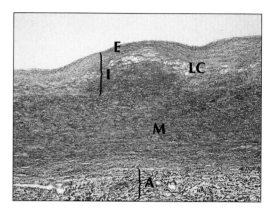

FIGURE 1-13.   Page 7

FIGURE 1-14A.   Page 7

FIGURE 1-14B.   Page 7

FIGURE 1-15A.   page 8

FIGURE 1-15B.   page 8

FIGURE 1-15C.   page 8

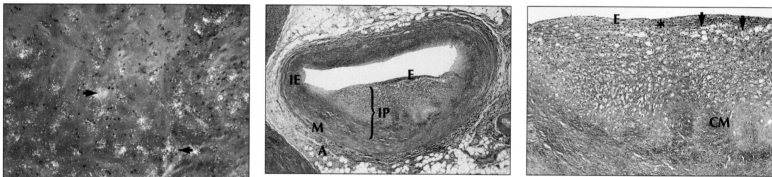

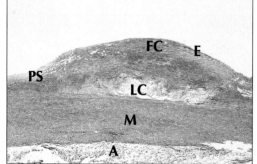 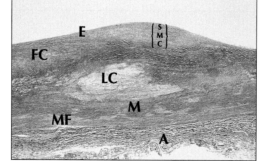 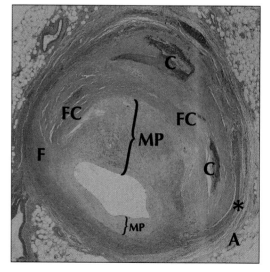

FIGURE 1-16.   page 8

FIGURE 1-17A.   page 9

FIGURE 1-17B.   page 9

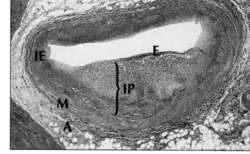

FIGURE 1-18A.   page 9

FIGURE 1-18B.   page 9

FIGURE 1-19A.   page 10

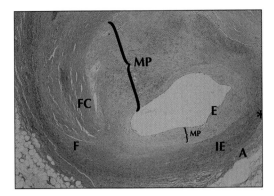

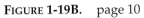

FIGURE 1-19B.   page 10

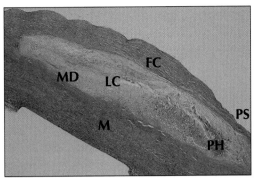

FIGURE 1-20.   page 10

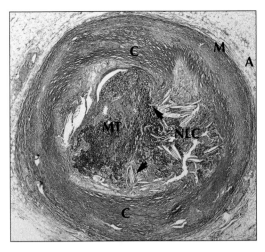

FIGURE 1-21.   page 11

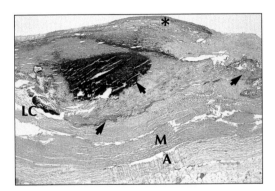

FIGURE 1-22.   page 11

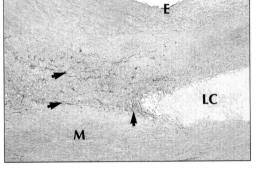

FIGURE 1-23A.   page 12

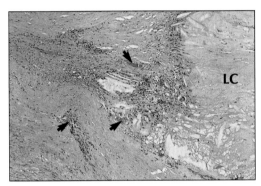

FIGURE 1-23B.   page 12

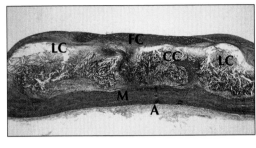

FIGURE 1-24.   page 12

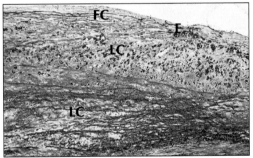

FIGURE 1-25A.   page 13

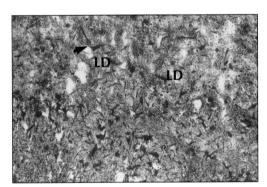

FIGURE 1-25B.   page 13

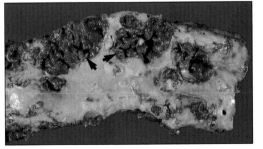

FIGURE 1-26A.   page 13

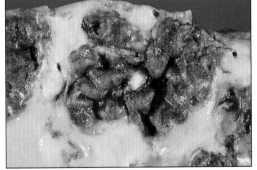

FIGURE 1-26B.   page 13

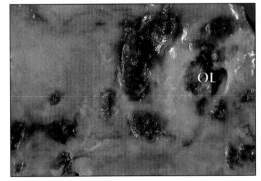

FIGURE 1-26C.   page 14

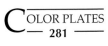

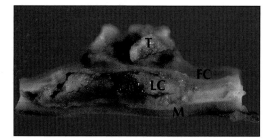

FIGURE 1-27A.   page 14

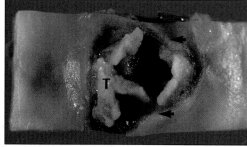

FIGURE 1-27B.   page 14

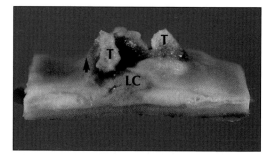

FIGURE 1-27C.   page 14

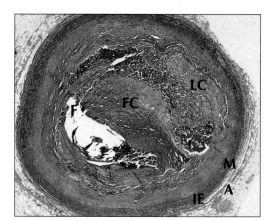

FIGURE 1-28.   page 15

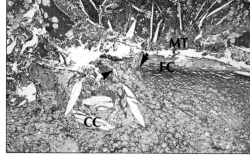

FIGURE 1-29.   page 15

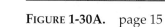

FIGURE 1-30A.   page 15

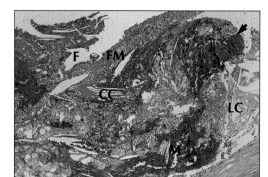

FIGURE 1-30B.   page 16

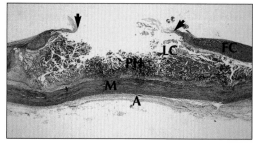

FIGURE 1-31A.   page 16

FIGURE 1-31B.
page 16

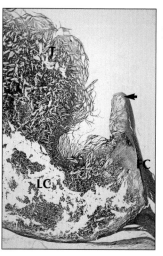

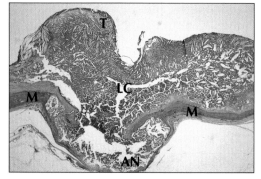

FIGURE 1-32A.   page 17

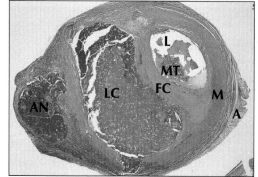

FIGURE 1-32B.   page 17

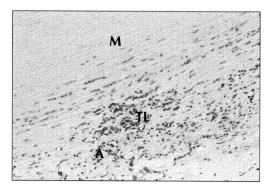

FIGURE 1-33A.   page 18

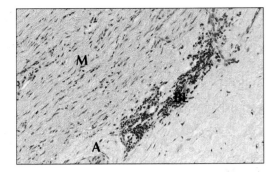

FIGURE 1-33B. page 18

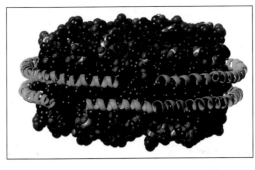

FIGURE 4-15A. Page 59

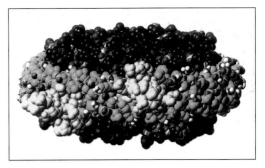

FIGURE 4-15B. Page 59

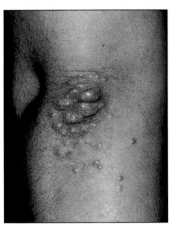

FIGURE 5-21.
Page 80

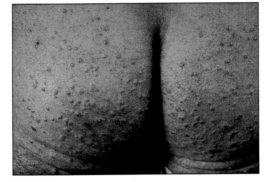

FIGURE 5-24. Page 80

FIGURE 6-18A. Page 104

FIGURE 6-18B. Page 104

FIGURE 6-18C. Page 104

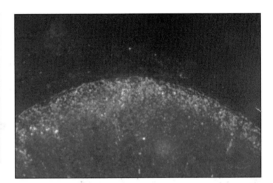

FIGURE 6-18D. Page 104

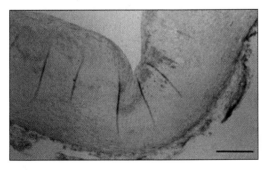

FIGURE 6-26A. Page 109

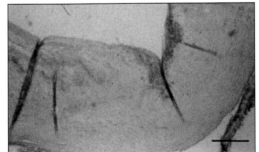

FIGURE 6-26B. Page 109

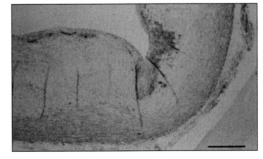

FIGURE 6-26C. Page 109

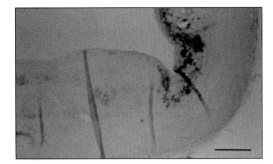

FIGURE 6-26D. Page 109

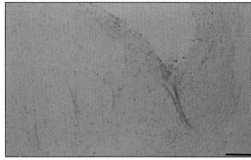

FIGURE 6-26E. Page 109

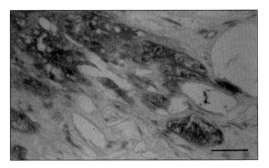

FIGURE 6-26F. Page 109

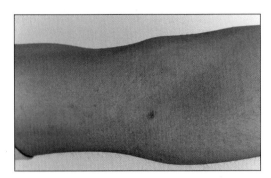

FIGURE 7-23. Page 125

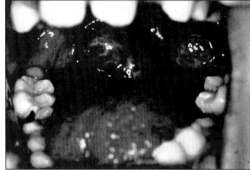

FIGURE 7-30. Page 127

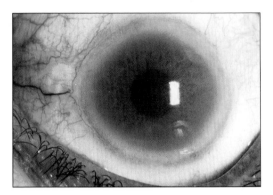

FIGURE 7-33. Page 128